ADVANCES IN PULMONARY DRUG DELIVERY

ADVANCES IN PULMONARY DRUG DELIVERY

edited by
PHILIP CHI LIP KWOK • HAK-KIM CHAN

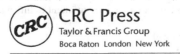

CRC Press
Taylor & Francis Group
Boca Raton London New York

CRC Press is an imprint of the
Taylor & Francis Group, an **informa** business

CRC Press
Taylor & Francis Group
6000 Broken Sound Parkway NW, Suite 300
Boca Raton, FL 33487-2742

First issued in hardback 2019

© 2017 by Taylor & Francis Group, LLC
CRC Press is an imprint of Taylor & Francis Group, an Informa business

No claim to original U.S. Government works

ISBN-13: 978-1-4987-5804-8 (hbk)

Visit the Taylor & Francis Web site at
http://www.taylorandfrancis.com

and the CRC Press Web site at
http://www.crcpress.com

Dedication

To my students

Hak-Kim Chan

To my family

Philip Chi Lip Kwok

Contents

Advances in Pulmonary Drug Delivery

The respiratory tract has been used to deliver biologically active chemicals into the human body for centuries. Inhaled volatile oils and herbal smokes have been employed by ancient civilizations for therapeutic and recreational purposes [1]. This demonstrates the efficiency of the lungs to absorb drugs into the systemic circulation, due to its large surface area and profuse blood supply. Inhalation is also the most effective route of administration for local diseases such as asthma, chronic obstructive pulmonary disease (COPD), and lung infections. The inhaled drug particles can target the site of action rapidly with a relatively low dose, thus reducing systemic adverse effects. However, the lungs are complex in their anatomy and physiology, which poses challenges to drug delivery. Therefore, inhaled formulations are generally more sophisticated than those for oral and parenteral administration. This book highlights the latest developments in this field.

Most classical inhaled drugs are small molecules (e.g., beta-2 agonists, anticholinergics, corticosteroids) for pulmonary diseases, but increasingly more biopharmaceuticals (e.g., proteins, peptides, nucleic acids) have been investigated or marketed for inhalation for both local and systemic delivery. This is a reflection of the global trend in the increasing use of biopharmaceutical formulations via other routes of administration. Wolff [2] provides an overview on various inhaled proteins and peptides such as insulin, alpha-1 antitrypsin, cyclosporine, human growth hormone, measles vaccine, and anti-IgE antibody for a variety of diseases. Of these agents, insulin and alpha-1 antitrypsin are further discussed by Patton and Miller [3]. The challenges of siRNA delivery and the use of nonviral vectors to enhance transfection efficiency are covered by Cun and Yang [4]. Advances in the understanding of the pathophysiology of asthma and COPD have led to the development of novel anti-inflammatory molecules (e.g., phosphoinositide-3-kinase-delta, dual phosphodiesterase-3 and -4, p38 mitogen-activated protein kinase, humanized antibodies, and chemokine receptor antagonists) [5]. Likewise, novel biopharmaceutical anticancer agents involving immunological and genetic agents are actively being investigated for lung cancer treatment [6]. Inhalation delivery is ideal for lung cancers to achieve local drug targeting and reduce potential systemic toxicity. The same rationale also applies to inhaled vaccines and antibiotics for pulmonary infections [7,8]. Liposomes have been used to effectively modify the release, and enhance the pharmacokinetics and pharmacodynamics, of inhaled antibiotics [9]. A novel trend for treating pulmonary diseases in China is the inhalation of traditional Chinese herbal formulae, which are usually administered orally or parenterally [10]. Although some effectiveness of inhaled traditional Chinese medicine has been demonstrated, more rigorously controlled clinical trials are required. Besides inhaling drugs to treat particular diseases, chemical trigger agents (e.g., mannitol, adenosine monophosphate, allergens) can also be delivered into the airways for asthma diagnosis and antiasthma drug evaluation in bronchoprovocation tests [11].

Pulmonary drug delivery is a specialized field because of its many unique issues and challenges. Rapid progress is being made and novel solutions are being offered to existing treatment problems. The major direction in which this field is headed is the use of biologically active macromolecules. These new drugs are generally more fragile and potentially more immunogenic than traditional small molecular drugs. Therefore, active research on their stability, safety, and efficacy is anticipated in the near future. Despite the setback caused by the withdrawal of Exubera® in 2007, the approval in 2014 of yet another dry powder inhaled insulin (Afrezza® by MannKind Corporation) [12] is likely to kindle more interests in the field.

Philip Chi Lip Kwok
Hak-Kim Chan

REFERENCES

1. Sanders M. Inhalation therapy: An historical review. *Primary Care Respiratory Journal.* 16(2), 71–81 (2007).
2. Wolff R. Chapter 1. Inhaled proteins and peptides.
3. Patton JS, Miller SR. Chapter 2. Inhaled insulin: More compelling than ever.
4. Cun D, Yang M. Chapter 4. Inhaled therapeutic siRNA for the treatment of respiratory diseases.
5. Hakim A, Usmani OS. Chapter 5. New molecules to treat asthma and COPD.
6. Dhand R. Chapter 6. Inhaled anti-cancer agents.
7. Tripp RA, Tompkins M. Chapter 7. Inhaled influenza vaccines.
8. Zhou Q, Chan H-K. Chapter 8. Pulmonary delivery of antibiotics for respiratory infections.
9. Cipolla D. Chapter 9. Inhaled liposomes.
10. Zhou J, Liao Y-H. Chapter 10. Inhaled traditional Chinese medicine for respiratory diseases.
11. Oliveria JP, Watson BM, Gauvreau GM. Chapter 11. Bronchoprovocation tests for evaluation of drug efficacy in asthma.
12. MannKind Corporation. *About MannKind.* http://www.mannkindcorp.com/. Accessed March 18, 2016.

Editors

Dr. Philip Chi Lip Kwok is an assistant professor at the Department of Pharmacology and Pharmacy, University of Hong Kong, Pokfulam, Hong Kong. He earned his BPharm (Hons) and PhD in 2002 and 2007, respectively, from the Faculty of Pharmacy, University of Sydney, Sydney, New South Wales, Australia. He was a research associate in the Advanced Drug Delivery Group in this faculty from 2007 to 2011. He has 45 peer-reviewed publications and 2 joint patents in pharmaceutical aerosols and respiratory drug delivery. He is an editorial board member of four scientific journals, including *the Journal of Aerosol Medicine and Pulmonary Drug Delivery*, which is the official journal of the International Society for Aerosols in Medicine. Dr Kwok co-hosted and chaired the inaugural Inhalation Asia conference in Hong Kong in June 2013. This was the first international conference of its kind in the Asian region. Following its success, he was an organizing committee member for the second one held in Shenyang, China, in September 2015.

Hak-Kim Chan, professor in pharmaceutics, is leading the Advanced Drug Delivery Group and Respiratory Disease Theme at the Faculty of Pharmacy, University of Sydney. He graduated from the NDMC in Taiwan (BPharm) and the University of Sydney (PhD, DSc) and did his postdoc training at the University of Minnesota. He worked as a scientist at Genentech Inc. His research focuses on inhalation drug delivery, ranging from powder production by novel processes, particle engineering and aerosol formulation to scintigraphic imaging of lung deposition and clinical outcomes. He has over 300 scientific publications on pharmaceutical formulation and drug delivery (with over 9500 citations) and holds seven patents in these areas. He is an executive editor of Advanced Drug Delivery Reviews and on the editorial advisory boards of various pharmaceutical journals, including *Pharmaceutical Research* and *International Journal of Pharmaceutics*. He is a fellow of the American Association of Pharmaceutical Scientists and of the Royal Australian Chemical Institute (RACI) and was chair of the NSW Pharmaceutical Science Group of the RACI and vice president of the Asian Federation for Pharmaceutical Sciences.

Contributors

Hak-Kim Chan
Faculty of Pharmacy
The University of Sydney
Sydney, New South Wales, Australia

David Cipolla
Aradigm Corporation
Hayward, California

Dongmei Cun
Department of Pharmaceutical Science
Shenyang Pharmaceutical University
Shenyang, Liaoning, People's Republic
of China

Rajiv Dhand
Department of Medicine
The University of Tennessee Graduate
School of Medicine
Knoxville, Tennessee

Gail M. Gauvreau
Department of Medicine
McMaster University
Hamilton, Ontario, Canada

Amir Hakim
National Heart and Lung Institute
Imperial College London and Royal
Brompton Hospital
London, United Kingdom

Jarod M. Hanson
Department of Infectious Diseases
University of Georgia
Athens, Georgia

Lan Wu
Department of Pharmaceutical Science
Shenyang Pharmaceutical University
Shenyang, Liaoning, People's Republic
of China

Yong-Hong Liao
Institute of Medicinal Plant
Development
Chinese Academy of Medical Sciences
and Peking Union Medical College
Haidian District, Beijing, People's
Republic of China

Samantha R. Miller
Dance Biopharm Inc.
Brisbane, California

John Paul Oliveria
Department of Medicine
McMaster University
Hamilton, Ontario, Canada

John S. Patton
Dance Biopharm Inc.
Brisbane, California

Li Qu
Monash Institute of Pharmaceutical
Sciences
Monash University
Parkville, Victoria, Australia

Brittany M. Salter
Department of Medicine
McMaster University
Hamilton, Ontario, Canada

Ralph A. Tripp
Department of Infectious Diseases
University of Georgia
Athens, Georgia

Omar S. Usmani
National Heart and Lung Institute
Imperial College London and Royal
Brompton Hospital
London, United Kingdom

Ron K. Wolff
Safety Consulting Inc.
Carbondale, Colorado

Mingshi Yang
Department of Pharmaceutical Science
Shenyang Pharmaceutical University
Shenyang, Liaoning, People's Republic
    of China

and

Department of Pharmacy
University of Copenhagen
Copenhagen, Denmark

Yun Zhao
Institute of Medicinal Plant Development
Chinese Academy of Medical Sciences
    and Peking Union Medical College
Haidian District, Beijing, People's
    Republic of China

Ying Zheng
State Key Laboratory of Quality
    Research in Chinese Medicine
University of Macau
Taipa, Macao SAR, People's Republic
    of China

Jing Zhou
Institute of Medicinal Plant
    Development
Chinese Academy of Medical Sciences
    and Peking Union Medical College
Haidian District, Beijing, People's
    Republic of China

Qi (Tony) Zhou
Department of Industrial and Physical
    Pharmacy
College of Pharmacy
Purdue University
West Lafayette, Indiana

1 Inhaled Proteins and Peptides

Ron K. Wolff

CONTENTS

INTRODUCTION

Inhaled proteins and peptides have undergone a great deal of study in the last two decades. However, at present, there is only one approved inhaled protein, Pulmozyme (DNase), for the treatment of cystic fibrosis. Exubera (inhaled insulin) was approved but was withdrawn from the market primarily due to a lack of commercial success, not due to a lack of efficacy. Pulmozyme is an example of using inhalation for local lung treatment, while Exubera is an example of using lung delivery for systemic administration. A number of nonclinical and clinical studies for either local treatment or systemic delivery have shown varying degrees of success for a range of proteins and peptides. Summary information is provided for inhalation programs with DNase, insulin, growth hormone, cyclosporine, alpha-1-antitrypsin (AAT), anti-IgE, and vaccines. Examination of the features of these various programs provides insights for future activities. This chapter will provide high-level information related to inhaled proteins and peptides. More details are available in recent review papers [1–6].

MECHANISMS OF ABSORPTION AND CLEARANCE

The major mechanisms for clearance of proteins from the lung have been reviewed by Patton and Byron [3] and Wolff [4]. Proteins that deposit on ciliated epithelium are not absorbed to a significant extent and are primarily cleared by mucociliary transport up the airways and then eliminated *via* the gastrointestinal tract where they are degraded and eliminated. Proteins that deposit in the alveolar region are cleared from the lung primarily *via* four routes: (1) phagocytosis by alveolar macrophages, (2) paracellular diffusion through tight junctions, (3) vesicular endocytosis or pino-cytosis, and (4) receptor-mediated transcytosis.

Phagocytosis by alveolar macrophages does not appear to be as important a clearance mechanism as absorption. This may occur because phagocytosis is most efficient for uptake of relatively insoluble particles. Therefore, this clearance pathway is likely to be of most importance if there is degradation of proteins to insoluble forms. It appears that soluble proteins effectively dissolve in lung fluids and distribute themselves in the surfactant and mucus layers of the lung.

For soluble proteins, clearance of protein from the lung closely parallels absorption into blood. The inverse dependence of absorption versus protein molecular weight, as shown in Figure 1.1, has been used to suggest that diffusion across alveolar epithelial membranes through tight junctions is a major absorption mechanism [3]. The available data also support the view that absorption of high-molecular-weight proteins the size of albumin (68 kDa) or greater is not likely to be extensive or rapid because they are generally too large to be absorbed *via* tight junctions. Antibodies that are frequently in the >150 kDa also show little absorption from the lung into blood.

These data (Figure 1.1) indicate for proteins less than or equal to the MW of human growth hormone (hGH; 22 kDa) that absorption is adequate enough that systemic delivery can be considered. However, the aerosol delivery system needs to be considered to maximize the overall efficiency. For larger proteins, certainly those greater than 68 kDa, absorption into the blood is low, half-life in the lung is relatively long, and so potential for utility in local lung treatment is enhanced.

More research is needed in this area, however, and it is clear that at present, the absorption and disposition of each protein being considered for therapeutic use must be studied individually, because there is not sufficient knowledge for accurate predictions with currently available data [4].

IMMUNOGENICITY

In the case of a biopharmaceutical, antidrug antibodies (ADAs) may be raised against the biomolecule. If the ADA response is sufficiently robust, this may result in immune complex formation and subsequent toxicity. Typically immune complexes

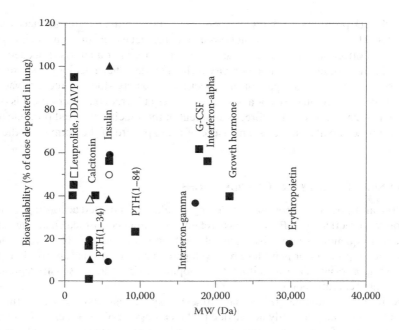

FIGURE 1.1 Bioavailability from the lung as a function of molecular weight calculated on the basis of the percentage of protein that is deposited in the lung and absorbed into the circulation.

are bound by red blood cells and then degraded in the spleen. However, immune complexes may result in inflammation and tissue damage following kidney deposition. ADA can have a direct effect on potency by preventing the antibody from binding to its ligand as well as a reduction in half-life *via* the clearance mechanisms involving neutralizing antibodies.

Assays for immunogenicity are able to measure the formation of ADA. However, these assays are typically unable to determine the impact of ADA on the potency of the drug; that is, they cannot differentiate between ADA and neutralizing antibody. For demonstration of neutralizing antibody, a cell-based potency assay may be necessary to clearly demonstrate a loss of drug potency in the presence of neutralizing antibody.

Nonclinical immunogenicity is not necessarily predictive of clinical immunogenicity but there are frequent parallels in relative immunogenicity between nonhuman primates (NHPs) and humans, particularly if there is close homology between these species. It is important to assess the pharmacokinetic/pharmacodynamic (PK/PD) exposure in terms of observed toxicities [7]. In practical terms, if the PK/PD profile of the biopharmaceutical is different between the first and last dose and/or there is evidence of immune-mediated toxicity, then ADA assessments can aid in the interpretation of the data. A dramatic decrease of C_{max} and AUC values after repeated doses is a major red flag that there may be antibody effects reducing the levels of the circulating protein. In this instance ADA measurements are definitely recommended. However, if the PK/PD profile is unchanged, then ADA measurements are not necessarily warranted. However, because it is not possible to predict events in advance, it is good practice to collect plasma samples that may be used for later analysis if needed.

For vaccine products, immunogenicity is the intended pharmacology and immune responses are an important part of the nonclinical toxicity studies. Because vaccine dosing is general single doses or a few repeat doses at infrequent intervals, it is often difficult to measure TK. Therefore, assessment of the vaccine-induced immune antibody response can also serve as a measure of the exposure of the animals to the test material.

Nonclinical Development Considerations

Nonclinical studies to support human dosing should be conducted according to Good Laboratory Practices (GLP) and must reflect the intended clinical use (e.g., dose level and frequency of administration) of the biopharmaceutical. However, studies for individual proteins or peptides are developed on a case-by-case approach to generate the appropriate data for clinical development. Consultations with regulatory agencies are recommended.

The ICH S6 guidelines [8] define a relevant species as "one in which the test material is pharmacologically active due to the expression of the receptor or an epitope (in the case of monoclonal antibodies)." Unlike small molecules, a single species may be sufficient if a second species is not suitable to predict risk in humans. For example, for many biopharmaceuticals, the human therapeutic target is expressed in the NHP and not in other species or target binding and pharmacology is only present within the NHP. However, where two pharmacologically relevant species exist (one rodent and one nonrodent), both should be used for initial safety assessment studies. The ICHS6 R1 addendum allows chronic studies to proceed only in rodents rather than nonrodents where adequate long-term exposure and pharmacology can be maintained.

The ICH S6 guidelines recommend that dose levels should be selected to provide information on a dose response that includes a toxic dose and a no observed adverse effect level (NOAEL). However, for some types of biologics where toxicity is a result of exaggerated pharmacology, the pharmacologically active dose, or PAD, may be a better indicator of observations of potential toxicity than NOAEL [9]. The high dose level in toxicity studies should ideally include a safety margin of at least 10× the maximum anticipated clinical dose; however, sometimes exaggerated pharmacological responses preclude dosing this high.

In repeat dose nonclinical safety studies, dosing frequency should be similar to that of proposed clinical trial. However, more frequent dosing may be required if the test item is more rapidly cleared in animals than humans [9]. Repeat dose studies should include toxicokinetics and a recovery phase (to detect regression of any pathological change and/or detect potential delayed toxic effects). Repeat dose toxicity studies of 6-month duration in rodents and nonrodents have been shown to be generally sufficient to predict potential human risks [10].

Pharmacodynamic endpoints: Since the toxicity of most biopharmaceuticals is related to their mechanism of action, then high doses may be associated with exaggerated pharmacology. Therefore, pharmacodynamic endpoints should be measured on studies to better understand adverse effects, such as glucose monitoring following insulin administration (discussed later).

EXAMPLES OF DEVELOPMENT CANDIDATES

INHALED rhDNase (PULMOZYME)

There is currently only one marketed inhaled protein, recombinant human(rh) DNase (Pulmozyme), developed for the treatment of cystic fibrosis. Inhalation toxicology studies were conducted in both rats and monkeys for durations of 28 days and 6 months [11]. The exposure concentrations and daily exposure durations spanned inhaled doses of 1.3–69 times the expected daily clinical inhaled dose. In the 28-day rat study, mild to moderate alveolitis was observed in the high-dose group. This lesion was not evident after 4 weeks of recovery. Bronchiolitis was observed in one of eight high-dose monkeys after 4 weeks of exposure, but, again, there were no lesions observed after 4 weeks of recovery. In the 6-month rat study, bronchiolitis was observed at the end of the treatment period but at a somewhat lower incidence than in the 4-week study. These data suggest that the mild lesion was not progressive in rats. In the 6-month monkey study, respiratory rates measured during aerosol exposure to monitor for anaphylactic or irritant responses were unchanged compared to preexposure values. Positive serum antibody titers to rhDNase were observed beginning at week 4 and persisting through the treatment period. Serum concentrations of rhDNase at 24 h postdose indicated that there was no accumulation of rhDNase throughout the 6-month treatment period. Histopathologically, there was increased perivascular lymphocytic cuffing, peribronchial lymphoid hyperplasia, terminal airway-related bronchiolitis/alveolitis with eosinophilic infiltrates, and increased siderophages. There appeared to be a close relationship between the severity of the pulmonary lesions and the antibody titer to rhDNase measured in serum. The lesions were consistent with an allergic or hypersensitivity (type I) response to a foreign protein. This is not unexpected, because there are considerable differences between animal and human DNases. There is only an 80% homology between the rat and human DNases; monkey DNase, although it has not been completely sequenced, also appears to be highly dissimilar to the human form (S. Shak, personal communication, 1997).

Some of the most persuasive data related to challenges of assessing immune reactions to inhaled therapeutic proteins in humans versus animals come from the development of rhDNase (Pulmozyme) for the treatment of cystic fibrosis. Pulmozyme involves the inhalation of a relatively large amount of rhDNase, which is an enzyme that cleaves DNA. The clinical summary portion of the Summary Basis of Approval for Pulmozyme (FDA, 1993) provides information related to immune responses. It was concluded that antibodies to rhDNase were of little consequence to the safety profile of rhDNase on patients because levels were generally low and there was no correlation between antibody levels and clinical responses. As noted previously, there were immune responses found in the rat and monkey inhalation toxicology studies in which the animals were exposed to a highly heterologous protein compared to their native DNases. There was no evidence of anaphylaxis in the animal studies; however, lung lesions that were observed were consistent with only mild alveolitis and were judged to be related to the immunological response to a foreign protein. Thus, the findings in the animal studies were deemed to be the result of immunological reaction to a nonhomologous foreign protein and not relevant to results in people. The clinical data indicate little concern for the homologous protein in humans [4].

INHALED INSULIN

Inhaled insulin is covered in detail in Chapter 7, and so it will be dealt with briefly here, concentrating mainly on safety issues. Inhaled insulin is attractive for the treatment of type 2 diabetes because it avoids the use of needles and may offer better outcomes through improved compliance. A large number of clinical trials have been carried with inhaled insulin by a number of companies, as thoroughly reviewed by Siekmeier and Scheuch [12] and Mastrandrea [13]. In controlled clinical trials, more than 13,000 patients have been treated with inhaled insulin on average for 1 year with some patients on Exubera® for up to 8 years. Overall, clinical trials have demonstrated that inhaled insulin is comparable to subcutaneous insulin for improving glycemic control. Also pharmacokinetics and pharmacodynamics were roughly similar, with the exception that inhaled regular insulin has faster absorption than subcutaneous regular insulin and it is comparable to fast-acting insulins.

Immunogenicity was studied extensively. In all major clinical programs, delivery of insulin by inhalation induced higher antibody levels in some patients than comparators. However, these antibodies were not shown to decrease the effectiveness, safety, or tolerability of inhaled insulin over time and did not affect clinical outcomes [14].

A number of inhaled insulin formulations have been developed but only Exubera received marketing authority. Most efforts were discontinued after Pfizer withdrew Exubera from the market but MannKind's inhaled insulin Afrezza continued in development. The major insulin development programs are cited in the following list, but a more complete list can be found in the publication of Siekmeier and Scheuch [12]:

- The only inhaled insulin that is approved is Afrezza (MannKind), a dry powder formulation, precipitated from fumaryl diketopiperazine solution.
- Exubera (insulin human [rDNA origin]) Inhalation Powder, a spray-dried dry powder formulation—withdrawn from the market by Pfizer.
- AERx (Novo Nordisk), an aqueous solution of insulin—discontinued after phase 3 studies.
- AIR (Eli Lilly), spray-dried dry powder formulation of insulin, dipalmitoyl phosphatidylcholine (DPPC), and sodium citrate—discontinued after phase 3 studies.
- Aerodose (Aerogen), liquid aerosol—development discontinued.

Preclinical study design considerations have to include both pharmacokinetics (measurement of serum insulin levels) and pharmacodynamics (onset and duration of the hypoglycemic effect). Hypoglycemia is a significant concern and has been mitigated by feeding animals immediately prior to insulin aerosol exposure, careful monitoring of the glucose response, and supplementation with food and/or glucose in episodes of severe hypoglycemia.

Of the major inhaled insulin toxicology programs, four have significant toxicology data available in the public domain [15–20]. In all four cases no adverse effects on lung were noted.

Pfizer/Nektar (two 1-month rat, one 6-month rat, one 1-month cynomolgus monkey, and one 6-month cynomolgus monkey studies): These studies, in addition to assessing standard toxicological parameters, also evaluated the potential toxicity of the complete formulation and the excipients alone to the respiratory tract. Investigations included respiratory and pulmonary function, lung cell proliferation indices, insulin antibody titers, and histopathology. There were no toxicological findings relevant to human systemic or pulmonary risk with the excipients or with the complete formulation at up to 40 times for rats and four times for monkeys compared to the clinical starting dose of 0.15 mg/kg/day. Maximum tolerated doses (MTDs) were limited by hypoglycemia. No evidence of exposure-related inflammatory or immune-mediated hypersensitivity reactions were observed in the respiratory tract. A weak antibody response to the insulin powder was observed in rat serum but anti-insulin antibodies were not detected in monkey serum or bronchoalveolar lavage fluid. Rat insulin differs from human insulin by three amino acids, pig and dog differ by one amino acid, and cynomolgus monkey insulin is identical to human insulin. A comparable weak antibody response in rats was also observed following subcutaneous injection. Assessment of respiratory and pulmonary function parameters revealed no exposure-related effects. No exposure-related histopathological responses were observed in the respiratory tract or in lung-associated lymph nodes in either species. Staining the bronchioles and alveoli with markers for cell proliferation showed no biologically significant differences in proliferation indices attributable to the complete formulation or excipients alone in either species [15,18].

AIR/Lilly (6 months, dogs): The purpose of this study was to characterize the toxicity, pharmacokinetics, and pharmacodynamics of daily human-inhaled insulin powder (HIIP) in beagle dogs *via* head-only exposures. The formulation was a dry powder composed of insulin, DPPC, and sodium citrate. Dogs were exposed 15 min/day to an air control, placebo, maximal placebo (3× the placebo dose), or one of three doses of HIIP (mean inhaled doses of 0.80, 0.24, or 0.70 mg/kg/day for the HIIP-low, HIIP-mid, and HIIP-high dose, respectively). Dose-related exposure (C_{max}, AUC) to inhaled insulin was observed with rapid absorption and there were no apparent gender differences or accumulation after repeated inhalation exposures for 26 weeks. The expected pharmacological effect of insulin was observed with dose-related decreases in serum glucose levels following HIIP administration. There were no toxic effects observed including no HIIP or placebo treatment–related effects on mean body weights, absolute body weight changes, clinical observations, food consumption, respiratory function parameters, ophthalmic examinations, electrocardiograms, heart rates, clinical pathology, or urinalysis. Similarly, there were no HIIP or placebo treatment–related effects on pulmonary assessments that included respiratory function parameters, bronchial alveolar lavage assessments, organ weights, or macroscopic and microscopic evaluations, including lung cell proliferation indices. HIIP was considered to have either low or no immunogenic potential in dogs. The NOAEL and MTD were the average inhaled dose of 0.70 mg insulin/kg/day [16], approximately fivefold greater than a typical clinical dose.

Aerogen (1 month, dogs): The inhalation safety of Humulin R U500 liquid insulin formulation was evaluated in a 28-day repeat dosing study in dogs. In addition to 500 IU/mL of human DNA-derived insulin, Humulin R contains glycerin 16 mg/mL, metacresol 2.5 mg/mL, and zinc oxide to supplement the endogenous zinc to obtain a total zinc content of 0.017 mg/100 units and water for injection. The pH was 7.0–7.8. Two pulmonary doses of insulin, a low dose, and the MTD were evaluated against water and placebo controls. After 28 days of daily exposure, the animals were killed and examined at necropsy. Respiratory tissues were examined microscopically. The mean pulmonary doses achieved were 2.3 and 8.3 U/kg/day for the low and MTD dose levels, respectively. The aerosols were highly respirable with 78% of the insulin aerosols being <3.8 μm. The treatments were well tolerated. No adverse in-life, necropsy, or histological findings were detected that were related to insulin or inhalation treatment [17].

MannKind/Sanofi (26-week rat, 39-week dogs; carcinogenicity studies, 104-week inhalation, rats; 26-week transgenic mice): In inhalation toxicology studies of AFREZZA, rats exposed to doses up to 1.91 mg/kg/day for 26 weeks and 1.23 mg/kg/day for 104 weeks, and dogs exposed to doses up to 1.92 mg/kg/day were well tolerated in all animals. There were no adverse findings including no microscopic findings in the lungs or evidence of carcinogenicity or proliferation. The main findings were, in rat 26-week study, goblet cell hyperplasia and eosinophilic globule accumulation of minimal severity in the olfactory/respiratory epithelium and, in dogs, neutrophil infiltration of minimal severity in lung. The TechnoSphere carrier controls at doses of 11.7 mg/kg also had similar lack of findings in the rat 26-week study, but also a slight increase in proliferating cell nuclear antigen in the bronchioles was observed [19].

In a 26-week carcinogenicity study, transgenic mice (Tg-ras-H2) exposed to doses up to 5 mg/kg/day of AFREZZA and to 75 mg/kg/day of TechnoSphere carrier had no increased incidence of tumors. AFREZZA also was not genotoxic in Ames bacterial mutagenicity assay and in the chromosome aberration assay, using human peripheral lymphocytes with or without metabolic activation. The TechnoSphere carrier alone was not genotoxic in the in vivo mouse micronucleus assay [20].

In a reproduction toxicity study, female rats given sc doses of 10, 30, and 100 mg/kg/day of TechnoSphere carrier starting 2 weeks before mating until gestation day 7 had no adverse effects on male fertility at doses up to 100 mg/kg/day (a systemic exposure 14–21 times that following the maximum daily AFREZZA dose of 99 mg based on AUC). Female rats at 100 mg/kg/day did have increased pre- and postimplantation loss but not at 30 mg/kg/day (14–21 times higher systemic exposure than the maximum daily AFREZZA dose of 99 mg based on AUC) [20].

In all of these extensive preclinical studies, at substantial multiples of clinical doses, no adverse effects on lung were found related to either insulin or the excipients. Potential still exists for inhaled insulin since it has been shown to be both safe and effective. However, its main advantage over sc delivery is convenience, which may result in better compliance. Two programs are currently conducting clinical trials (Mannkind and Dance) and so there should be indications in the near future if inhaled insulin will be part of the diabetes treatment arsenal.

INHALED HUMAN GROWTH HORMONE

Inhaled hGH was under development by Alkermes/Lilly [5]. One-month and 6-month inhalation toxicology studies were carried out in cynomolgus monkeys with no adverse effects in the lung observed. These studies supported clinical trials in normal volunteers. The trial was a crossover design in 12 young adult subjects, each subject receiving both subcutaneous and inhaled hGH on separate days. Inhaled hGH was well tolerated with no coughing or adverse taste issues. Pulmonary function and vital signs were measured with no apparent changes of clinical significance. The PK profiles for sc injection (4 mg hGH) and inhalation delivery (92 mg hGH in 4 dry powder capsules) were quite similar as seen in Figure 1.2 Overall delivery efficiency was approximately 5% compared to sc delivery, somewhat less than the approximately 10% values observed for a similar dry powder formulation and delivery system for inhaled insulin. The decreased efficiency with respect to inhaled insulin was expected because of the greater molecular weight of hGH.

Following the demonstration of safety in normal young adults, a similar crossover study was carried out in pediatric patients. Again, there were no adverse clinical outcomes for inhaled delivery, PK profile was similar to that from sc delivery, but overall delivery efficiency was less than the business development goal of 5% relative to sc delivery. With this result, the program was terminated.

If manufacturing costs of hGH can be reduced, inhaled delivery of hGH could be considered to improve compliance in children and increase the willingness of parents to start therapy in their children since reluctance to start injections is a negative factor in initiating growth hormone therapy.

PTH1-34

Development of inhaled PTH1-34 to treat osteoporosis was also considered. Feasibility data from intratracheal instillation studies in rats had shown that PTH1-34 was well absorbed from the lung into blood with similar bioavailability to that of insulin (Figure 1.1). Then a single-dose PK study in monkeys was carried out. The PK of PTH1-34 delivery by inhalation and subcutaneous (sc) administration was studied in a crossover manner in three anesthetized rhesus monkeys (Figure 1.3). Aerosol was delivered from an ultrasonic nebulizer through an endotracheal tube to intubated monkeys. The PK profiles from the sc and inhalation routes were similar and indicated a bioavailability of approximately 40% for inhaled delivery compared to sc. T_{max} values were approximately 0.5 h and half-lives were approximately 1 h for each delivery mode. This type of pulsatile delivery is important to provide the desired anabolic effect on bone since constant delivery actually results in hypercalcemia and bone resorption.

Subsequently, a 2-week inhalation toxicity study was conducted in rhesus monkeys. No adverse effects were noted in any of the measured endpoints, including no test-article-related effects on lung histopathology. PK profiles were similar on the

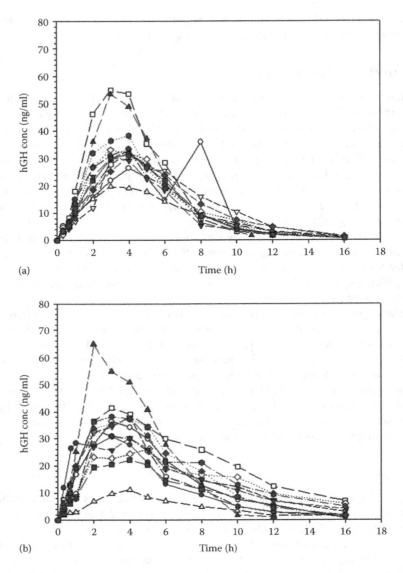

FIGURE 1.2 Pharmacokinetic profiles in healthy volunteers following Inhalation (a) and sc (b) administration of human growth hormone.

first and last day of exposure, indicating no accumulation of the compound and also no indication of neutralizing antibody production. Further, there was clear indication of efficacy. The time scale was too short for increases in bone density but there were clear significant increases in 1,25 di-hydroxyvitamin D3 levels indicating a positive bone formation response. Despite these positive findings, further development was not carried out because there was no clear therapeutic benefit of PTH1-34 inhalation

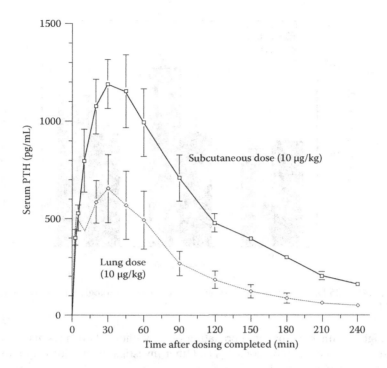

FIGURE 1.3 Single-dose inhalation studies of PTH1-34 in monkeys show good absorption and similar pharmacokinetics to sc delivery.

delivery over sc administration other than more convenience. In a motivated population suffering from osteoporosis, it was deemed that there was limited additional market potential for an inhaled product (Figure 1.4).

CYCLOSPORINE

Cyclosporine is a cyclic peptide with potent immunosuppressive properties. Inhaled cyclosporine has been investigated over a large number of years to aid in the postoperative treatment of lung transplant patients to reduce the incidence of rejection [21]. The inhaled formulation had no unexpected systemic toxicity or clinically limiting findings in the respiratory tract in 28-day rat and dog studies [22] and 9-month dog studies with exposures 3 days a week [23]. In phase 2 clinical trials, the inhaled formulation improved overall survival [24]. Recent data have shown that inhalation of cyclosporine in solution with propylene glycol given in addition to conventional immunosuppression appeared to improve important pulmonary function parameters in lung transplant recipients compared to patients receiving aerosol placebo or conventional immunosuppression alone. It was also shown to improve overall survival in phase 2 clinical trials [24]. However, recently completed phase 3 trials showed no efficacy beyond that of standard of care when used as supplemental targeted therapy [25]. The authors noted that "administering a cyclosporine aerosol

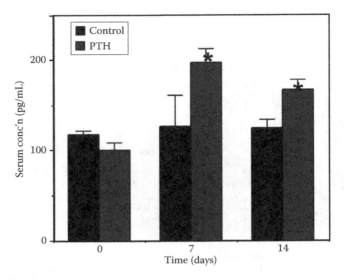

FIGURE 1.4   1,25 Dihydroxyvitamin D3 levels show positive biological response to inhaled PTH1-34.

to this highly vulnerable patient population is not without challenges and this may have influenced the study outcome" [17]. Other investigators are looking into possible uses to treat asthma [1].

ALPHA-1 ANTITRYPSIN

Alpha-1 antitrypsin is an enzyme that can be used to treat protease–antiprotease imbalance in the lung. For patients with alpha-1 antitrypsin deficiency, this is a serious issue since because of the low levels of antiproteases in the lung, proteases predominant and lead to lung inflammation, tissue destruction, and a predisposition to emphysema. Currently, there are three FDA-approved alpha-1 antitrypsins for IV administration: Prolastin (Grifols), Zemaira (Aventis-Behring), and Aralast (Alpha Therapeutic Corp.). All of these products are derived by purification from human serum.

Inhaled alpha-1 antitrypsin has been studied as a potential therapy with generally encouraging results [26]. Siekmeier [27] summarized that "the data demonstrate the feasibility of alpha-1 antitrypsin inhalation for restoration of the impaired protease antiprotease balance, attenuation of the inflammation and neutralization of the excess activity of neutrophil elastase." Inhaled alpha-1 antitrypsin may well be useful to COPD and CF as well as pure alpha-1 antitrypsin deficiency since protease–antiprotease imbalances have been suggested to contribute to both these respiratory diseases. Siekmeier [27] also noted that potentially the inhalation route may provide cheaper therapy than that for IV administration since only about 2% is delivered to the lung following IV delivery as compared to possibly 20%–30% that could be delivered to the lung following inhalation. The 20%–30% aerosol deposition value can only be achieved with optimized devices and formulations. Kamada [28] is developing inhaled alpha-1 antitrypsin as potential therapy for AAT deficiency and announced results from their European phase 2/3 clinical study in September 2014. These failed to meet either the primary "time to the first moderate or severe exacerbation event" or secondary exacerbation endpoints with the intent to treat (ITT) population. However, there were clinically relevant changes in various lung function measurements in the ITT population, as well as in the Most Frequent Exacerbators population, of which some were statistically significant. Inhaled AAT was also safe and well tolerated in the patients. Based on the strength of the lung function changes, especially in the Most Frequent Exacerbators population, Kamada still plans to file for approval in Europe and the United States. The complete data set from the phase 2/3 clinical study was presented in May 2015 [28]. The benefit of inhaled AAT treatment is also being evaluated in other patient populations including cystic fibrosis [28].

One additional opportunity that could enhance inhaled alpha-1 antitrypsin usage would be the availability of a recombinant human protein to reduce immunogenicity potential, increase product reproducibility, and potentially reduce costs if an appropriate manufacturing process can be developed.

INHALED VACCINES

Inhaled vaccines, particularly measles vaccines, have received considerable attention. There has been the thought that delivery of the vaccine to the respiratory tract, the natural entry route for the pathogen, might provide an attractive therapy by engaging mucosal immunological mechanisms. Inhaled delivery is attractive for use in developing countries because of lack of suitably trained staff to administer injections and problems in disposal of used needles and syringes. Early work by Albert Sabin [29] demonstrated the feasibility followed by a mass vaccination campaign in 4 million children between 1988 and 1990 [30].

In 2002 the Measles Aerosol Vaccine Project was initiated by the WHO, CDC, and American Red Cross in order to develop a practical inhaled measles vaccine using liquid aerosol delivery [31]. Phase 1 studies showed that the aerosolized vaccine was safe and well tolerated and produced an appropriate immune response. Phase 2/3 studies were completed and showed results equivalent to sc delivery for children ages 10–35 months, but for ages 9–10 months, immune response was not as good as for sc delivery [32]. Challenges with getting good lung deposition in nose-breathing infants likely contributed to these findings. The conclusion by WHO was that for children greater than 10 months aerosol delivery should be effective. In addition, there have been efforts to develop a dry powder aerosolized vaccine using carbon dioxide–assisted bubble drying [33]. This effort was spearheaded by Aktiv-Dry with key support from a Grand Challenges grant from the Gates foundation. Preclinical studies in monkeys with the dry powder vaccine showed no adverse effects and the production of an immune response was similar to that from sc delivery [34]. Phase 1 clinical trials have been completed in healthy men with preexisting immunity to measles [35]. No adverse events were reported and the inhaled dry powder vaccine produced serologic responses generally similar to subcutaneous vaccination; however, these results are difficult to interpret because of the high baseline antibody levels.

One of the key hopes of the inhaled measles vaccines efforts is to provide access to therapies in developing countries where infrastructure for needle injection delivery systems is problematical. Another key hope is that ultimately more cost-effective therapies might also be possible [36]. This may be challenging, but with continued technological innovation, it appears to be feasible.

Anti-IgE

In the late 1990s there was a very interesting drug development plan by Genentech to investigate the possibility of using inhaled anti-IgE to treat asthma. The rationale was that there was evidence for both local and systemic effects of IgE in the etiology of asthma. The hypothesis was that local delivery of anti-IgE to the lung would inhibit IgE-mediated inflammation in the lung and provide improved asthma therapy. Both nonclinical [37] and clinical studies [38] were undertaken. The definitive data from the clinical trials showed that inhaled anti-IgE were well tolerated. It was concluded "that aerosol administration of an anti-IgE monoclonal antibody does not inhibit the airway responses to inhaled allergen in allergic asthmatic subjects." The nonclinical studies had demonstrated that aerosol delivery did result in good deposition of the anti-IgE in lungs. It was also found that only <0.1% of the IgE delivered to lungs was absorbed into blood. These data confirm that local deposition was indeed achieved and the low absorption into blood, consistent with the high molecular weight of anti-IgE, suggested a potential long-term residence in lung. In this case, systemic delivery of anti-IgE by subcutaneous injection produces superior therapeutic results for treating asthma than local delivery by inhaled administration.

The results of this program suggest that for new initiatives with inhaled antibodies, there needs to be careful consideration of target receptors, receptor affinities, and relative influence of systemic and local effects. Although not discussing inhaled therapies, Catley et al. [39] have reviewed potential use of monoclonal antibodies to treat asthma. There has been some conjecture that future targets with relatively high-affinity receptors in the lung and high lung specificity might be attractive opportunities. Another factor supporting inhaled use for future therapies would be if there were no systemic delivery alternative for the proposed therapy or if the only systemic therapy is intravenous delivery.

INHALED GENE THERAPY

Inhaled gene therapy approaches to treat cystic fibrosis have been largely unsuccessful using approaches such as attenuated adenovirus vectors to deliver the CFTR gene [40]. There is broad consensus that treatment of CF lung disease will require prolonged expression of CFTR for many months. However, only three trials using adenovirus and adeno-associated virus vectors [41–43] have assessed duration in the lung. These vectors were shown to be unsuitable because of adaptive immune responses to these viral vectors [44].

However, newer approaches using lipid-based carriers of CFTR DNA are underway. An inhalation study was carried out in mice to determine the efficacy and safety of administering of cationic lipid formulation GL67A complexed with pGM169, a CpG-free plasmid encoding human CFTR complementary DNA [45]. Twelve biweekly inhalation exposures were carried out over a period of 6 months. Results showed that repeated administration of pGM169/GL67A to murine lungs resulted in a NOAEL at the lowest dose of 1.2 mg pGM169/kg and 6.7 mg GL67A/kg that was estimated to be approximately fivefold the anticipated clinical dose. Reproducible, dose-related, and persistent gene expression (>140 days after each dose) was achieved using an aerosol generated by a clinically relevant nebulizer. This study supported progression into the first nonviral multidose lung trial in CF patients [46].

Approaches have also been used with polyethylenimine (PEI) carriers. The intermittent exposure of Balb/c mice (sex not reported) to PEI (branched)–DNA *via* an aerosol delivery system resulted in a higher expression of DNA in the lungs of treated animals compared to control aerosol mice (no exposure) or to mice exposed to lipid–DNA vectors [47]. Treatment involved exposure of the mice to 1 min of aerosol followed by a 9 min delay to allow the animals to breathe the aerosol before beginning the cycle again; this cycle was repeated until all of the nebulizer fluid (40 mL in total) was used (approximately 16 h).

While clinical signs of toxicity were not reported in the previous study, a similar study in which female Balb/c mice were exposed to a PEI (branched)–DNA vector *via* an aerosol delivery system for 30 min did not result in any signs of lung toxicity (including any signs of acute inflammation) [48]. Following the 30 min exposure period, gene expression (as measured by the levels of chloramphenicol acetyl transferase [CAT] in the lung) persisted for 10 days postexposure, although CAT levels decreased to approximately 50% of peak levels at 7 days postexposure [48]. These data suggest that aerosol administration of branched PEI results in lung deposition but does not result in clinical signs of acute toxicity.

A study in which PEI (branched)–DNA or lipid–DNA complexes were delivered to female C57BL/6 mice *via* an aerosol delivery system (duration of exposure was 30 min) reported a lower level of lung and serum cytokines (specifically, tumor necrosis factor-α [TNF-α] and interleukin-1β [IL-1β] levels) in these mice compared to mice receiving an equivalent amount of PEI (branched)–DNA *via* the IV route (at a level from 6.45 μg of branched PEI to 5 μg of DNA in a 200 μL solution, based on a PEI–DNA weight ratio of 1.29:1) or compared to mice exposed to the lipid–DNA complex [49]. Additionally, the levels of TNF-α and IL-1β in the lungs peaked at 5–8 h postaerosol exposure and resolved to control levels within 24 h postaerosol exposure, while levels in the bronchoalveolar lavage fluid (BALF) peaked at 24 h and resolved to control levels within 48 h postaerosol exposure. There was no neutrophil infiltration into the BALF at the timepoints evaluated, suggesting that the cytokine levels in the BALF may not be high enough to stimulate an acute inflammatory response. The data suggest that the aerosol delivery of genetic material using branched PEI as a vector decreases the cytokine responses associated with plasmid delivery when compared to cytokine levels *via* the IV route or *via* aerosol delivery of genetic material using lipid vectors.

There were no significant differences noted in the levels of CAT in the liver, spleen, kidney, thymus, brain, and blood compared to untreated controls following aerosol delivery of a PEI (branched)–DNA complex to female Balb/c mice for 30 min, suggesting a lack of systemic gene delivery and, by inference, PEI delivery following aerosol exposure to the vector [48]. Delivery of an aerosolized labeled PEI (branched)–DNA complex to female Balb/c mice (exposure duration of 30–120 min) resulted in localization of the label mainly in the epithelial cells lining the airways, suggesting that PEI is concentrated in the lung tissue following aerosol administration [48,50].

Repeated administration of a branched PEI complex also did not result in signs of toxicity [51]. Following the injection of B16-F10 cells (a metastatic melanoma cell line) *via* the lateral tail vein, male nude mice (strain not reported) received PEI (branched)–p53 *via* an aerosol delivery system twice a week for 5 weeks, starting at 6 weeks postinoculation of the cancer cells [52]. Control groups included untreated mice, mice treated with PEI (branched; alone) or with PEI (branched)–CAT complexes. There were no signs of acute inflammatory responses, including neutrophil infiltration or tissue damage, in any of the tissues examined from any of the treatment groups (tissues that were examined included lung, liver, kidney, spleen, brain, and heart). In addition, there was no significant loss of body weight in treated animals when compared to the control animals [52].

Intranasal administration of PEI (branched)–DNA at a level from 51.6 μg of PEI (branched) to 40 μg of DNA (based on a PEI–DNA weight ratio of 1.29:1) to female Balb/c mice resulted in a higher expression of DNA in the lungs of treated animals compared to the control (no aerosol exposure) or compared to mice exposed to lipid–DNA vectors [47]. Note that nasal delivery of droplets in mice results in good lung delivery of the solution. Clinical signs of toxicity were not reported in this study; however, it is unclear if the study authors examined the animals for signs of toxicity.

For novel gene therapy vectors, information on biodistribution measurements is needed to determine PK/PD of vector. Usually qPCR is measured in tissues including blood, liver, kidneys, heart, brain, testes, ovaries, and spleen as suggested in FDA guidance [53]. Levels in reproductive organs are important since to assess possible risk of transmission of gene therapy vectors from parent to offspring. These measurements can be conducted along with measurement of the desired transcribed therapeutic protein carried by the vector.

FORMULATION APPROACHES

Appropriate formulations and devices are crucial for delivering proteins and peptides to the lung. There have been many advances that have been recently reviewed [54–57] (Weers, Sakagami, Lechuga, Muralidharan). Novel molecular or formulation approaches, for example, spray-drying (PulmoSphere®, ARCUS®, iSPERSE®), TechnoSphere®, Fc-/scFv-fusion protein, PEGylation, and polymeric or lipid-based micro-/nanoparticles and liposomes, offer opportunities to improve lung absorption and therapeutic duration of many biotherapeutics. The dry powder spray-dried formulations that have been developed are particularly flexible and produce highly dispersible engineered particles that, with the appropriate excipient components, also afford substantial stability for proteins and peptides [54].

Fortunately the array of excipients that can now be used for inhalation delivery has expanded in recent years. Excipients that can now be considered for use in inhalation products include distearyl phospatidylcholine (DSPC), DPPC mannitol, glycine, and fumaryl diketopiperazine. Other agents, such as other amino acids, are also being increasingly used in inhaled drugs in develop. If the excipients in an inhaled drug candidate are novel, that is, they have not been used in previously approved inhaled drug products, then toxicological characterization of the novel excipients will be required [58,59]. The toxicology studies needed for novel excipients depend on the nature of the excipient. If the excipient is a sugar, similar to lactose that is an approved inhalation excipient or if the excipient is an endogenous material, the types of studies needed might be relatively minor. This is especially the case for endogenous compounds where the administered dose results in small increments in preexisting levels. For instance, for mannitol and glycine in Exubera (inhaled insulin) formulation and DPPC in Lilly's inhaled insulin formulation, a placebo control group containing excipients was included in addition to an air breathing control group into the subchronic and chronic inhalation toxicity studies. Thus, the studies used a total of five groups instead of the more usual four groups as there were air control, placebo control, and low-, mid-, and high-dose treatment groups. This approach, as well as literature review of these agents, was considered sufficient by regulatory agencies for approval. Similar approaches have been used for the use of DSPC in spray-dried powder formulations. A less familiar excipient has been used in Afrezza inhaled insulin, namely, fumaryl diketopiperazine, which is used to produce TechnoSphere particles. In this case more extensive studies were needed, including a 2-year inhalation carcinogenicity study in rats, a 6-month subcutaneous transgenic mouse study (Tg.rasH2), as well as the study of fumaryl diketopiperazine pharmacokinetics [19,20].

PEGylation involving the attachment of high-molecular-weight polyethylene glycol (PEG) to molecules is an approach that offers the possibility of altering biodistribution and clearance times [57]. PEGylation increases drug stability and the retention time and reduces proteolysis and renal excretion. PEGylation is also an approach that has a considerable database related to its relatively low toxicity as evidenced by the large numbers of marketed PEGylated proteins and also a long history of toxicology studies that have been extensively reviewed by Working [60]. PEGylation of therapeutic proteins has significantly improved the treatment of several chronic diseases, including hepatitis C, leukemia, severe combined immunodeficiency disease, rheumatoid arthritis, and Crohn disease. The most important PEGylated drugs include pegademase bovine, pegaspargase, pegfilgrastim, interferons, pegvisomant, pegaptanib, and certolizumab pegol [61]. The successful use of this strategy for parenterally delivered drugs makes it a reasonable candidate for use inhaled drugs.

An example is provided here that demonstrates the potential for pegylation to increase half-life of inhaled compounds. Insulin was used as a model compound and PEG compounds of increasing molecular weight from 2000 (2K) to 5000 (5K) were used. Further modification of the PEGS with diacyl groups was also explored. Following preliminary intratracheal studies in rats, inhalation studies were carried out in anesthetized dogs to study the effect of the PEGs in increasing the time of glucose suppression. As seen in Figure 1.5 the order of increase in glucose response was PEG5K diacyl > PEG5K > PEG2K diacyl > PEG2K > insulin. The time course of insulin response for the PEG5K diacyl and PEG5K was similar to that of neutral protamine Hagedorn (NPH) insulin. The lengthening of glucose response was closely correlated with the longer half-lives of insulin detected in blood. Two-week inhalation toxicity studies were subsequently carried out and it was found that PEG2K

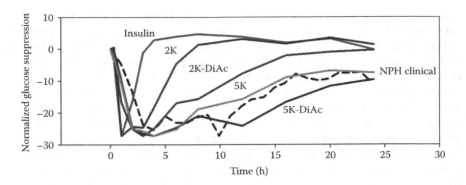

FIGURE 1.5 Increasing polyethylene glycol molecular weight increases glucose lowering action time following inhalation of 2K–5K PEGylated insulins in anesthetized dogs. (Response to sc NPH insulin in humans is shown in the dotted line.)

insulin was well tolerated at inhaled doses that would support clinical investigation, whereas higher-molecular-weight PEG insulins produced some mild inflammation, which made them unsuitable for clinical development.

FUTURE DIRECTIONS

Although inhaled proteins and peptides have shown limited success thus far, there are a number of opportunities for future success. Appropriate situations must be assessed to determine if there is an unmet medical need that can be addressed with inhaled therapies. It seems only a matter of time before some inhaled antibodies are developed to treat some forms of local respiratory disease. Of course, the correct receptors and time action need to be addressed, and so this is not a simple endeavor. Other proteins or peptides may also be good candidates to treat local respiratory disease, such as dealing with protease–antiprotease imbalances.

Modified proteins or peptides have been developed to improve pharmacokinetics for systemic delivery. In my personal opinion, pegylation provides the most promising approach for increasing systemic half-lives. It has been demonstrated that by using PEGs in the molecular weight range of 2–5 kDa, lung disappearance half-lives of the order of 7–12 h can be achieved [62], which is excellent for many therapies since it allows optimal once or twice a day dosing. PEGs greater than 5K tended to show a long-lived component in the lung and are unlikely to be compatible with once a day dosing.

Further use of inhaled proteins and peptides has definite promise. There should be careful consideration of dealing with clear unmet clinical needs and validated target selection. In addition, cost needs to be considered. Advances in protein manufacture to reduce cost will help. High-efficiency delivery systems are needed with careful consideration of aerosol properties for reproducible delivery to the lung with high deposition efficiency in the alveolar region. Excellent vibrating mesh devices for liquid delivery such as those by Aerogen and Pari should be considered. Engineered dry powder formulations advances such as those by Novartis (PulmoSphere), Civitas (ARCUS), and Pulmatrix (iSPERSE) can also aid inhaled protein development.

SUMMARY

- The development of Pulmozyme and Exubera has shown that both local and systemic use of inhaled proteins can be safe and efficacious.
- There are a number of opportunities for future success including inhaled antibodies, approaches to address protease–antiprotease imbalances contributing to lung disease, and PEGylated proteins and peptides to improve pharmacokinetics.
- Future therapies should concentrate on unmet medical needs and validated targets.
- High-efficiency delivery systems are needed with careful consideration of aerosol properties for reproducible delivery to the lung with high deposition efficiency in the alveolar region.
- Cost needs to be considered. Advances in protein manufacture and biosimilars to reduce cost will help.

REFERENCES

1. Depreter F, Picher C, Amighi K. Inhaled proteins: Challenges and perspectives. *International Journal of Pharmaceutics* 447: 251–280 (2013).
2. Kane C, O'Neil K, Conk M, Picha K. Inhalation delivery of protein therapeutics. *Inflammation & Allergy—Drug Targets* 12(2): 81–87 (2013).
3. Patton JS, Byron PR. Inhaling medicines: Delivering drugs to the body through the lungs. *Nature Reviews—Drug Discovery* 6: 67–74 (2007).
4. Wolff RK. Safety of inhaled proteins for therapeutic use. *Journal of Aerosol Medicine* 11(4): 197–219 (1998). http://online.liebertpub.com/doi/abs/10.1089/jam.1998.11.197.
5. McElroy MC, Kirton C, Gliddon D, Wolff RK. Inhaled biopharmaceutical drug development: Non-clinical considerations and case studies. *Inhalation Toxicology* 5(4): 219–232 (2013).
6. Siekmeier R, Scheuch S. Systemic treatment by inhalation of macromolecules—Principles, problems and examples. *Journal of Physiology and Pharmacology* 59(Suppl. 6): 53–79 (2008).
7. Ponce R, Abad L, Amaravadi L, Gelzleichter T, Gore E, Green J et al. Immunogenicity of biologically-derived therapeutics: Assessment and interpretation of nonclinical safety studies. *Regulatory Toxicology and Pharmacology* 54: 164–182 (2009).
8. ICH S6 (R1). Preclinical safety evaluation of biotechnology-derived pharmaceuticals (2011). http://www.ich.org/fileadmin/Public_Web_Site/ICH_Products/Guidelines/Safety/S6_R1/Step4/S6_R1_Guideline.pdf. Accessed Jan, 2016.
9. Cavagnaro J. The principles of the ICH S6 and the case-by-case approach. In *Preclinical Safety Evaluation of Biopharmaceuticals: A Science-Based Approach to Facilitating Clinical Trials*, Cavagnaro J, ed. John Wiley & Sons, Hoboken, NJ, pp. 45–65 (2008).
10. Clarke J, Hurst C, Martin P, Vahle J, Ponce R, Mounho B, Heidel S, Andrews L, Reynolds T, Cavagnaro J. Duration of chronic toxicity studies for biotechnology-derived pharmaceuticals: Is 6 months still appropriate? *Regulatory Toxicology and Pharmacology* 50: 2–22 (2008).
11. Green JD. Pharmaco-toxicological expert report: Pulmozyme™, rhDNase, Genentech, Inc. *Human & Experimental Toxicology* 13(Suppl.): S1–S42 (1994).
12. Siekmeier R, Scheuch G. Inhaled insulin—Does it become reality? *Journal of Physiology and Pharmacology* 59(Suppl. 6): 81–113 (2008).

13. Mastrandrea LD. Inhaled insulin: Overview of a novel route of insulin administration. *Vascular Health and Risk Management* 3(6): 47–58 (2010).
14. Fineberg SE, Kawabata T, Finco-Kent D, Liu C, Krasner A. Antibody response to inhaled insulin in patients with type 1 or type 2 diabetes. *Journal of Clinical Endocrinology & Metabolism* 90: 3287–3294 (2005).
15. McConnell WR, Finch GL, Elwell MR, Kawabata T, Moutvic R, Shaw M, Stammberger I. Toxicological investigations on inhaled insulin. *Society of Toxicology Annual Meeting*, San Diego (2006).
16. Vick A, Wolff R, Koester A, Reams R, Deaver D, Heidel S. A 6-month inhalation study to characterize the toxicity, pharmacokinetics, and pharmacodynamics of human insulin inhalation powder (HIIP) in Beagle dogs. *Journal of Aerosol Medicine* 20: 112–126 (2007).
17. Gopalakrishnan V, Uster P, Cow G, McDonald P. Four week repeat dose inhalation safety of insulin in dogs. *Journal of Aerosol Medicine* 14: 379–421 (2001).
18. FDA. Pharmacological/toxicological evaluation—Exubera®, NDA 21-868 (2005). http://www.fda.gov/ohrms/dockets/ac/05/briefing/2005–4169B1_02_04-FDA-ClinPharm-Toxicology.pdf. Accessed Jan, 2016.
19. Greene S, Nikula K, Poulin D, McInally K, Reynolds J. Assessment of long-term nonclinical safety of Technosphere® particles and AFREZZA® inhalation powder. Presented at the *Society of Toxicology 52th Annual Meeting*, San Antonio, TX (March 10–14, 2013); *Toxicological Sciences* 132(Suppl. 1): 263 (2013).
20. AFREZZA. Medication guide and instructions for use (2014). http://www.mannkind-corp.com/Collateral/Documents/English-US/Afrezza_PrescribingInformation.pdf. Accessed Jan, 2016.
21. Muggenburg BA, Hoover MD, Griffith BP, Haley PJ, Snipes MB, Wolff RK, Yeh HC, Burckart GJ, Mauderly JL. Administration of cyclosporine by inhalation: A feasibility study in beagle dogs. *Journal of Aerosol Medicine* 3(1): 1–13 (1990).
22. Wang T, Noonberg S, Steigerwalt R, Lynch M, Kovelesky RA, Rodríguez CA, Sprugel K, Turner N. Preclinical safety evaluation of inhaled cyclosporine in propylene glycol. *Journal of Aerosol Medicine* 20: 417–428 (2007).
23. Niven R, Lynch M, Moutvic R, Gibbs S, Briscoe C, Raff H. Safety and toxicology of cyclosporine in propylene glycol after 9-month aerosol exposure to beagle dogs. *Journal of Aerosol Medicine and Pulmonary Drug Delivery* 24: 205–212 (2011).
24. Groves S, Galazka M, Johnson B, Corcoran T, Verceles A, Britt E, Todd N, Griffith B, Smaldone GC, Iacono A. Inhaled cyclosporine and pulmonary function in lung transplant recipients. *Journal of Aerosol Medicine and Pulmonary Drug Delivery* 23: 31–39 (2010).
25. Niven RW, Verret W, Raff H, Corcoran TE, Dilly SG. The challenges of developing an inhaled cyclosporine product for lung transplant patients. *Respiratory Drug Delivery* 1: 51–60 (2012).
26. Hubbard RC, McElvaney NG, Sellers SE, Healy JT, Czerski DB, Crystal RG. Recombinant DNA-produced alpha 1-antitrypsin administered by aerosol augments lower respiratory tract antineutrophil elastase defenses in individuals with alpha 1-antitrypsin deficiency. *Journal of Clinical Investigation* 84(4): 1349–1354 (1989).
27. Siekmeier R. Lung deposition of inhaled alpha-1-proteinase inhibitor (alpha 1-P1)—Problems and experience of alpha 1-P1 inhalation therapy in patients with hereditary alpha 1-P1 deficiency and cystic fibrosis. *European Journal of Medical Research* 15: 164–174 (2010).
28. Kamada. http://www.kamada.com/news_item.php?ID=244. Kamada meets primary endpoint of U.S. Phase 2 study of inhaled alpha-1 antitrypsin for the treatment of alpha-1 antitrypsin deficiency. www.kamada.com/events.php. Accessed Aug 30, 2016.

29. Sabin AB. Immunization against measles by aerosol. *Reviews of Infectious Diseases* 5: 514–523 (1983).
30. Valdespino-Gomez JL, de Lourdes Garcia-Garcia M, Fernandez-de-Castro J, Henao-Restrepo AM, Bennett J, Sepulveda-Amor J. Measles aerosol vaccination. *Current Topics in Microbiology and Immunology* 304: 165–193 (2006).
31. Henao-Restrepo AM, Greco M, Laurie X, John O, Aguado T. Measles aerosol vaccine project. *Proceedia in Vaccinology* 2: 147–150 (2010).
32. WHO. Measles aerosol vaccine project: Report to SAGE (2012). www.who.int/immunization/.../3_MeaslesAerosolVaccineProject-report. Accessed Jan, 2016.
33. Burger JL, Cape SP, Braun CS, McAdams DH, Best JA, Bhagwat P, Pathak P, Rebits LG, Sievers RE. Stabilizing formulations for inhalable powders of live-attenuated measles virus vaccine. *Journal of Aerosol Medicine and Pulmonary Drug Delivery* 21(1): 25–34 (2008).
34. Lin WH, Griffin DE, Rotab PA, Papania M, Cape SP, Bennett D et al. Successful respiratory immunization with dry powder live-attenuated measles virus vaccine in rhesus macaques. *Proceedings of the National Academy of Sciences of the United States of America* 108(7): 2987–2992 (2011). www.pnas.org/content/early/2011/01/26/1017334108.full.pdf.
35. Agarkhedkar S, Kulkarni SP, Winston S, Sievers R, Dhere RM, Gunale B, Powell K, Rota PA, Papania M. Safety and immunogenicity of dry powder measles vaccine administered by inhalation: A randomized controlled Phase I clinical trial. *Vaccine* 32: 6791–6797 (2014).
36. Garrison Jr LP, Bauch CT, Bresnahan BW, Hazlet TK, Kadiyala S, Veenstra DL. Using cost-effectiveness analysis to support research and development portfolio prioritization for product innovations in measles vaccination. *Journal of Infectious Diseases* 204: S124–S132 (2011).
37. Sweeney TD, Marian M, Achilles M, Bussiere J, Ruppel J, Shoenhoff M, Mrsny RJ. Biopharmaceutics of immunoglobin transport across lung epithelium. In *Respiratory Drug Delivery VII*, P Byron et al., eds. Serentec Press, Raleigh, NC, pp. 59–66 (2000).
38. Fahy JV, Cockcroft DW, Boulet LP, Wong HH, Deschesnes F, Davis EE, Ruppel J, Su JQ, Adelman DC. Effect of aerosolized anti-IgE (E25) on airway responses to inhaled allergen in asthmatic subjects. *American Journal of Respiratory and Critical Care Medicine* 160(3): 1023–1027 (1999).
39. Catley MC, Coote J, Bari M, Tomlinson KL. Monoclonal antibodies for the treatment of asthma. *Pharmacology & Therapeutics* 132: 333–351 (2011).
40. Moss RB, Milla C, Colombo J, Accurso F, Zeitlin PL, Clancy JP et al. Repeated aerosolized AAV-CFTR for treatment of cystic fibrosis: A randomized placebo-controlled phase 2b trial. *Human Gene Therapy* 18: 726–732 (2007).
41. Zabner J, Ramsey BW, Meeker DP, Aitken ML, Balfour RP, Gibson RL et al. Repeat administration of an adenovirus vector encoding cystic fibrosis transmembrane conductance regulator to the nasal epithelium of patients with cystic fibrosis. *Journal of Clinical Investigation* 97: 1504–1511 (1996).
42. Harvey BG, Leopold PL, Hackett NR, Grasso TM, Williams PM, Tucker AL et al. Airway epithelial CFTR mRNA expression in cystic fibrosis patients after repetitive administration of a recombinant adenovirus. *Journal of Clinical Investigation* 104: 1245–1255 (1999).
43. Moss RB, Rodman D, Spencer LT, Aitken ML, Zeitlin PL, Waltz D et al. Repeated adeno-associated virus serotype 2 aerosol-mediated cystic fibrosis transmembrane regulator gene transfer to the lungs of patients with cystic fibrosis: A multicenter, double-blind, placebo-controlled trial. *Chest* 125: 509–521 (2004).
44. Griesenbach U, Alton EW. Expert opinion in biological therapy: Update on developments in lung gene transfer. *Expert Opinion on Biological Therapy* 13: 345–360 (2013).

45. Alton EW, Boyd AC, Cheng SH, Davies JC, Davies LA, Dayan A et al. Toxicology study assessing efficacy and safety of repeated administration of lipid/DNA complexes to mouse lung. *Gene Therapy* 21(1): 89–95 (2014). Accessed May, 2014.

46. DNA Science Blog: A Checklist for Gene Therapy from the UK Cystic Fibrosis Trial (2014). http://blogs.plos.org/dnascience/2014/05/22/checklist-gene-therapy-uk-cystic-fibrosis-trial/. Accessed May, 2014.

47. Densmore CL, Orson FM, Xu B, Kinsey BM, Waldrep JC, Hua P et al. Aerosol delivery of robust polyethyleneimine-DNA complexes for gene therapy and genetic immunization. *Molecular Therapy* 1: 180–188 (2000).

48. Gautam A, Densmore CL, Xu B, Waldrep JC. Enhanced gene expression in mouse lung after PEI-DNA aerosol delivery. *Molecular Therapy* 2: 63–70 (2000).

49. Gautam A, Densmore CL, Waldrep JC. Pulmonary cytokine responses associated with PEI-DNA aerosol gene therapy. *Gene Therapy* 8: 254–257 (2001).

50. Gautam A, Densmore CL, Golunski E, Xu B, Waldrep JC. Transgene expression in mouse airway epithelium by aerosol gene therapy with PEI-DNA complexes. *Molecular Therapy* 3: 551–556 (2001).

51. Densmore CL, Kleinerman ES, Gautam A, Jia S-F, Xu B, Worth LL et al. Growth suppression of established human osteosarcoma lung metastases in mice by aerosol gene therapy with PEI-p53 complexes. *Cancer Gene Therapy* 8: 619–627 (2001).

52. Densmore CL. Polyethyleneimine-based gene therapy by inhalation. *Expert Opinion on Biological Therapy* 3: 1083–1092 (2003).

53. FDA. Guidance for industry: Gene therapy clinical trials—Observing subjects for delayed adverse events. FDA, Rockville, MD (2006).

54. Weers JG, Miller DP. Formulation design of dry powders for inhalation. *Journal of Pharmaceutical Sciences* 104(10): 3259–3288 (2015).

55. Sakagami M. Systemic delivery of biotherapeutics through the lung: Opportunities and challenges for improved lung absorption. *Therapeutic Delivery* 4(12): 1511–1525 (2013).

56. Lechuga-Ballesteros D, Miller DP. Advances in respiratory and nasal drug delivery. *Molecular Pharmaceutics* 12(8): 2561 (2015).

57. Muralidharan P, Mallory E, Malapit M, Hayes Jr D, Mansour HM. Inhalable PEGylated phospholipid nanocarriers and PEGylated therapeutics for respiratory delivery as aerosolized colloidal dispersions and dry powder inhalers. *Pharmaceutics* 6: 333–353 (2014).

58. DeGeorge J, Ahn CH, Andrews PA, Brower ME, Choi YS, Chun MY et al. Considerations for toxicology studies of respiratory drug products. *Regulatory Toxicology and Pharmacology* 25: 189–193 (1997).

59. FDA. Draft guidance for industry and staff: Nonclinical evaluation of reformulated drug products and products intended for administration by an alternate route (2008). http://www.fda.gov/downloads/drugs/guidancecomplianceregulatoryinform-ation/guidances/ucm079245.pdf+&cd=1&hl=en&ct=clnk&gl=us. Accessed Jan, 2016.

60. Working PK, Newman MS, Johnson J, Cornacoff JB. Safety of poly(ethylene glycol) and poly(ethylene glycol) derivatives. In *Poly(Ethylene Glycol): Chemistry and Biological Applications*, Harris M, Zalipsky S, eds. Division of Polymer Chemistry Symposium, *213th National Meeting of the ACS*, San Francisco, CA (April 13–17, 1997). American Chemical Society (ACS), Washington, DC, pp. 45–57 (1998) (ACS Symposium Series, No. 680).

61. Veronese FM, Mero A. The impact of PEGylation on biological therapies. *BioDrugs* 22(5): 315–329 (2008).

62. Gursahani H, Riggs-Sauthier J, Pfeiffer J, Lechuga-Ballesteros D, Fishburn CS. Absorption of polyethylene glycol (PEG) polymers: The effect of PEG size on permeability. *Journal of Pharmaceutical Sciences* 98(8): 2847–2856 (2009).

2 Inhaled Insulin
More Compelling than Ever

John S. Patton and Samantha R. Miller

CONTENTS

INTRODUCTION

According to the International Diabetes Federation in its 2013 report, roughly 382 million people worldwide suffer from diabetes of which 85%–95% or more are type 2 diabetes patients [1]. The number of patients is expected to grow to 592 million in less than 25 years [1]. Approximately 26% of type 2 diabetes patients currently take daily insulin injections in the United States [1–3]. Insulin is currently underutilized by type 2 diabetes patients due to resistance to daily injections [4–7]. Insulin injections are generally viewed unfavorably by patients, leading those with poor glycemic control to postpone insulin for up to 7 years. Approximately 73% of type 2 diabetes patients delay insulin injection therapy, and of those approximately 25% refuse insulin despite their physician's recommendation and some are needle phobic. Patients avoid and delay insulin therapy partially due to the inconvenience, pain, and the social stigma of daily injections. Of patients who finally accept treatment, 70% resist increasing the number of injections, and we believe a significant portion regularly skip insulin treatment at mealtime [4–8]. Despite these drawbacks, according to BCC Research, global sales of insulin and insulin devices were estimated to reach approximately $26 billion in 2013 and are projected to grow to $40 billion by 2018 [2].

UNMET NEED

CURRENT GUIDELINES

Lifestyle modification and metformin, an inexpensive noninsulin therapy, are preferred in the early stages of type 2 diabetes treatment [9]. Over time, additional medications become necessary and combinations of drugs, including metformin plus other oral agents, GLP-1 receptor agonists, or injectable insulin, can be effective. In patients with chronically high blood glucose levels, oral medication alone is unlikely to adequately control blood glucose, and insulin therapy is often recommended. Studies indicate that insulin is the most effective way to treat type 2 diabetes as it has durable effects in all patients, offers the greatest reduction in blood glucose, and reduces the decline of insulin-producing cell function [9].

INSULIN TREATMENT NOW RECOMMENDED EARLIER IN THE TREATMENT REGIME

Traditional treatment guidelines following diagnoses of type 2 diabetes recommended that patients start insulin therapy approximately 10 years after initial diagnosis. However, the latest ADA and European Association for the Study of Diabetes guidelines in 2009 recommend earlier use of insulin by patients who are unable to adequately maintain appropriate blood glucose with noninsulin therapy [10]. In 2013, the American Association of Clinical Endocrinologists recommended that if patients present with blood glucose above a certain concentration and are showing symptoms of diabetes complications, they should be placed on insulin immediately [11].

Patient preference studies have concluded that most diabetes patients strongly prefer inhaled insulin to injections. According to the multiple studies conducted at the Harvard School of Public Health, people with type 2 diabetes were almost three times as likely to choose insulin therapy if inhaled insulin was available than if they could only select injectable insulins [12–14]. The preference for inhaled insulin was also strong among type 1 diabetes patients [15].

Several studies have been conducted showing strong patient preference for Exubera inhaled insulin over insulin injections among patients who had experience with both modes of therapy. The graph in Figure 2.1 summarizes the results of a 2002 study demonstrating satisfaction with Exubera over injectable insulin after 6 months and across 298 type 2 diabetes patients [14].

THE FIRST GENERATION

There have been many attempts to deliver insulin without the use of injections. The most promising noninjection route of insulin delivery is via the deep lung, where insulin is readily absorbed [16]. Over 20 years of research has demonstrated that inhaled insulin can be a safe, effective, and reliable alternative to injections. Inhaled insulin has been studied extensively in over 10,000 patients across more than 100 clinical trials, demonstrating safety and efficacy. The most advanced of these products,

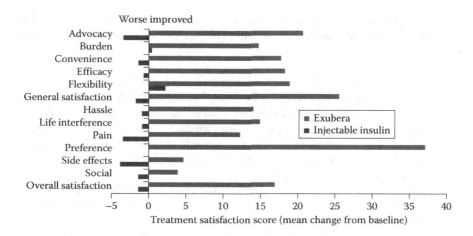

FIGURE 2.1 Satisfaction after 6 months on Exubera or injectable insulin.

Exubera, was approved for use in adults with type 1 and type 2 diabetes in the United States, Europe, and other countries in January 2006 [17]. It was front-page headlines all over the world. The Wall Street Journal named it 2006 Medical Innovation of the Year. Patients preferred it by a large margin to injections [12–15]. In October 2007, Pfizer voluntarily withdrew Exubera from the market for business reasons. Subsequently, Lilly and Novo Nordisk discontinued the development of their respective inhaled insulin products, AIR and AERx. None of the first-generation inhaled insulin products are currently on the market. However, one company, MannKind, persisted to develop its inhaled insulin, Afrezza, which was approved by the FDA in July 2014.

There were many reasons for the withdrawal of Exubera. The new senior management at Pfizer expected the product to take off but initial sales were sluggish. Pfizer also expected to be able to sell at a significant premium over injections, but having shown noninferiority, payers were not willing to allow a significant premium. Taking a tax write-off for the program added significant money to Pfizer's bottom line. Despite its reliability and efficacy, Exubera was approximately a foot long, cumbersome to handle, and conspicuous in public places. Inhalation of a high dose of insulin required a time-consuming procedure involving the insertion of a series of blister packets containing a dry powder formulation of insulin, activation of the air pump in the inhaler, and inhalation of the standing cloud from the delivery chamber. In addition, Exubera was dosed in milligram units rather than international units (IUs), the standard measurement used for insulin doses.

Clinical Efficacy of Inhaled Insulin

Published clinical data for Exubera, AIR, and AERx show that inhaled insulin was noninferior to injected mealtime insulin in most studies based on an average measurement of overall blood glucose control based on HbA1c, the generally accepted biomarker, glycosylated hemoglobin, formed when red blood cells are exposed to blood glucose. The extensive inhaled insulin clinical data also indicate improvement in terms of the following:

- *Greater patient preference.* Most type 1 and type 2 diabetes patients strongly preferred inhaled insulin over injected insulin [12–15].
- *Lower blood glucose.* Several phase 3 studies conducted by third parties showed lower fasting blood glucose with inhaled insulin, 8 h after a meal, and postmeal blood glucose, 2 h after a meal, which are real-time immediate blood glucose measures versus the average-over-time blood glucose measurement, HbA1c [18–20].
- *Fewer occurrences of hypoglycemia.* Studies conducted by third parties found fewer occurrences of hypoglycemia in type 2 diabetes patients using inhaled insulin compared to injected insulin [17].
- *Less weight gain.* Inhaled insulin resulted in less weight gain as seen in five phase 3 studies [21].

When Exubera received FDA approval, a collective analysis of 16 phase 3 controlled trials of inhaled insulin efficacy from 1999 to 2006 was published in 2006 in the Annals of Internal Medicine by the Tufts-New England Medical Center [22]. This analysis, which included 4023 patients, concluded that inhaled insulin is similar to injected insulin in lowering blood glucose and showed superior efficacy compared to oral agents, as measured by reduction in HbA1c, for type 2 diabetes patients. In some of these trials inhaled insulin also demonstrated statistically significant improvements in fasting blood glucose relative to injectable insulin.

RELIABILITY OF DOSING

Many large controlled clinical studies assessed inhaled insulin dose-to-dose variability between patients and within individual patients and found that inhaled insulin produced similar variability to that obtained with traditional insulin injections. Inaccurate dosing of insulin can cause low blood glucose, known as hypoglycemia, or high blood glucose, known as hyperglycemia. Severe hypoglycemia can cause loss of consciousness, which can result in emergency room admission. Mild to moderate forms of hypoglycemia can cause dizziness, which can be quickly treated with sugar pills or fruit juices among other things. Hyperglycemia indicates that patients are not taking enough insulin, which can be adjusted accordingly. Hyperglycemia is not immediately dangerous like hypoglycemia and is accompanied by drowsiness and loss of energy. Concerns about reliability of inhaled insulin have focused primarily on hypoglycemia.

In almost all prior published studies, blood glucose control with inhaled insulin was noninferior to injected regular insulin in both type 1 and 2 diabetes patients [22]. The efficacy of inhaled insulin was maintained for a prolonged period of time and was preferred by patients to injected insulin and oral regimes [22]. The similarity with injections was notable because the dosing unit with Exubera, 3 and 8 IU increments or combinations, is considerably less than the 1 IU increment typically available with pen injection insulin. Despite Exubera's larger dosing unit, rates of hypoglycemia were lower among type 2 diabetes patients using Exubera than those using injections and declined with use over time [17].

In a 3-month study conducted by Novo Nordisk, the AERx inhaled insulin product candidate and insulin injections demonstrated similar rates of overall blood glucose control and hypoglycemia in type 2 diabetes patients [23]. A 6-month study conducted by Lilly with AIR demonstrated that there were no statistical differences in efficacy or episodes of hypoglycemia among type 2 diabetes patients receiving AIR therapy or injected insulin [24]. AIR insulin powder was available to patients in either 2 or 6 IU increments.

In summary, the previous concerns regarding inhaler dosing reliability for inhaled insulin were repeatedly addressed using a variety of inhaler systems [13]. These studies demonstrate that insulin administration by inhalation had similar or improved repeatability to injectable insulin.

CLINICAL SAFETY OF INHALED INSULIN

Inhaled insulin has been studied extensively in over 10,000 patients across more than 100 clinical trials demonstrating safety and efficacy. Numerous nonclinical and clinical publications have demonstrated the safety of inhaled insulin. Concern regarding first-generation inhaled insulin focused on the incidence of hypoglycemia and pulmonary safety.

PULMONARY SAFETY

During more than 20 years of inhaled insulin development, investigators primarily focused on three pulmonary safety issues.

Changes in lung function. 1- to 2-year trials observed small, reversible, non-progressive changes of 1%–2% in one or two measurements of lung function [22]. These effects were not deemed clinically significant, were not detectable by the patients, and were not associated with any pathology. In the 8-year study, patients on Exubera had lung function similar to or better than patients treated with injections [25]. No signs of pulmonary inflammation were observed in two subsequent 7-month studies of Exubera [26]. Insulin is an anabolic hormone and has been shown to be beneficial to the lungs in animal models of pulmonary injury and disease [27–30].

Antibody levels. The delivery of insulin, whether by injection or inhalation, leads to the formation of circulating insulin antibodies in some patients [31]. In prior clinical development programs, the delivery of insulin by inhalation induced higher antibody levels in some patients than comparators; however, these antibodies were not associated with any adverse events and did not decrease the effectiveness, safety, or tolerability of inhaled insulin over time and were similar in type to those generated by injection [32–34]. In both injections and inhalation of insulin, the immune response does not produce an allergic reaction or inflammation except in very rare cases with injections.

Incidence of lung cancer. In the phase 3 trials conducted by Pfizer, a numeri-cally larger but not statistically significant number of incidents of lung cancer were seen in Exubera patients who were former heavy smokers compared to former heavy smokers who used injected insulin. In a 2-year observational follow-up on the preva-lence of lung cancer in Exubera patients completed in 2012, the Follow Up Study of Exubera (FUSE) study, an apparent imbalance was seen in lung cancer diagno-sis between patients who were former smokers and took Exubera and those who were treated with multiple comparators [35]. After reviewing the results of the FUSE study, an independent scientific steering committee recommended that no special screening for lung cancer be conducted for patients exposed to Exubera beyond what is currently recommended. In a 2-year phase 3 clinical trial involving 385 patients conducted with another inhaled insulin product, five cases of lung neoplasia (abnor-mal mass of lung tissue) were seen in the injected group as compared to the three cases in the inhaled group [36]. To date, MannKind Corporation has not reported any increased risk of lung cancer during clinical trials conducted with its inhaled insulin. We are not aware of any other published studies of lung cancer incidences with inhaled insulin. High circulating insulin concentrations in diabetes, known as hyperinsulinemia, are not associated with an increase in lung cancer incidence [37]. The literature on cancer, diabetes, and insulin is long and extensive and suggests that although there is an increased incidence of some cancers in diabetes (but not lung cancer), insulin use may be associated with a decrease in cancer incidence in diabe-tes patients, presumably through the lowering of blood glucose [38,39].

SUMMARY

- The need for noninvasive insulin is clear.
- More than 100 clinical trials conducted over the past 25 years in many thousands of patients over years of exposure have provided a level of com-fort for the safety and efficacy of inhaled insulin across a variety of delivery devices and formulations.
- The case for making inhaled insulin available to patients suffering from diabetes remains more compelling than ever.
- The key challenges for introducing a commercially successful inhaled insu-lin product are to develop
  - A device that is equally reliable as the first-generation devices, but smaller, more discrete, and easier to use
  - An insulin formulation that is equally safe and even more comfortable for daily inhalation
  - A product that is robust and inexpensive to manufacture at high scale

REFERENCES

1. http://www.idf.org/diabetesatlas/.
2. http://www.bccresearch.com/market-research/healthcare/insulin-drug-delivery-devices-hlc149a.html.
3. http://diabetes.niddk.nih.gov/dm/pubs/statistics/#Treatment.

4. Hauber AB, Johnson FR, Sauriol L, Lescrauwaet B. Risking health to avoid injections: Preferences of Canadians with type 2 diabetes. *Diabetes Care*, 28(9):2243–2245 (2005).

5. Peyrot M, Rubin RR, Khunti K. Addressing barriers to initiation of insulin in patients with type 2 diabetes. *Prim Care Diabetes*, 4(Suppl. 1):S11–S18 (2010).

6. Peyrot M et al. Resistance to insulin therapy among patients and providers: Results of the cross-national Diabetes Attitudes, Wishes, and Needs (DAWN) study. *Diabetes Care*, 28(11):2673–2679 (2005).

7. Polonsky WH, Fisher L, Guzman S, Villa-Caballero L, Edelman SV. Psychological insulin resistance in patients with type 2 diabetes: The scope of the problem. *Diabetes Care*, 28(10):2543–2545 (2005).

8. Zambanini A, Newson RB, Maisey M, Feher MD. Injection related anxiety in insulin-treated diabetes. *Diabetes Res Clin Pract*, 46(3):239–246 (1999).

9. Ismail-Beigi F. Clinical practice: Glycemic management of type 2 diabetes mellitus. *N Engl J Med*, 366(14):1319–1327 (2012).

10. Nathan DM et al. Medical management of hyperglycemia in type 2 diabetes: A consensus algorithm for the initiation and adjustment of therapy: A consensus statement of the American Diabetes Association and the European Association for the Study of Diabetes. *Diabetes Care*, 32(1):193–203 (2009).

11. Garber AJ. AACE comprehensive diabetes management algorithm 2013. *Endocr Pract*, 19:327–336 (2013).

12. Freemantle N et al. Availability of inhaled insulin promotes greater perceived acceptance of insulin therapy in patients with type 2 diabetes. *Diabetes Care*, 28(2):427–428 (2005).

13. Rosenstock J, Cappelleri JC, Bolinder B, Gerber RA. Patient satisfaction and glycemic control after 1 year with inhaled insulin (Exubera) in patients with type 1 or type 2 diabetes. *Diabetes Care*, 27(6):1318–1323 (2004).

14. Testa MA et al. Patient satisfaction with insulin therapy in type 2 diabetes randomized trial of injectable and inhaled insulin. *Diabetes*, 51(Suppl. 2):A135 (2002).

15. Gerber RA, Cappelleri JC, Kourides IA, Gelfand RA. Treatment satisfaction with inhaled insulin in patients with type 1 diabetes: A randomized controlled trial. *Diabetes Care*, 24(9):1556–1559 (2001).

16. Patton, Bukar JG, Eldon MA. Clinical pharmacokinetics and pharmacodynamics of inhaled insulin. *Clin Pharmacokinet*, 43(12):781–801 (2004).

17. http://www.fda.gov/ohrms/dockets/ac/05/briefing/2005–4169B1_01_01-Pfizer-Exubera.pdf.

18. Quattrin T, Bélanger A, Bohannon NJ, Schwartz SL; Exubera Phase III Study Group. Efficacy and safety of inhaled insulin (Exubera) compared with subcutaneous insulin therapy in patients with type 1 diabetes: Results of a 6-month, randomized, comparative trial. *Diabetes Care*, 27(11):2622–2627 (2004).

19. Skyler JS et al. Use of inhaled insulin in a basal/bolus insulin regimen in type 1 diabetic subjects: A 6-month, randomized, comparative trial. *Diabetes Care*, 28(7):1630–1635 (2005).

20. Hollander PA et al. Efficacy and safety of inhaled insulin (Exubera) compared with subcutaneous insulin therapy in patients with type 2 diabetes: Results of a 6-month, randomized, comparative trial. *Diabetes Care*, 27(10):2356–2362 (2004).

21. Hollander PA et al. Body weight changes associated with insulin therapy. *Diabetes Care*, 30(10):2508–2510.

22. Ceglia L, Lau J, Pittas AG. Meta-analysis: Efficacy and safety of inhaled insulin therapy in adults with diabetes mellitus. *Ann Intern Med*, 145(9):665–675 (2006).

23. Hermansen K, Rönnemaa T, Petersen AH, Bellaire S, Adamson U. Intensive therapy with inhaled insulin via the AERx insulin diabetes management system: A 12-week proof-of-concept trial in patients with type 2 diabetes. *Diabetes Care*, 27(1):162–167 (2004).

24. Gross JL et al. Initiation of prandial insulin therapy with AIR inhaled insulin or insulin lispro in patients with type 2 diabetes: A randomized noninferiority trial. *Diabetes Technol Ther*, 11(Suppl. 2):S27–S34 (2009).

25. Burge M et al. Sustained long-term efficacy and safety of inhaled human insulin (Exubera®) following at least 8 years of continuous therapy, in *43rd EASD*, Amsterdam, the Netherlands (2007).

26. Liu MC et al. Effects of inhaled human insulin on airway lining fluid composition in adults with diabetes. *Eur Respir J*, 32(1):180–188 (2008).

27. Fan W et al. Inhaled aerosolized insulin ameliorates hyperglycemia-induced inflammatory responses in the lungs in experimental model of acute lung injury. *Crit Care*, 17:R83 (2013).

28. Zhang WF, Zhu XX, Hu DH, Xu CF, Wang YC, Lv GF. Intensive insulin treatment attenuates burn-initiated lung injury in rats: Role of protective endothelium. *J Burn Care Res*, 32:51–58 (2011).

29. Di Petta A et al. Insulin modulates inflammatory and repair responses to elastase-induced emphysema in diabetic rats. *Int J Exp Path*, 92:392–399 (2011).

30. Guazzi M et al. Diabetes worsens pulmonary diffusion in heart failure, and insulin counteracts this effect. *Am J Respir Crit Care Med*, 166:978–982 (2002).

31. Schernthaner G. Immunogenicity and allergenic potential of animal and human insulins. *Diabetes Care*, 16(Suppl. 3):155–165 (1993).

32. Fineberg SE, Kawabata T, Finco-Kent D, Liu C, Krasner A. Antibody response to inhaled insulin in patients with type 1 or type 2 diabetes. An analysis of initial phase II and III inhaled insulin (Exubera) trials and a two-year extension trial. *J Clin Endocrinol Metab*, 90(6):3287–3294 (2005).

33. Fineberg SE, Kawabata TT, Finco-Kent D, Fountaine RJ, Finch GL, Krasner AS. Immunological responses to exogenous insulin. *Endocr Rev*, 28(6):625–652 (2007).

34. Teeter JG, Riese RJ. Dissociation of lung function changes with humoral immunity during inhaled human insulin therapy. *Am J Respir Crit Care Med*, 173(11):1194–1200 (2006).

35. http://clinicaltrials.gov/ct2/results?term=FUSE+Study&Search=Search.

36. Garg SK et al. Two-year efficacy and safety of AIR inhaled insulin in patients with type 1 diabetes: An open-label randomized controlled trial. *Diabetes Technol Ther*, 11(Suppl. 2):S5–S16 (2009).

37. Balkau B, Kahn HS, Courbon D, Eschwège E, Ducimetière P; Paris Prospective Study. Hyperinsulinemia predicts fatal liver cancer but is inversely associated with fatal cancer at some other sites: The Paris Prospective Study. *Diabetes Care*, 24(5):843–849 (2001).

38. Jee SH, Ohrr H, Sull JW, Yun JE, Ji M, Samet JM. Fasting serum glucose level and cancer risk in Korean men and women. *JAMA* 293:194–202 (2005).

39. Yang X et al. et al. Associations of hyperglycemia and insulin usage with the risk of cancer in type 2 diabetes: The Hong Kong diabetes registry. *Diabetes* 59:1254–1260.

3 Inhaled Therapeutic siRNA for the Treatment of Respiratory Diseases

Dongmei Cun, Lan Wu, and Mingshi Yang

CONTENTS

INTRODUCTION

The expression of gene can be silenced in a highly specific and effective way via the RNA interference (RNAi) pathway, a sequence-specific post-transcriptional gene silencing mechanism that occurs intracellularly to degrade target mRNA and regulates endogenous RNA level.[1] Fire and Mello were awarded the Nobel Prize in physiology in 2006 for their discovery of RNAi pathway. RNAi pathway could be triggered by introducing the molecule of chemically synthesized 21–23 bp small interfering RNA (siRNA). siRNA is assembled into the RNA-induced silencing complex (RISC) and cleaved upon activation of RISC in cytoplasm of target cells. In the activated RISC, the sense strand is removed and degraded by nucleases, whereas the antisense strand guides the RISC to the base-complementary sequence of the target mRNA and induces the degradation of complementary mRNA and eventually downregulates the target gene expression.[2]

Since the discovery of RNAi, the therapeutic potential of siRNAs has been rapidly recognized. Compared to conventional therapeutic approaches using small molecules, proteins, and monoclonal antibodies and even compared to other antisense strategies such as antisense DNA oligonucleotides and ribozymes, RNAi-based therapy may provide several advantages, including high selectivity and potency, possibility of providing personalized therapy, and easy synthesis.[3] In 2004, the first human clinical trial of RNAi-based therapy was initiated for the treatment of age-related macular degeneration with a siRNA targeting VEGF-receptor 1 delivered via ophthalmic route.[4] But unfortunately, until now, more than 10 years after the initiation of the first clinical trial, the clinical use of siRNA is still not very successful. The bottleneck that hinders the advancing of this process is delivery of siRNA, not only intracellular delivery of siRNA across biological barriers in general but also delivery to target cells in particular, which is not straightforward at all. siRNA is negatively charged hydrophilic macromolecules with a molecular weight of around 13 kDa; therefore, the naked siRNAs cannot bind to the cell surface or cross the cell membrane by passive diffusion (the term "naked siRNAs" refers to the delivery of siRNAs without any delivery vectors). Furthermore, there are some other problems such as rapid degradation by nucleases, off-target gene silencing, and immune stimulatory effects that also need to be resolved. Currently, it is widely believed that the successful translating of RNAi machinery into an applicable therapy in the clinic is highly dependent on the development of efficient and safe delivery vehicles that can overcome extracellular and intracellular barriers and that improve the currently inefficient targeting of siRNA to the desired organs and cell types.[5–7]

DELIVERY OF THERAPEUTIC siRNA TO THE LUNG

Just like eyes and skin, lung epithelium and macrophages are anatomically accessible to therapeutic agents through inhalation. Local delivery of siRNA into the lung allows for noninvasive access and avoids interactions with serum proteins that degrade siRNA after i.v. administration,[5] from which the delivery of siRNA could be more efficient. In fact, many studies have been conducted over the past few years involving the delivery of siRNAs to the lungs for the treatment of various lung diseases. Delivery of siRNA to the lung may expedite translation of siRNA technology to clinics. On the other hand, because of the prevalence and lethality of various respiratory disorders, the lung is emerging as an attractive target organ for siRNA-mediated cures. According to the World Health Organization, lung cancer is the top eight cause of death worldwide, tuberculosis number 7, chronic obstructive pulmonary disease (COPD) number 4, and lower respiratory infections number 3.[8] Thus, the clinical utility of siRNA as inhaled therapeutics is under intensive investigation. Furthermore, pulmonary administration also brings higher local concentration, reduced systemic exposure, and lower risk of enzymatic degradation compared to other administration routes such as oral and injection.[9] The lung also offers other advantages over systemic administration such as the large alveolar surface area with high vascularization and the thin air–blood barrier, which are beneficial factors for absorption. Obviously, all of these are beneficial for the treatment of lung-confined diseases. The completion of phase IIb clinical trial of ALN-RSV01 (details shown in Table 3.1) has demonstrated the feasibility of this administration route.

TABLE 3.1

Examples of siRNA-Based Therapeutics in Clinical Trials for Lung Diseases

Product Name	Delivery Agent/ Route of Administration	Indication	Sponsor	Latest Development Status
ALN-RSV01	Naked siRNA/ intranasal	RSV infection	Alnylam pharmaceuticals	IIb (completed)
Excellair™	Unknown/inhalation	Asthma	Zabecor pharmaceuticals	II

BARRIERS TO siRNA DELIVERY TO THE LUNG

As illustrated in Figure 3.1, there are generally five steps that siRNA go through when administered via pulmonary route. Although local delivery of siRNA could obviate the need for targeting and the interaction with serum nuclease to minimize degradation, the lung itself possesses some intrinsic anatomic, physiologic, immunologic, and metabolic hurdles for efficient siRNA delivery. The specific barriers to lung

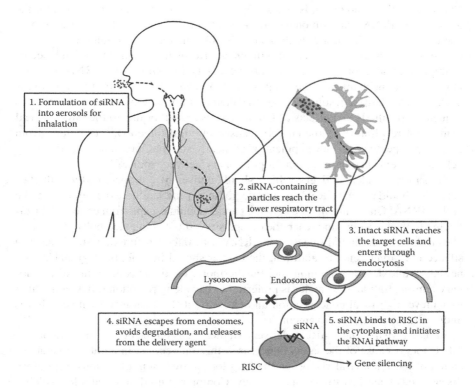

1. Formulation of siRNA into aerosols for inhalation

2. siRNA-containing particles reach the lower respiratory tract

3. Intact siRNA reaches the target cells and enters through endocytosis

Lysosomes   Endosomes

4. siRNA escapes from endosomes, avoids degradation, and releases from the delivery agent

siRNA

5. siRNA binds to RISC in the cytoplasm and initiates the RNAi pathway

RISC   Gene silencing

FIGURE 3.1   Schematic illustrates steps involved in the delivery of siRNA into the lungs. (Reproduced from Lam, J.K.-W. et al., *Adv. Drug Deliv. Rev.*, 64(1), 1, 2012. With permission.)

administration include highly branched anatomic structure ranging from the trachea to the alveoli, phagocytosis by macrophages, and the presence of mucus on the surface of conducting airway, which could effectively capture and remove the inhaled foreign particles by the beating of the cilia and mucociliary clearance. In addition, depending on the region of deposition, siRNA might be absorbed into the systemic circulation, which would adversely decrease local concentration, decrease therapeutic effect, and raise potential side effects.[10]

It was well known that the size, density, shape, and surface of the particle in which the siRNA is formulated and the patient's pulmonary function are two main factors determining the fate of siRNA-incorporated particle in lung.[11] Carefully screening and optimizing the aerosolization properties of the formulation could facilitate the overcoming of the lung-specific barriers mentioned earlier to ensure siRNA reaches its target site in the lung (the first two steps shown in Figure 3.1). But the remaining processes of entering the target cell, escaping from endosome, and being released from the delivery agent are still needed to go through before siRNA starts to trigger the RNAi pathway.

NONVIRAL FORMULATIONS FOR PULMONARY siRNA DELIVERY

Considering these biological barriers, appropriate carrier systems are critical for the delivery of siRNA via pulmonary administration. In contrast, the success in producing gene silencing effect with naked siRNA, such as the inhibition of respiratory syncytial virus (RSV) and parainfluenza virus by nasal administration,[12] seems to imply that additional carriers are not necessary for pulmonary siRNA delivery. However, the mechanism of how naked siRNAs can enter cells to initiate RNAi is unclear. Indeed, these results may be attributed to immune stimulation rather than to sequence-specific RNAi effects as Olivia has discussed[8] or due to the physiological damage of respiratory epithelial cells caused by viral infection.[13] Therefore, from today's perspective, the development of clinically suitable, safe, and effective drug delivery systems is required even for pulmonary delivery route.[5,13]

Generally, an ideal delivery vehicle should deliver siRNA specifically to the target cells, should protect siRNA against degradation, and facilitate the cellular uptake of the siRNA. Once entering the cell, the carrier should escape from endosomal trafficking to the lysosome and reach the cytoplasm without being metabolized. In cytoplasm, the carrier should release the siRNA with intended function and efficiently silence the target gene. In addition, the carrier should be safe, biodegradable, and neither cytotoxic nor immunogenic. Furthermore, for the specific route of pulmonary administration, the carrier is preferred to have long retention times in the lung to achieve high local concentration and circumvent the clearance by macrophages and/or the mucociliary movement.

In recent years, many siRNA delivery studies focus on the development of nonviral vectors because of the safety concerns with viral vectors. In addition, the application of these nonviral vectors in the lung for the treatment of various respiratory diseases has been investigated extensively. Commonly used nonviral siRNA delivery vectors can be generally divided into three types including lipid-, polymer-, and peptide-based delivery systems.

POLYMER-BASED siRNA DELIVERY SYSTEMS

Polymer-based nonviral vectors were shown to be very promising for siRNA delivery *in vitro* as well as *in vivo*. Their versatile natures allow a variety of structural modifications, resulting in the modulation of their delivery properties to fit different purposes. In addition, it has been suggested that polymers generally do not evoke as strong an immune response as liposomes.[14] The majority of the polymers applied for siRNA delivery are hydrophilic polycations, such as polyethylenimine (PEI), chitosan, and their derivatives, which generally form the so-called polyplexes with siRNA through the spontaneous electrostatic interaction. The size of polyplexes is normally in the range of 50–200 nm and affected by the molecular weight of polymers, the charge ratio, and the pH and ionic strength of the medium.[15] Apart from polyplex, siRNA also could be entrapped in the solid matrix of polymeric nanoparticles that were made from some hydrophobic polymers, such as poly(D,L-lactide-co-glycolide) (PLGA).[16]

It is relatively easy to produce polyplexes, and the overall positive surface charges of polyplexes facilitate the cellular uptake of siRNA and influence subsequent intracellular process. However, the positive charge is also believed to contribute to the cytotoxicity of cationic polymers, and the complex based on electrostatic interactions tends to disassemble or aggregate over time due to the possible interaction with the airway surface liquid covering the airway epithelial cells, which are negatively charged.[17] In addition, polyplexes do not render prolonged release profiles for siRNAs, which is essential because of the transient nature of the RNAi therapeutic effect.[18] In contrast, solid polymeric nanoparticles may offer improved colloidal stability and controlled release of their payloads. However, how to increase the encapsulation efficiency of siRNA in hydrophobic polymer matrix is one of the main challenges in utilizing this delivery system. In the following paragraphs, both hydrophilic and hydrophobic polymer-based vectors will be discussed.

Polyethylenimine

Synthetic polymer PEI represents the most extensively studied cationic polymer for nonviral gene delivery, especially with respect to pulmonary application.[19] The transfection efficiency and cytotoxicity of PEI are affected by many factors, such as molecular weight, degree of branching, cationic charge density, molecular structure, sequence, and the ratio between PEI and siRNA. The highly cationic property and the powerful ability to compact nucleic acid and trigger endosomal release through proton sponge effect make PEI the "gold standard" for *in vitro* gene delivery. PEI is often used in proof-of-principle studies or setups where a method is optimized. Gene expression in lung epithelium downregulated by the polyplexes of siRNA and PEI has also been demonstrated *in vivo*.[20] Despite the excellent performance of PEI, its clinical application is severely hampered by its poor biocompatibility and cytotoxicity. Linking PEI with other polymers, mostly polyethylene glycol (PEG), with the possibility of further conjugation to other polymers is the common strategy to reduce the cytotoxicity of PEI. With respect to siRNA delivery to the lungs, it would appear that the higher the degree of PEGylation and the shorter the PEG chain length, the fewer the cytotoxic effects that were observed.[21] Subsequently, Beyerle et al.[22]

compared lung toxicity, inflammation, and efficiency of siRNA nanocomplex with two types of PEG-modified PEI derivatives on ubiquitously enhanced green fluorescent protein (EGFP) expressing transgenic in BALB/c mice models after intratracheal administration. It was found that the PEG modification reduced cytotoxicity but elevated the immune response and proinflammatory effects. Therefore, further chemical modifications on PEI backbone, aimed at increasing the biocompatibility, specificity, and efficacy of PEI-based nanocarriers, are needed in future studies.

To address the issue of poor physical stability of polyplex, Kedinger et al. modified the structure of siRNA and designed the so-called sticky siRNAs that polymerize via their complementary 3′ overhangs. The polyplexes formed between "sticking" siRNAs and linear PEI exhibited better stability than usually obtained siRNA/PEI complexes and showed enhanced gene silencing efficiency both *in vitro* and *in vivo*.[23] For long-term storage, Terry et al. proposed a lyophilization method in which the two components (polymer and siRNA) were flash frozen and lyophilized as separate droplets in the same reaction tube and rapidly formed polyplexes upon addition of water. This formulation step did not have any adverse effects on the particle size of polyplexes or transfection efficiency and the knockdown efficiency of up to 90% was maintained.[15]

Chitosan

Chitosan, a product of partial deacetylation of chitin, is a natural nontoxic polysaccharide comprising copolymers of glucosamine and *N*-acetylglucosamine. The biodegradable, mucoadhesive, and mucosa permeation properties make cationic chitosan particularly suitable for pulmonary siRNA delivery. Nielsen et al. have evaluated the feasibility of aerosolized chitosan/siRNA polyplexes for pulmonary siRNA delivery.[24] In their study, aerosolized chitosan/siRNA nanoparticles were pneumatically formed using a nebulizing catheter. Noninvasive intratracheal insertion of the catheter was also used to study nanoparticle deposition and gene silencing in transgenic EGFP mouse lungs. The *in vitro* gene knockdown experiment proved that the nebulization process has negligible effects on the transfection efficiency of chitosan/siRNA polyplexes, and the polyplexes was found to deposit throughout the entire lung in both alveoli and bronchiolar regions and show significant EGFP gene silencing. Three years later, in a study by Okuda et al.,[25] the authors fabricated an inhalable chitosan/siRNA dry powder by using a supercritical CO_2 technique and manual grinding.[25] A lung metastasis model was established and the silencing efficiency of the delivered siRNA was measured by luciferase knockdown in the lung metastases. This study somehow proved the effectiveness of this delivery system even though the *in vivo* study they performed is not a real pharmacodynamics study.

However, poor water solubility and low transfection efficiency posed a limitation for its clinical application, even though the transfection efficiency could be improved to some extent by formulation optimization. Structure modification could be another strategy to improve the gene silencing efficiency of chitosan. For example, the development of imidazole-modified chitosan[26] and conjugation of chitosan to both PEG and a polyarginine cell-penetrating peptide (CPP)[27] have been found to increase gene knockdown, with improved cell viability compared to that of unmodified chitosan.

Poly (D,L-Lactide-co-Glycolide)

PLGA is a biodegradable and biocompatible polymer that has a long history of safe use for both medical applications and drug delivery. Many therapeutic macromolecules such as peptides, proteins, and nucleic acids have been encapsulated into PLGA microparticles or nanoparticles to achieve a prolonged and controlled release profiles to reduce the frequency of administration.[28] SiRNA also has been successfully entrapped into the matrix of PLGA with relatively high loading efficiency,[16] and the siRNA-loaded PLGA nanoparticles were further spray-dried with mannitol into inhalable nanocomposite microparticles.[29] The integrity and biological activity of siRNA was successfully preserved during the spray-drying process and the physicochemical properties of the particles are suitable for inhalation. However, this system did not show significant gene silencing efficiency on lung cancer cell lines probably due to the anionic surface charge of PLGA nanoparticles and too slow release rate of payload. The incorporation of some cationic polymer or lipid such as dioleoyltrimethylammoniumpropane (DOTAP) showed to be a promising strategy to potentiate the gene silencing capability, and again it was demonstrated by the same group that spray-drying is an excellent technique to formulate siRNA nanoparticles into inhalable dry powders, thus enabling local delivery of biologically active siRNA directly to the lung tissue.[30] Nevertheless, their results also clearly indicated that the excellent safety profile of PLGA had been compromised with the incorporation of DOTAP. A DOTAP of 5% (w/w) did not affect the cell viability in the tested DOTAP/PLGA concentration range, whereas nanoparticles modified with more than 5% (w/w) DOTAP reduced the cell viability in a nanoparticle- and DOTAP-concentration-dependent way. Therefore, it was essential to understand the delivery dynamics of this DOTAP/PLGA hybrid nanocarriers (lipid–polymer hybrid nanoparticles, LPNs) to improve their design for therapeutic applications. Recently, Foged et al. investigated the carrier structure–function relationship of LPNs.[31] The results suggested that the siRNA-loaded LPNs are characterized by a core–shell structure consisting of a PLGA matrix core coated with lamellar DOTAP structures with siRNA localized both in the core and in the shell. Release studies in TE buffer and serum-containing medium combined with *in vitro* gene silencing and quantification of intracellular siRNA suggested that this self-assembling core–shell structure influenced the siRNA release kinetics and the delivery dynamics. A main delivery mechanism appears to be mediated via the release of transfection-competent siRNA–DOTAP lipoplexes from the LPNs. Based on these results, a model for the nanostructural characteristics of the LPNs was suggested, in which the siRNA is organized in lamellar superficial assemblies and/or as complexes entrapped in the polymeric matrix.

Another strategy to address the low transfection efficiency of PLGA nanoparticles is to modify the structure of PLGA to endow it some favorable properties. For example, the polyester of tertiary-amine-modified polyvinyl alcohol backbones grafted PLGA showed faster degrading rate than PLGA. It is also biodegradable and achieved 80%–90% knockdown of a luciferase reporter gene *in vitro*.[32] It will be interesting to see the performance of these PLGA-based siRNA delivery systems *in vivo*.

Other Polymers

Apart from the commonly used polymers mentioned earlier, other polymers such as atelocollagen, cationic bovine serum albumin, spermine, polymethacrylates, and poly(amidoamine) dendrimer also have been exploited to design carriers for pulmonary siRNA delivery.[5,33] The work conducted by Conti et al.[33] has tested the ability of generation four, amine-terminated poly(amidoamine) dendrimer (G4NH2)–siRNA complexes (dendriplexes) to silence the EGFP gene on A549 lung epithelial cells stably expressing EGFP. Subsequently, the encapsulated dendriplexes in mannitol and also in a biodegradable and water-soluble cooligomer were dispersed in hydrofluoroalkane (HFA) to obtain HFA-based pressurized metered-dose inhalers (pMDIs) with favorable aerosol properties suitable for oral inhalation.

To the best of our knowledge, this is the first work to report the formulation of inhalable siRNA using pMDIs devices that are the least expensive and most widely used portable inhalers. This pMDI formulation and the other two dry powder inhaler formulations, i.e. chitosan dry powder (25) and DOTAP/PLGA hybrid nanoparticles based dry powder(31), need to be highlighted as the studies that could potentially be administered to patients.

LIPID-BASED DELIVERY SYSTEMS FOR siRNA

Similar to cationic polymer, the positive charges of cationic lipid or liposome allow an efficient interaction with siRNAs to form complexes that are referred to as lipoplexes. Lipoplexes can bind onto cell plasma membrane and be endocytosed and produce significant target gene knockdown effects. There are some cationic lipids commercially available such as Lipofectamine 2000®, which are routinely used in lab to deliver siRNA intracellularly to cells including lung cell lines. But the major problems with lipoplexes are their toxicity and the activation of inflammation responses. Since the adverse effects are mainly due to the positive charge, most of the strategies to overcome the drawbacks of cationic lipid concentrate on shielding the charge with PEG[34] or switching to neutral lipid cholesterol[35] or some lipid-like molecules such as lipidoids.[36] Although some of these alternatives, such as the covalent conjugate of siRNA with cholesterol, showed extended gene knockdown effects at mRNA level as compared to naked siRNA, they still need to be further optimized to improve their efficiency.

Recently, a multifunctional system based on nanostructured lipid carrier was developed to efficiently deliver anticancer drugs and siRNA simultaneously into the lungs by inhalation for the treatment of lung cancer.[37] Excitingly, the multifunctional system showed enhanced antitumor activity when compared to intravenous treatment.

PEPTIDES

A variety of CPPs and derivatives have been frequently employed to facilitate the membrane translocation of siRNA, but their application in the area of pulmonary delivery of siRNA is limited. Only a few such as HIV-derived TAT trans-activator proteins and polyarginine peptides have been assessed for their suitability as a vector for pulmonary siRNA delivery. In most of the cases, CPPs are formulated with siRNA in the way of either forming nanocomplexes based on the electrostatic interaction or covalently attaching to siRNA. In addition, CPPs also could be used to modify lipid- or polymer-based siRNA delivery systems, for example, the conjugation of octa-arginine and TAT to neutral lipids to increase cellular uptake. Despite the 30%–45% gene knockdown obtained when siRNA was conjugated to cholesterol and TAT and delivered intratracheally to BALB/c mice, it was also found that the incorporation of CPP could elicit inflammatory response.[35] Nevertheless, in another more recent study, CPP–siRNA complexes condensed by calcium promisingly offer high (up to 93%) target gene silencing effects in the human epithelial lung cell line (i.e., A549-luc-C8) with little to no evidence of cytotoxicity,[38] suggesting it is worth putting more efforts in promoting this vector in the clinical application of siRNA.

RNAi-BASED THERAPY FOR THE TREATMENT OF LUNG CANCER

Lung is very susceptible to many severe diseases because of its anatomical location and physiological function. Respiratory diseases are a major world health problem in the twenty-first century. Some severe respiratory diseases include lung cancer, asthma, COPD, a-1-antitrypsin deficiency, and cystic fibrosis, along with bacterial and viral respiratory infections such as tuberculosis and RSV. Given that lung cancer is the most lethal respiratory disease, we will mainly focus on the application of RNAi therapy in the treatment of lung cancer in the following section.

Lung cancer is the most common cancer and the leading cause of cancer mortality worldwide. Although there are various therapeutic strategies, including surgery, chemotherapy, radiotherapy, and molecular targeted therapies available in clinic, the mortality of this disease still keeps very high. Most patients die in less than 12 months. Patients who initially respond to the treatment often relapse and succumb to therapy-resistant tumors.[18] The overall prognosis is very poor, despite the increase in knowledge of the genetic and molecular basis of lung cancer. Novel and more effective therapeutic strategies are desperately needed to combat lung cancer.

One promising alternative to the conventional therapeutic approaches currently available may be the RNAi-based therapy. Theoretically, siRNA can cure the cancer by silencing the expression of any gene involved in tumor initiation, growth, and metastasis formation as long as it could be delivered to its target site. So far, various therapeutic target genes for lung cancer therapy have been identified and the anticancer effects of the matching therapeutic siRNA has been tested on various animal models via either systemic or pulmonary administration route.[39] Most of the target genes, such as survivin, Mdm2, BCL_2, NPT2b, and signal transducer and activator of transcription 3 (STAT3), which encode the proteins that play an important role in cell cycle progression, apoptosis, and cellular transformation, are overexpressed in lung cancer and many other types of cancer too. For example, BCL_2 is a key regulator among the antiapoptotic proteins, which was found in the mitochondrial outer membrane and related to the mitochondrial pathway of apoptosis. The knockdown of these genes by means of RNAi could induce apoptosis and suppress the progression of lung cancer consequently.

Apart from these apoptosis-relevant gene, there are some other genes like multidrug resistance–associated protein 1 (MRP1) mRNA, which could also be the potential target of RNAi therapy for lung cancer. Although the silencing of MRP1 would not lead to the death of cancer cells directly, it can significantly enhance the efficiency and avoid the severe side effects of codelivered anticancer drugs by suppressing the resistance mechanism.[40] In fact, the enthusiasm of combining anticancer drugs with siRNA to overcome the anticancer drugs–associated problems such as high toxicity and tumor resistance is rapidly growing in the field of anticancer research.[41] The main mechanisms of this resistance are common to most cancers, which includes *pump* and *nonpump* resistance. Membrane efflux transporters pump out the anticancer agents from the cancer cells, hence decreasing the efficacy of the treatment, that is, pump resistance. Regarding nonpump resistance, there are different mechanisms, and the main one is the activation of cellular antiapoptotic defense. As mentioned earlier, siRNA has significant gene silencing effect by binding and degrading complementary mRNA. Cancer cells will become more sensitive to anticancer drugs when siRNA is codelivered with anticancer drugs since both the *pump* and *nonpump* resistance-relevant genes can be silenced by siRNA.[42] Taratula et al. have reported a combined therapy with the combination of doxorubicin or cisplatin and two types of siRNAs against the mRNA of MRP1 (pump cellular resistance) and B-cell lymphoma 2 (BCL2) mRNA (nonpump cellular resistance), respectively. The *in vivo* distribution study showed the preferential accumulation of nanoparticles in the mouse lungs and limited accumulation in other organs. But unfortunately, the data about the *in vivo* anticancer effects on animal models were missing. Afterward, the same group applied the same strategy to enhance the cytotoxicity of doxorubicin or paclitaxel and the evaluation on mouse orthotopic model of human lung cancer demonstrating that codelivery of anticancer drugs with siRNA exhibited better therapeutic effects than delivery of anticancer alone when both of them were administered via inhalation route.[37] SiRNA-based therapeutics for lung cancer treatment in *in vivo* studies are summarized in Table 3.2.

Mainelis et al. have reported a similar work in which they combined the anticancer drug doxorubicin, antisense oligonucleotides (ASOs), and siRNA. The results showed that the therapeutic effect of inhalation delivery of DOX and ASO targeted to MRP1 and BCL2 mRNA is more efficient compared to inhalation delivery of DOX alone formulated in liposomes.[40] Ganesh et al.[58] also reported the combined therapy of cisplatin and siRNA to silence survivin and BCL-2, which are overexpressed in cisplatin-resistant cancer cells. That the combined therapy can increase the sensitivity of cancer cells to anticancer drugs may be an effective way for overcoming MDR effects.

Besides anticancer resistance, synergistic anticancer effects could be achieved when anticancer drugs were codelivered with siRNAs. For example, Zhang et al. have showed that coentrapment of VEGF against siRNA and gemcitabine monophosphate (GMP) into hybrid lipid/calcium/phosphate (LCP) nanoparticles could lead to better performance in controlling tumor growth and tumor vessel density. Their explanation for the enhanced anticancer effects was that VEGF-targeted siRNA destroyed the established tumor endothelium and increased the vessel permeability of cancer cells by inhibiting the mRNA of VEGF; therefore, the GMP can inhibit the cell proliferation more effectively.[59] Similarly, Xia et al.[60] have combined hematoporphrphyrin derivative–mediated photodynamic therapy with siRNA against APE1 (purinic/apyrimidinic endonuclease), which is a DNA damage repairer and cell damage reducer.

TABLE 3.2
siRNA-Based Therapeutics for Lung Cancer Treatment in *In Vivo* Studies

Target Gene	Route of Administration	siRNA Delivery Vector	Animal Models	Reference
B-cell lymphoma 2 (BCL2)	Intratracheal	PEI-CA-DOX/siRNA complex (CA pH-sensitive linker)	B16F10 melanoma-bearing mice	[43]
Ribophorin II (RPN2)	Intratracheal	Naked nucleic acids	A549-luc-C8 cells lung cancer xenograft tumor in C.B-17/Icr-scid/scidJcl mice	[44]
Myeloid cell leukemia sequence 1 (*Mcl1*)	Intratracheal	Ethylphosphocholine-based lipoplexes	B16F10 or LLC cells xenograft tumor in female BALB/c mice (metastatic model)	[45]
Multidrug resistance–associated protein 1 (MRP1)	Inhalation	Liposomes	A549 cells xenograft tumor in Nude nu/nu mice	[40]
Sodium-dependent phosphate cotransporter 2b (*NPT2b*)	Inhalation	Glycerol propoxylate triacrylate-spermine	Female K-ras^LA1 mice	[46]
c-Myc	Intratracheal instillation	Arginine-glycine-aspartic acid (RGD) gold nanoparticles	C57BL/6 female mice induced with LA-4 adenocarcinoma cells	[47]
MRP1 and *Bcl-2*	Inhalation	Luteinizing hormone–releasing hormone-modified mesoporous silica nanoparticles	A549 cells xenograft tumor in NCR nude mice	[48]
v-Akt murine thymoma viral oncogene homolog 1 (*Akt1*)	Inhalation	Glycerol propoxylate triacrylate-spermine copolymer	Female K-ras^LA1 mice	[49]
Insulin-like growth factor receptor 1 (*IGF-1R*)	Intravenous	Magnetic lipoplexes	A549 cells xenograft tumor in male BALB/cAnNCrj-nu mice	[50]
Survivin	Intravenous	Liposomes	H292 cells xenograft tumors in nude mice	[42]
Bcl-2	Intravenous	Cationic bovine serum albumin	B16 lung metastasis model	[51]

(Continued)

TABLE 3.2 (*Continued*)

siRNA-Based Therapeutics for Lung Cancer Treatment in *In Vivo* Studies

Target Gene	Route of Administration	siRNA Delivery Vector	Animal Models	Reference
Mouse double minute 2 (*MDM2*)	Intravenous	pH-responsive diblock copolymer of poly(methacryloyloxy ethyl phosphorylcholine)-block-poly(diisopropanolamine ethyl methacrylate) (PMPC-b-PDPA)	H2009 xenograft tumor in nude mice	[52]
Signal transducer and activator of transcription 3 (*STAT3*)	Intraperitoneal	PEI–poly(lactide-co-glycolide) nanoparticles	Carcinogen fed induced lung cancer in Balb/c mice	[53]
Codelivery of MDM2, c-myc, VEGF	Intravenous	An LCP nanoparticle	B16F10 cells xenograft tumor in female C57BL/6 mice (metastatic model)	[54]
Osteopontin (OPN) gene	Intravenous	Low-molecular-weight branched PEI (bPEI) cross-linked with sorbitol diacrylate	H460 cells or A549 cells xenograft tumor in male nude mice (BALB/c-nu)	[55]
Polo-like kinase (PLK1)	Intratumoral injections	Cationic multiwalled carbon nanotubes	Calu6 xenografts tumor in female Swiss nude mice	[56]
Prohibitin1 (PHB1)	Intravenous	Nanostructure comprising PLGA polymer core and a lecithin/lipid-PEG shell	Cancer cells A549 xenograft tumor in BALB/C nude mice	[57]

The siRNA against APE1 could prevent the damaged cancer cells from self-repairing, thus increasing the effect of hematoporphrphyrin derivative–mediated photodynamic therapy.

In general, the site-specific delivery of siRNA to the lung for the treatment of lung cancer can be achieved through systemic administration or local administration as shown in Table 3.2. However, it is increasingly being recognized that pulmonary delivery is the preferable route of administration for the treatment of lung-confined diseases and also lung cancer (even though it is not really a lung-confined disease). Recently, Caina Xu et al.[43] designed pH-sensitive nanoparticles as the carrier of siRNA for pulmonary codelivery of doxorubicin and siRNA. Here, DOX is conjugated onto PEI by using cis-aconitic anhydride (CA, a pH-sensitive linker) to obtain PEI-CA-DOX conjugates. The PEI-CA-DOX/siRNA complex nanoparticles are formed spontaneously via electrostatic interaction between cationic PEI-CA-DOX and anionic siRNA. When the codelivery systems in liquid state are directly sprayed into the lungs of B16F10 melanoma-bearing mice, the PEI-CA-DOX/BCL-2 siRNA complex nanoparticles show a long-term retention in the lungs, and a considerable number of the drugs and siRNAs accumulate in the tumor tissues of the lungs but rarely in normal lung tissues compared to systemic delivery of this formulation. Their work strongly supports the feasibility of using the route of pulmonary to delivery siRNA for lung cancer therapy. Gayong Shim et al. have also developed a cationic nanolipoplex as a pulmonary cellular delivery system for siRNA.[45] In their studies, six nanoliposomes differing in cationic lipids were formulated and screened *in vitro* and *in vivo* for cellular delivery functions in lung cells/tissues. Among the six nanoliposomes, cationic dioleoyl-sn-glycero-3-ethylphosphocholine and cholesterol (ECL)-based nanoliposomes showed the highest pulmonary cellular delivery *in vivo* and the lowest cytotoxicity *in vitro*. In metastatic lung cancer mouse models induced by B16F10 or Lewis lung carcinoma (LLC) cells, intratracheal administration of siMcl1 in ECL nanolipoplexes significantly silenced Mcl1mRNA and protein levels in lung tissue. Reduced formation of melanoma tumor nodules was observed in the lung. Besides these promising results, an important lesson we learned from this literature is that lack of correlation between *in vitro* and *in vivo* fluorescent dsRNA delivery efficiencies and lack of correlation between pulmonary cellular delivery efficiency and whole lung tissue delivery would happen sometimes. So it is risky to make any decision simply on the basis of *in vitro* data. We think the complex lung structure and *in vivo* microenvironments could be attributed to this poor correlation.

FUTURE PERSPECTIVE

Herein we introduced some obstacles in pulmonary siRNA delivery and some strategies to overcome the challenges. However, we need to be aware that there is still a long way to go before real inhalable siRNA products are available in the clinic. First of all, the cell-type specificity should be improved because of the diversity of lung cells. The introduction of targeting moieties such as ligands or antibody could be an effective way to lead siRNA to the selected cell types and reduce the undesired side effects in nontarget cells. Second, better understanding of the biodistribution of siRNA in the lung being administered and the vector materials after the release of its payload is crucial. Third, the safety issue in light of siRNA itself and toxicity of delivery materials needs to be addressed before RNAi-based drugs are used for clinical use. Last but not the least, the manufacturability of inhaled siRNA products should not be overlooked. Most of the current strategies for effective siRNA delivery tend to exploit complex formulation compositions and multiple preparation procedures. The consistence of critical quality attributes of these inhaled products, the cost, and the patient compliance can also be important factors that would need to be considered in the development of future siRNA-based therapeutics.

SUMMARY

- The therapeutic application of RNAi machinery opened an innovative way for the treatment of some severe respiratory diseases.
- Delivery is the primary hurdle to translate this technique from lab to clinic.
- Polymer-, lipid-, and peptide-based nonviral siRNA delivery systems showed promising gene silencing capacity *in vitro* and *in vivo*.
- Challenges remain for the development of effective, safe, targeted, and stable delivery systems for siRNA therapeutic application.

ACKNOWLEDGMENTS

Dongmei Cun acknowledges the support from the National Nature Science Foundation of China (No. 81302720) and Liaoning Provincial Education Officer's Excellent Talents Supporting Plan.

Mingshi Yang acknowledges the support from the National Nature Science Foundation of China (No. 81573380) and Liaoning Province Pan Deng Xue Zhe grant.

REFERENCES

1. Fire, A.; Xu, S.; Montgomery, M. K.; Kostas, S. A.; Driver, S. E.; Mello, C. C., Potent and specific genetic interference by double-stranded RNA in Caenorhabditis elegans. *Nature* **1998**, *391* (6669), 806–811.
2. Agrawal, N.; Dasaradhi, P. V. N.; Mohmmed, A.; Malhotra, P.; Bhatnagar, R. K.; Mukherjee, S. K., RNA interference: Biology, mechanism, and applications. *Microbiology and Molecular Biology Reviews* **2003**, *67* (4), 657–685.
3. Kumar, L. D.; Clarke, A. R., Gene manipulation through the use of small interfering RNA (siRNA): From *in vitro* to *in vivo* applications. *Advanced Drug Delivery Reviews* **2007**, *59* (2–3), 87–100.
4. Kaiser, P. K.; Symons, R. C. A.; Shah, S. M.; Quinlan, E. J.; Tabandeh, H.; Do, D. V.; Reisen, G. et al., RNAi-based treatment for neovascular age-related macular degeneration by sirna-027. *American Journal of Ophthalmology* **2010**, *150* (1), 33–39.e2.
5. Merkel, O. M.; Rubinstein, I.; Kissel, T., siRNA delivery to the lung: What's new? *Advanced Drug Delivery Reviews* **2014**, *75*, 112–128.
6. Higuchi, Y.; Kawakami, S.; Hashida, M., Strategies for *in vivo* delivery of siRNAs recent progress. *Biodrugs* **2010**, *24* (3), 195–205.

7. Kumar, L. D.; Clarke, A. R., Gene manipulation through the use of small interfering RNA (siRNA): From *in vitro* to *in vivo* applications. *Advanced Drug Delivery Reviews* **2007**, *59* (2–3), 87–100.

8. Merkel, O. M.; Kissel, T., Nonviral pulmonary delivery of siRNA. *Accounts of Chemical Research* **2012**, *45* (7), 961–970.

9. Garbuzenko, O. B.; Saad, M.; Betigeri, S.; Zhang, M.; Vetcher, A. A.; Soldatenkov, V. A.; Reimer, D. C.; Pozharov, V. P.; Minko, T., Intratracheal versus intravenous liposomal delivery of siRNA, antisense oligonucleotides and anticancer drug. *Pharmaceutical Research* **2009**, *26* (2), 382–394.

10. Lam, J. K.-W.; Liang, W.; Chan, H.-K., Pulmonary delivery of therapeutic siRNA. *Advanced Drug Delivery Reviews* **2012**, *64* (1), 1–15.

11. Cun, D.; Wan, F.; Yang, M., Formulation strategies and particle engineering technologies for pulmonary delivery of biopharmaceuticals. *Current Pharmaceutical Design* **2015**, *21* (19), 2599–2610.

12. Bitko, V.; Musiyenko, A.; Shulyayeva, O.; Barik, S., Inhibition of respiratory viruses by nasally administered siRNA. *Nature Medicine* **2005**, *11* (1), 50–55.

13. Fujita, Y.; Takeshita, F.; Kuwano, K.; Ochiya, T., RNAi therapeutic platforms for lung diseases. *Pharmaceuticals (Basel)* **2013**, *6* (2), 223–250.

14. Brower, V., RNA interference advances to early-stage clinical trials. *Journal of the National Cancer Institute* **2010**, *102* (19), 1459–1461.

15. Steele, T. W.; Zhao, X.; Tarcha, P.; Kissel, T., Factors influencing polycation/siRNA colloidal stability toward aerosol lung delivery. *European Journal of Pharmaceutics and Biopharmaceutics* **2012**, *80* (1), 14–24.

16. Cun, D. M.; Jensen, D. K.; Maltesen, M. J.; Bunker, M.; Whiteside, P.; Scurr, D.; Foged, C.; Nielsen, H. M., High loading efficiency and sustained release of siRNA encapsulated in PLGA nanoparticles: Quality by design optimization and characterization. *European Journal of Pharmaceutics and Biopharmaceutics* **2011**, *77* (1), 26–35.

17. Rosenecker, J.; Naundorf, S.; Gersting, S. W.; Hauck, R. W.; Gessner, A.; Nicklaus, P.; Muller, R. H.; Rudolph, C., Interaction of bronchoalveolar lavage fluid with polyplexes and lipoplexes: Analysing the role of proteins and glycoproteins. *Journal of Gene Medicine* **2003**, *5* (1), 49–60.

18. Raemdonck, K.; Vandenbroucke, R. E.; Demeester, J.; Sanders, N. N.; De Smedt, S. C., Maintaining the silence: Reflections on long-term RNAi. *Drug Discovery Today* **2008**, *13* (21–22), 917–931.

19. Di Gioia, S.; Conese, M., Polyethylenimine-mediated gene delivery to the lung and therapeutic applications. *Drug Design, Development and Therapy* **2009**, *2*, 163–188.

20. Gunther, M.; Lipka, J.; Malek, A.; Gutsch, D.; Kreyling, W.; Aigner, A., Polyethylenimines for RNAi-mediated gene targeting *in vivo* and siRNA delivery to the lung. *European Journal of Pharmaceutics and Biopharmaceutics: Official Journal of Arbeitsgemeinschaft fur Pharmazeutische Verfahrenstechnik e.V* **2011**, *77* (3), 438–449.

21. Beyerle, A.; Merkel, O.; Stoeger, T.; Kissel, T., PEGylation affects cytotoxicity and cell-compatibility of poly(ethylene imine) for lung application: Structure-function relationships. *Toxicology and Applied Pharmacology* **2010**, *242* (2), 146–154.

22. Beyerle, A.; Braun, A.; Merkel, O.; Koch, F.; Kissel, T.; Stoeger, T., Comparative *in vivo* study of poly(ethylene imine)/siRNA complexes for pulmonary delivery in mice. *Journal of Controlled Release: Official Journal of the Controlled Release Society* **2011**, *151* (1), 51–56.

23. Kedinger, V.; Meulle, A.; Zounib, O.; Bonnet, M. E.; Gossart, J. B.; Benoit, E.; Messmer, M. et al., Sticky siRNAs targeting survivin and cyclin B1 exert an antitumoral effect on melanoma subcutaneous xenografts and lung metastases. *BMC Cancer* **2013**, *13*, 338.

24. Nielsen, E. J.; Nielsen, J. M.; Becker, D.; Karlas, A.; Prakash, H.; Glud, S. Z.; Merrison, J. et al., Pulmonary gene silencing in transgenic EGFP mice using aerosolised chitosan/siRNA nanoparticles. *Pharmaceutical Research* **2010**, *27* (12), 2520–2527.

25. Okuda, T.; Kito, D.; Oiwa, A.; Fukushima, M.; Hira, D.; Okamoto, H., Gene silencing in a mouse lung metastasis model by an inhalable dry small interfering RNA powder prepared using the supercritical carbon dioxide technique. *Biological and Pharmaceutical Bulletin* **2013**, *36* (7), 1183–1191.

26. Ghosn, B.; Singh, A.; Li, M.; Vlassov, A. V.; Burnett, C.; Puri, N.; Roy, K., Efficient gene silencing in lungs and liver using imidazole-modified chitosan as a nanocarrier for small interfering RNA. *Oligonucleotides* **2010**, *20* (3), 163–172.

27. Noh, S. M.; Park, M. O.; Shim, G.; Han, S. E.; Lee, H. Y.; Huh, J. H.; Kim, M. S. et al., Pegylated poly-l-arginine derivatives of chitosan for effective delivery of siRNA. *Journal of Controlled Release* **2010**, *145* (2), 159–164.

28. Panyam, J.; Labhasetwar, V., Biodegradable nanoparticles for drug and gene delivery to cells and tissue. *Advanced Drug Delivery Reviews* **2003**, *55* (3), 329–347.

29. Jensen, D. M.; Cun, D.; Maltesen, M. J.; Frokjaer, S.; Nielsen, H. M.; Foged, C., Spray drying of siRNA-containing PLGA nanoparticles intended for inhalation. *Journal of Controlled Release* **2010**, *142* (1), 138–145.

30. Jensen, D. K.; Jensen, L. B.; Koocheki, S.; Bengtson, L.; Cun, D. M.; Nielsen, H. M.; Foged, C., Design of an inhalable dry powder formulation of DOTAP-modified PLGA nanoparticles loaded with siRNA. *Journal of Controlled Release* **2012**, *157* (1), 141–148.

31. Colombo, S.; Cun, D.; Remaut, K.; Bunker, M.; Zhang, J.; Martin-Bertelsen, B.; Yaghmur, A.; Braeckmans, K.; Nielsen, H. M.; Foged, C., Mechanistic profiling of the siRNA delivery dynamics of lipid-polymer hybrid nanoparticles. *Journal of Controlled Release* **2015**, *201*, 22–31.

32. Nguyen, J.; Steele, T. W.; Merkel, O.; Reul, R.; Kissel, T., Fast degrading polyesters as siRNA nano-carriers for pulmonary gene therapy. *Journal of Controlled Release* **2008**, *132* (3), 243–251.

33. Conti, D. S.; Brewer, D.; Grashik, J.; Avasarala, S.; da Rocha, S. R. P., Poly(amidoamine) dendrimer nanocarriers and their aerosol formulations for siRNA delivery to the lung epithelium. *Molecular Pharmaceutics* **2014**, *11* (6), 1808–1822.

34. Griesenbach, U.; Kitson, C.; Escudero Garcia, S.; Farley, R.; Singh, C.; Somerton, L.; Painter, H. et al., Inefficient cationic lipid-mediated siRNA and antisense oligonucleotide transfer to airway epithelial cells *in vivo*. *Respiratory Research* **2006**, *7*, 26.

35. Moschos, S. A.; Jones, S. W.; Perry, M. M.; Williams, A. E.; Erjefalt, J. S.; Turner, J. J.; Barnes, P. J.; Sproat, B. S.; Gait, M. J.; Lindsay, M. A., Lung delivery studies using siRNA conjugated to TAT(48-60) and penetratin reveal peptide induced reduction in gene expression and induction of innate immunity. *Bioconjugate Chemistry* **2007**, *18* (5), 1450–1459.

36. Akinc, A.; Zumbuehl, A.; Goldberg, M.; Leshchiner, E. S.; Busini, V.; Hossain, N.; Bacallado, S. A. et al., A combinatorial library of lipid-like materials for delivery of RNAi therapeutics. *Nature Biotechnology* **2008**, *26* (5), 561–569.

37. Taratula, O.; Kuzmov, A.; Shah, M.; Garbuzenko, O. B.; Minko, T., Nanostructured lipid carriers as multifunctional nanomedicine platform for pulmonary co-delivery of anticancer drugs and siRNA. *Journal of Controlled Release* **2013**, *171* (3), 349–357.

38. Baoum, A.; Ovcharenko, D.; Berkland, C., Calcium condensed cell penetrating peptide complexes offer highly efficient, low toxicity gene silencing. *International Journal of Pharmaceutics* **2012**, *427* (1), 134–142.

39. Fujita, Y.; Kuwano, K.; Ochiya, T., Development of small RNA delivery systems for lung cancer therapy. *International Journal of Molecular Sciences* **2015**, *16* (3), 5254–5270.

40. Mainelis, G.; Seshadri, S.; Garbuzenko, O. B.; Han, T.; Wang, Z.; Minko, T., Characterization and application of a nose-only exposure chamber for inhalation delivery of liposomal drugs and nucleic acids to mice. *Journal of Aerosol Medicine and Pulmonary Drug Delivery* **2013**, *26* (6), 345–354.
41. Gandhi, N. S.; Tekade, R. K.; Chougule, M. B., Nanocarrier mediated delivery of siRNA/miRNA in combination with chemotherapeutic agents for cancer therapy: Current progress and advances. *Journal of Controlled Release: Official Journal of the Controlled Release Society* **2014**, *0*, 238–256.
42. Tian, H.; Liu, S.; Zhang, J.; Zhang, S.; Cheng, L.; Li, C.; Zhang, X. et al., Enhancement of cisplatin sensitivity in lung cancer xenografts by liposome-mediated delivery of the plasmid expressing small hairpin RNA targeting Survivin. *Journal of Biomedical Nanotechnology* **2012**, *8* (4), 633–641.
43. Xu, C.; Wang, P.; Zhang, J.; Tian, H.; Park, K.; Chen, X., Pulmonary codelivery of doxorubicin and siRNA by pH-sensitive nanoparticles for therapy of metastatic lung cancer. *Small* **2015**, *11* (34), 4321–4333.
44. Fujita, Y.; Takeshita, F.; Mizutani, T.; Ohgi, T.; Kuwano, K.; Ochiya, T., A novel platform to enable inhaled naked RNAi medicine for lung cancer. *Scientific Reports* **2013**, *3*, 3325.
45. Shim, G.; Choi, H. W.; Lee, S.; Choi, J.; Yu, Y. H.; Park, D. E.; Choi, Y.; Kim, C. W.; Oh, Y. K., Enhanced intrapulmonary delivery of anticancer siRNA for lung cancer therapy using cationic ethylphosphocholine-based nanolipoplexes. *Molecular Therapy: The Journal of the American Society of Gene Therapy* **2013**, *21* (4), 816–824.
46. Hong, S. H.; Minai-Tehrani, A.; Chang, S. H.; Jiang, H. L.; Lee, S.; Lee, A. Y.; Seo, H. W.; Chae, C.; Beck, G. R., Jr.; Cho, M. H., Knockdown of the sodium-dependent phosphate co-transporter 2b (NPT2b) suppresses lung tumorigenesis. *PLOS ONE* **2013**, *8* (10), e77121.
47. Conde, J.; Tian, F.; Hernandez, Y.; Bao, C.; Cui, D.; Janssen, K. P.; Ibarra, M. R.; Baptista, P. V.; Stoeger, T.; de la Fuente, J. M., *In vivo* tumor targeting via nanoparticle-mediated therapeutic siRNA coupled to inflammatory response in lung cancer mouse models. *Biomaterials* **2013**, *34* (31), 7744–7753.
48. Taratula, O.; Garbuzenko, O. B.; Chen, A. M.; Minko, T., Innovative strategy for treatment of lung cancer: Targeted nanotechnology-based inhalation co-delivery of anticancer drugs and siRNA. *Journal of Drug Targeting* **2011**, *19* (10), 900–914.
49. Jiang, H.-L.; Hong, S.-H.; Kim, Y.-K.; Islam, M. A.; Kim, H.-J.; Choi, Y.-J.; Nah, J.-W. et al., Aerosol delivery of spermine-based poly(amino ester)/Akt1 shRNA complexes for lung cancer gene therapy. *International Journal of Pharmaceutics* **2011**, *420* (2), 256–265.
50. Wang, C.; Ding, C.; Kong, M.; Dong, A.; Qian, J.; Jiang, D.; Shen, Z., Tumor-targeting magnetic lipoplex delivery of short hairpin RNA suppresses IGF-1R overexpression of lung adenocarcinoma A549 cells *in vitro* and *in vivo*. *Biochemical and Biophysical Research Communications* **2011**, *410* (3), 537–542.
51. Han, J.; Wang, Q.; Zhang, Z.; Gong, T.; Sun, X., Cationic bovine serum albumin based self-assembled nanoparticles as siRNA delivery vector for treating lung metastatic cancer. *Small* **2014**, *10* (3), 524–535.
52. Yu, H.; Zou, Y.; Jiang, L.; Yin, Q.; He, X.; Chen, L.; Zhang, Z.; Gu, W.; Li, Y., Induction of apoptosis in non-small cell lung cancer by downregulation of MDM2 using pH-responsive PMPC-b-PDPA/siRNA complex nanoparticles. *Biomaterials* **2013**, *34* (11), 2738–2747.
53. Das, J.; Das, S.; Paul, A.; Samadder, A.; Bhattacharyya, S. S.; Khuda-Bukhsh, A. R., Assessment of drug delivery and anticancer potentials of nanoparticles-loaded siRNA targeting STAT3 in lung cancer, *in vitro* and *in vivo*. *Toxicology Letters* **2014**, *225* (3), 454–466.

54. Yang, Y.; Li, J.; Liu, F.; Huang, L., Systemic delivery of siRNA via LCP nanoparticle efficiently inhibits lung metastasis. *Molecular Therapy* **2012**, *20* (3), 609–615.

55. Cho, W.-Y.; Hong, S.-H.; Singh, B.; Islam, M. A.; Lee, S.; Lee, A. Y.; Gankhuyag, N. et al., Suppression of tumor growth in lung cancer xenograft model mice by poly(sorbitol-co-PEI)-mediated delivery of osteopontin siRNA. *European Journal of Pharmaceutics and Biopharmaceutics* **2015**, *94*, 450–462.

56. Guo, C.; Al-Jamal, W. T.; Toma, F. M.; Bianco, A.; Prato, M.; Al-Jamal, K. T.; Kostarelos, K., Design of cationic multiwalled carbon nanotubes as efficient siRNA vectors for lung cancer xenograft eradication. *Bioconjugate Chemistry* **2015**, *26* (7), 1370–1379.

57. Zhu, X.; Xu, Y.; Solis, L. M.; Tao, W.; Wang, L.; Behrens, C.; Xu, X. et al., Long-circulating siRNA nanoparticles for validating prohibitin1-targeted non-small cell lung cancer treatment. *Proceedings of the National Academy of Sciences of the United States of America* **2015**, *112* (25), 7779–7784.

58. Fehring, V.; Schaeper, U.; Ahrens, K.; Santel, A.; Keil, O.; Eisermann, M.; Giese, K.; Kaufmann, J., Delivery of therapeutic siRNA to the lung endothelium via novel Lipoplex formulation DACC. *Mol Ther* **2014**, *22* (4), 811–820.

59. Zhang, Y.; Schwerbrock, N. M.; Rogers, A. B.; Kim, W. Y.; Huang, L., Codelivery of VEGF siRNA and gemcitabine monophosphate in a single nanoparticle formulation for effective treatment of NSCLC. *Molecular Therapy* **2013**, *21* (8), 1559–1569.

60. Xia, L.; Guan, W.; Wang, D.; Zhang, Y.-S.; Zeng, L.-L.; Li, Z.-P.; Wang, G.; Yang, Z.-Z., Killing effect of Ad5/F35-APE1 siRNA recombinant adenovirus in combination with hematoporphrphyrin derivative-mediated photodynamic therapy on human nonsmall cell lung cancer. *BioMed Research International* **2013**, *2013*, 957913.

4 New Molecules to Treat Asthma and COPD

Amir Hakim and Omar S. Usmani

CONTENTS

INTRODUCTION

Asthma and chronic obstructive pulmonary disease (COPD) are chronic inflammatory diseases that account for substantial global morbidity and mortality and financial costs to healthcare institutions [1–5]. Chronic inflammation in asthma and COPD is characterized and orchestrated by distinct inflammatory cells, cytokines, chemokines, adhesion molecules, enzymes, and receptors. The mainstay of current treatments includes inhaled bronchodilators, inhaled corticosteroids (ICS), antileukotriene receptor antagonists, and combinations of bronchodilators with corticosteroids in a single inhaler. However, in severe asthmatics and COPD patients, corticosteroids fail to alter the decline in lung function and reduce the underlying inflammation [6–9]. This presents an urgent medical need to develop novel anti-inflammatory drugs. Recent advancements in our understanding of the pathogenesis and molecular biology underlying asthma and COPD have led to the identification of novel therapeutic targets that offer hope in reducing the underlying inflammation and consequently improving quality of life [3,10].

ASTHMA

Asthma affects 5%–16% of the worldwide population, with varying rates of prevalence in different countries [2]. Globally, healthcare costs for asthma have increased, with drug treatment accounting for the majority of asthma costs [11]. Asthma is characterized by recurrent episodes of reversible airway obstruction, bronchial hyperresponsiveness, and chronic airway inflammation. Reversal of airway obstruction may occur either spontaneously or after use of medication. Fortunately, most asthmatic patients respond well to ICS alone or in combination with long-acting β2-adrenoceptor agonists, as recommended by the Global Initiative for Asthma guidelines [12]. In contrast, at the severe end of the asthma spectrum, reversibility of airway obstruction to medication is poor and patients with severe asthma account for a high proportion of total asthma costs [7,13]. Patients with severe asthma often remain uncontrolled and have frequent exacerbations, even with high doses of ICS and long-acting beta2-agonists (LABA), and this highlights the pressing need for effective treatments.

Over the last decade, our understanding of the immunopathology and pathogenesis underlying asthma has notably improved. In particular, the importance of different subsets of T cells that may initiate different inflammatory profiles and, consequently, determine different structural changes has been recognized [10]. Classically, asthma has been considered as a T-helper type 2 (Th2) cell-dependent, IgE-mediated allergic disease. Th2 cells secrete a number of cytokines including interleukin (IL)-4, IL-5, and IL-13 that coordinate an allergic inflammatory response (Figure 4.1) [10,14]. Activation of Th2 cells leads to mucus-cell hyperplasia and infiltration of inflammatory cells, including eosinophils, mast cells, and CD4+ T cells. However, it is important to acknowledge that asthma has been recognized as a heterogeneous condition that comprises several different phenotypes (Figure 4.2) [15]. These phenotypes are associated with distinct patterns of inflammation and different clinical characteristics. Better characterization of these clinical and molecular phenotypes is likely to lead to the research and development of more successful treatments tailored toward specific spectrums of the disease.

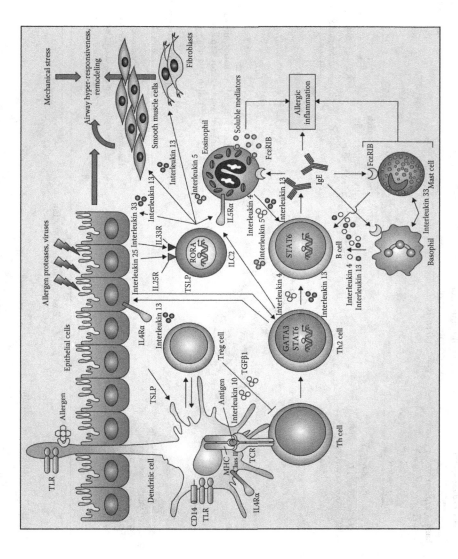

FIGURE 4.1 Innate and adaptive allergic mechanisms in asthma. (From Martinez, F.D. and Vercelli, D., *Lancet*, 382(9901), 1360, October 19, 2013.)

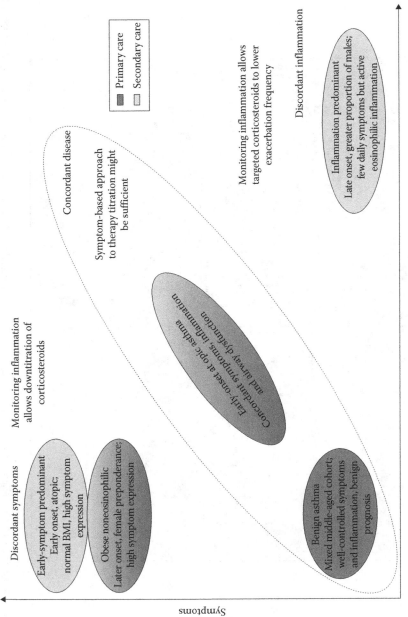

FIGURE 4.2 Clinical phenotypes of adult asthma.

COPD

COPD is the fourth most common cause of mortality and is projected to rank fifth in global burden of disease according to the World Health Organization [1,16]. The general prevalence of COPD is 10%, although there are reports of a much higher prevalence [17]. Clinically, the hallmark of the disease is progressive airflow limitation that is not fully reversible, which manifests itself primarily as breathlessness in the patient [3,18]. Biologically, COPD is an inflammatory disease of the lungs, characterized by an abnormal inflammatory response to noxious particles and gases, and the extent of pulmonary inflammation in COPD correlates to disease severity. Chronic inflammation in COPD is predominantly characterized by macrophages, neutrophils, and T-lymphocytes. These cells release a variety of chemotactic factors, pro-inflammatory cytokines, and growth factors that further amplify the abnormal inflammatory response in COPD patients [18].

Oxidative stress is an important feature in COPD, where an imbalance between the production of harmful reactive oxygen species (ROS) and the ability to repair the resulting damage is believed to be important. The increased burden of inhaled oxidants is enhanced by activated macrophages and neutrophils in the lungs of smokers [19]. This abnormal inflammatory response to noxious particles and gases, orchestrated by a cascade of inflammatory cells and mediators, leads to narrowing and structural changes of the small airways and destruction of the lung parenchyma (emphysema) [20]. These structural changes include increased bronchial wall thickness and smooth muscle tone, mucus hypersecretion, and loss of elastic structure (Figure 4.3) [18], and it is these key pathological changes of the lungs that lead to progressive airflow limitation, the hallmark of COPD. It is also recognized that there are significant extrapulmonary effects and comorbidities in COPD patients that contribute to the severity of the disease [3]. Several clinical trials have shown that existing medications do not reverse the decline in lung function, the key feature of the disease [6]. According to the Global Initiative for Chronic Obstructive Lung Disease, patients should be treated with bronchodilators in all stages of the disease, with the addition of ICS in severe (stage III) to very severe (stage IV) COPD [4].

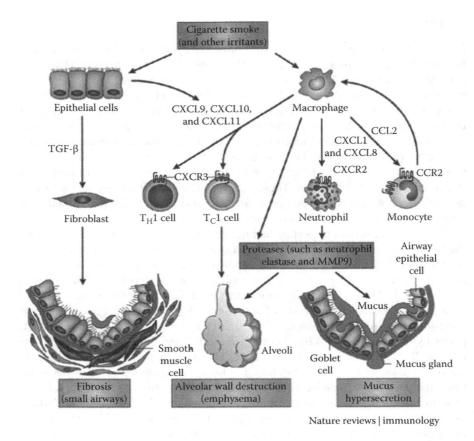

Nature reviews | immunology

FIGURE 4.3 The immunopathology in chronic obstructive pulmonary disease. (From Barnes, P.J., *Nat. Rev. Immunol.*, 8(3), 183, March 2008.)

NEW MOLECULES TO TREAT ASTHMA AND COPD

Significant advances in our understanding of the pathogenesis of asthma and COPD have identified new molecular targets. This offers great hope for the development of new, targeted therapies for patients with asthma and COPD who are poorly managed with current treatments. This chapter aims to discuss some of the most promising new therapeutic targets and the current status of the development of anti-inflammatory drugs for asthma and COPD (Table 4.1).

CHEMOKINE AND CYTOKINE INHIBITORS

Disease progression in asthma and COPD is driven by a multitude of inflammatory mediators, including chemokines, cytokines, lipids, and growth factors. Inhibiting or preventing their synthesis would seem a logical therapeutic approach to improve the underlying inflammation, as observed in rheumatoid arthritis (RA) [21]. Currently,

TABLE 4.1
Novel Anti-Inflammatory Treatments in the Development for Asthma and Chronic Obstructive Pulmonary Disease

Drug Class	Drugs under Development
PDE4 inhibitors	Roflumilast
	GSK256066
	RPL554
p38 MAPK inhibitors	SD-282
	Dilmapimod
	PH797804
NF-κB inhibitors	BMS-345541
	PS-1145
Chemokine and cytokine antagonists	ADZ8309 (CXCR2 antagonist)
	Navarixin (CXCR2 antagonist)
	CXCR3 antagonist
	Infliximab (TNF-α inhibitor)
	Mepolizumab
	Lebrikizumab
	Tocilizumab
Phosphoinositide-3-kinase inhibitors	TG100-115
	AS605240
Antiproteases	AZ11557272
	MMP-9 inhibitors
	AZD1236
Antimicrobials	Moxifloxacin
	Ciprofloxacin
	EM-703
Antioxidants	Sulforaphane
	Bardoxolone methyl
	Dimethyl fumarate
Antiageing molecules	SIRT2172
	Resveratrol

Abbreviations: PDE4, phosphodiesterase-4; MAPK, mitogen-activated protein kinase; MMP, matrix metalloprotease; NF, nuclear factor; TNF, tumor necrosis factor.

several inhibitors of inflammatory mediators are in early clinical development, including antagonists of CXCR2, a receptor that mediates the chemotactic roles of chemokine ligand (CXCL)-8, CXCL-1, and CXCL-5 on monocytes and neutrophils [22]. Potentially, blockade of chemokine receptors would inhibit leukocyte recruitment (a process that is corticosteroid resistant in COPD patients) and therefore dampen down the inflammatory response that drives asthma and COPD.

Several asthma subphenotypes prone to exacerbations and associated with sputum eosinophilia have considerable levels of IL-5, the most potent chemoattractor for eosinophils [23]. In patients with severe asthma and evidence of eosinophilic inflammation, mepolizumab, a humanized monoclonal antibody against IL-5, significantly reduced exacerbation rates, although no improvement in lung function was observed [24]. In healthy volunteers challenged with lipopolysaccharide (LPS), oral administration of ADZ8309, a CXCR-1/2 receptor antagonist, inhibited neutrophil inflammation in the lungs [25]. Additionally, in ozone-induced sputum neutrophilia in healthy volunteers, navarixin, an allosteric antagonist of CXCR2, effectively inhibited sputum neutrophilia, although in several large clinical studies in COPD, navarixin had no beneficial effect [26]. Another chemokine receptor, CXCR3, is increased in the sputum of COPD patients compared with nonsmokers. It mediates the role of CXCL-9, CXCL-10, and CXCL-11 chemokines, which may be involved in T-lymphocyte recruitment in the small airways and lung parenchyma. CXCR3 antagonists are currently under development for COPD [3,27].

Several antibodies inhibiting cytokines or their receptors are under development for asthma and COPD [28–31]. These include humanized monoclonal antibodies against IL-4 and IL-13, cytokines central to disease progression in asthma. In asthmatic patients with high levels of serum periostin, a biomarker of IL-13 activation, lebrikizumab, a monoclonal antibody against IL-13, significantly improved lung function, compared to patients with low serum levels of periostin [31]. The cytokines tumor necrosis factor (TNF)-α and IL-6 are both found in increased levels in sputum and in the systemic circulation of patients with asthma and COPD. TNF-α is important in propagating the inflammatory response in patients with severe asthma and COPD. Infliximab, an effective TNF-α inhibitor in RA, has no beneficial effect on clinical outcomes in severe asthma and COPD [32]. More worryingly in this study, patients on infliximab developed severe lung infections and lung cancer. A study of tocilizumab, a potent IL-6 inhibitor that is currently used in patients with RA, is planned and may be effective in patients with severe respiratory disease ($\leq 50\%$ forced expiratory volume in 1 second (FEV$_1$)/forced vital capacity (FVC)) as it will also target the autoimmune component of COPD [33]. Finally, novel therapeutic inhibitors of IL-17, a family of cytokines that are involved in numerous immune regulatory functions, such as inducing and mediating pro-inflammatory responses and neutrophil recruitment, are also currently under development for COPD [34]. Indeed, targeting a single mediator may have little or no major clinical benefit in asthma and COPD as both diseases are characterized by a plethora of inflammatory mediators.

ANTIPROTEASES

In COPD, emphysema is predominantly due to an imbalance between proteases that digest elastin and other structural proteins and antiproteases [35]. Epithelial cells, macrophages, and neutrophils secrete proteases, neutrophil elastase (NE), and matrix metalloproteases (MMPs), which not only break down connective tissue but also stimulate mucus hypersecretion. An increase in elastic activity in COPD patients also contributes to neutrophilic inflammation through production of matrikines [36]. Several low-molecular-weight NE inhibitors have shown great promise in animal models; however, they have failed to show benefit in early-stage clinical trials in COPD patients [3].

Inhibitors of MMPs have also shown great promise in animal models. In guinea pigs exposed to daily cigarette smoke for up to 6 months, AZ11557272, a novel dual MMP-9 and MMP-12 inhibitor, suppressed desmosine from bronchoalveolar lavage, a marker of elastin breakdown [37]. Additionally, TNF-α levels in lavage were significantly reduced in AZ11557272-treated guinea pigs, and furthermore, AZ11557272 reversed approximately 70% of cigarette smoke–induced airspace enlargement and prevented cigarette smoke–induced small airway wall thickness as observed by Churg and colleagues [37]. In a clinical study in COPD patients, AZD1236, a novel dual MMP-9 and MMP-12 inhibitor, was well tolerated and had an acceptable safety profile [38]. Further studies need to be conducted to assess their importance in protecting against further airway remodeling.

Antioxidants

Oxidative stress is increased in patients with asthma who smoke and those with COPD. Oxidative stress drives and amplifies chronic inflammation in COPD. Cigarette smoke, a major risk factor for COPD, is abundant in ROS and also activates endogenous mechanisms, such as inflammatory cells, that further contribute to intracellular ROS. Oxidative stress is also associated with corticosteroid insensitivity in smoking asthmatics and COPD patients [19,39]. Therefore, antioxidants have the potential to reduce inflammation and restore corticosteroid insensitivity. However, to date, currently available antioxidants such as N-acetylcysteine have failed to be effective due to poor bioavailability and inactivation by oxidative stress. Several more potent and stable antioxidants are currently in preclinical development [3].

Mitochondria are a major source of intracellular ROS and their function in respiratory muscle cells has been reported to be abnormal in COPD patients [40]. Indeed, endogenous intracellular mechanisms that protect against oxidative stress have been shown to be defective in COPD, namely, nuclear factor erythroid 2–related factor 2 (NRF2) [41]. A randomized, proof-of-principle trial in COPD patients is currently in progress to assess changes in basal levels of NRF2 after 4 weeks treatment of sulforaphane (ClinicalTrials.gov identifier: NCT01335971). In a phase III clinical study, dimethyl fumarate (BG-12), an NRF2 activator, reduced relapse rates in patients with multiple sclerosis [42]. In light of this, a clinical trial to assess whether BG-12 may also provide clinical benefit in COPD patients may be sensible. There is a need to develop more specific NRF2 activators with better safety profiles. In diabetic patients, bardoxolone methyl treatment was associated with an increase in albuminuria, blood pressure, and liver enzyme levels [43]. Accumulating evidence also suggests aldose reductase inhibitors (ARIs) may play a central role in inflammatory disorders that are associated with oxidative stress. In in vitro and in vivo studies, ARIs have been shown to attenuate ROS production and lead to a subsequent reduction cytokine and chemokine production [44].

PDE Inhibitors

Phosphodiesterase (PDE)4 are a family of enzymes responsible for hydrolyzing cAMP and are most commonly expressed in macrophages, neutrophils, and T-lymphocytes, which are immune cells that drive inflammation in COPD [45]. In a 4-week crossover, placebo-controlled study in 38 COPD patients, a once-daily selective PDE4 inhibitor, roflumilast 500 μg, significantly improved postbronchodilator FEV_1 compared with placebo. In sputum, roflumilast significantly reduced the absolute numbers of eosinophils and neutrophils, as well as CXCL8 and NE. In blood cells, roflumilast suppressed TNF-α levels to a far greater extent than placebo [46]. In a 52-week placebo-controlled study in severe COPD patients, with frequent exacerbations and mucus hypersecretion, roflumilast improved FEV_1 by 48 mL and reduced exacerbations by approximately 15%. However, adverse effects were more common with roflumilast than placebo [47]. Roflumilast has also been shown to improve clinical benefit when combined with bronchodilators, salmeterol, and tiotropium. In two double-blind studies in moderate-to-severe COPD patients, oral roflumilast 500 μg daily significantly improved mean prebronchodilator FEV_1 in patients treated with either salmeterol or tiotropium. However, as reported earlier, adverse effects were more common in patients treated with roflumilast [48]. The development of inhaled delivery of roflumilast may limit systemic adverse effects associated with oral administration, as well as allowing greater therapeutic doses of roflumilast to be tolerated. GSK256066, an inhaled PDE4 inhibitor, has completed a randomized, double-blind, placebo-controlled phase II study to investigate the safety and tolerability in mild-to-moderate COPD patients [49].

Several different selective isoenzyme inhibitors of PDE4 are under development, and current evidence suggests PDE4-D inhibition, as opposed to PDE4-B inhibition, may be responsible for the adverse effects observed with roflumilast [50,51]. Interestingly, the development of mixed PDE3/PDE4 inhibitors that display a combination of bronchodilator (PDE3) and anti-inflammatory activity (PDE3 and PDE4) may be beneficial [52]. RPL554, a PDE3/PDE4 inhibitor, has completed a favorable phase I/IIa study in patients with asthma and allergic rhinitis. Extension of the study in COPD patients is currently planned [53]. In severe asthma, which is associated with neutrophilic inflammation, theoretically PDE4 inhibitors may prove to be effective in reducing inflammation.

PI3K INHIBITORS

Phosphoinositide-3-kinase (PI3K) inhibitors are a family of lipid kinases that regulate a number of cellular functions, such as cell growth, intracellular trafficking, proliferation, and innate and adaptive immune responses. The pharmacological development of isoform-selective inhibitors of PI3K has not only allowed better understanding of the role of each member of this family but may also serve as future therapeutic agents to treat poorly managed COPD. PI3K-γ and phosphoinositide-3-kinase-delta (PI3K-δ) are predominantly found in leukocytes, where knockout of PI3K-γ leads to reduced macrophage and T-lymphocyte function and impaired neutrophil activation and migration [54]. As highlighted previously, PI3K-δ inhibitors have improved corticosteroid sensitivity by restoring histone deacetylase (HDAC)-2 levels that have been reduced due to oxidative stress [55]. In mice exposed to either LPS or inhaled smoke, TG100-115, a small-molecule inhibitor of PI3K-γ and PI3K-δ, inhibited pulmonary neutrophilia [56]. Furthermore, a PI3K-γ-selective inhibitor, AS605240, reduced polymorphonuclear leukocyte infiltration into the lung in an LPS-induced lung injury murine model [57]. Inhibitors of PI3K-γ and PI3K-δ are currently under development; however, adverse effects such as hypotension are a concern, as PI3Ks are involved in a spectrum of cellular functions [58,59].

p38 MITOGEN-ACTIVATED PROTEIN KINASE INHIBITORS

The p38 mitogen-activated protein kinase (MAPK) are a class of MAPKs that respond to cellular stress stimuli, such as inflammatory cytokines and growth factors, and regulate inflammatory responses and cell differentiation. In surgical lung specimens from 18 COPD patients, significantly greater amounts of phosphory-lated p38 (phospho-p38), the active form of p38 MAPK, were observed in alveolar macrophages and alveolar walls than in smoking and nonsmoking control subjects. Furthermore in this study, increased levels of phospho-p38 inversely correlated to FEV_1 and FEV_1/FVC values [60]. In an 11-day cigarette smoke–induced pulmonary inflammation study in mice resistant to dexamethasone, SD-282 (a novel inhibitor of p38 MAPK) reduced phospho-p38. This reduction was associated with significantly lower levels of macrophage and neutrophil numbers and IL-6 production [61]. In a 4-week study in COPD patients, dilmapimod reduced sputum neutrophil and serum fibrogen levels, which were associated with an improvement in FVC, but not in FEV_1 [62]. However, another p38 MAPK inhibitor, PH797804, at 3, 6, and 10 mg/day in a 6-week clinical study in COPD patients significantly improved FEV_1 levels [63]. All these data suggest p38 MAPK inhibitors may be potential therapeutic targets for dampening down inflammation in corticosteroid-resistant COPD patients, but similar to PI3K and PDE4 inhibitors, inhaled p38 MAPK inhibitors may need to be developed to reduce systemic side effects and toxicity from oral agents. Additionally, the risk of short-term efficacy due to feedback mechanisms needs to be addressed. Therefore, it is important to ascertain whether treatment should be targeted either up- or downstream of p38 itself and also whether such treatment should be used acutely, for example, during exacerbations, as opposed to the chronic management of stable disease.

NUCLEAR FACTOR KAPPA-B INHIBITORS

Nuclear factor kappa-B (NF-κB) is a pro-inflammatory redox-sensitive transcription factor and is highly expressed in epithelial and macrophage cells of COPD patients, especially during exacerbations [64]. It is central to the expression of numerous pro-inflammatory genes and pathogenesis of COPD [18]. In LPS-challenged animal models, IκB kinase (IKK)-2 inhibitors of NF-κB blocked NF-κB DNA binding, which is essential for transcriptional activity of NF-κB-sensitive genes, which was associated with a decrease in TNF-α and IL-1β secretion and neutrophil and eosino-phil numbers [65]. In airway smooth muscle cells, BMS-345541, a highly selective inhibitor of IKK, inhibited TNF-α-induced expression of IL-6, CXCL-8, and eotaxin in a concentration-dependent manner [66]. PS-1145, another IKK inhibitor, in airway

smooth muscle cells, also suppressed inflammatory markers and NF-κB activation
[67]. There is concern about the effects on the immune system of long-term administration of NF-κB inhibitors. In a study involving NF-κB knockout mice, septicemia
was a major adverse event [68].

ANTIMICROBIALS

Susceptibility to asthma and COPD seems to be associated with microbial colonization of the respiratory tract. In the lower airways of COPD patients, bacterial
colonization is found in at least 50% of patients, especially in severe and exacer-
bating COPD patients. Regular antibiotic therapy would seem an ideal therapeutic strategy; however, antibiotic resistance cautions against this. Furthermore, in a
clinical study, a 5-day treatment with moxifloxacin every 8 weeks had no effect on
exacerbation rates and lung function; however, a benefit was observed in patients
with purulent sputum. Inhaled liposomal formulations of antibiotics are also being
developed to minimize adverse effects. Moreover, the effects of liposomal formulations on drug deposition in the lung are currently being explored. Inhaled ciprofloxacin is currently under clinical development. Long-term use of antibiotic
therapy, macrolides, has shown to significantly reduce exacerbation rates in COPD
patients, particularly in patients with purulent sputum. In addition to their antibiotic
effects, macrolides have also shown to have anti-inflammatory effects. In hypoxia
and oxidative stress–induced reduction in HDAC-2 activity, EM-703, a nonantibac-
terial erythromycin derivative, restored HDAC-2 activity. This resulted in reduced
NF-κB-driven inflammation [69]. Several macrolides are currently under development as anti-inflammatory drugs [70].

ANTIAGEING MOLECULES

COPD is an age-related disease that shows evidence of accelerated lung ageing [3,71].
It is believed to be due to defective function of endogenous antiageing molecules,
such as sirtuins and forkhead box proteins [72]. Oxidative stress has been shown to
directly reduce sirtuin 1 activity and expression [72]. In rodent models, resveratrol, a
weak sirtuin activator, has been shown to prolong the life span of mice [73]. In macrophages from COPD patients and healthy epithelial cells, resveratrol suppressed
the inflammatory response [74]. A more potent sirtuin activator SRT2172 reversed
the effects of cigarette smoke on MMP-9 activity in mice [71]. Sirtuin activators are
currently in preclinical development for COPD.

CONCLUSION

Asthma and COPD contribute significantly to global rates of morbidity and mortality. Current treatments, including corticosteroids and LABA, provide little or
no clinical benefit in patients with severe asthma and COPD. Fortunately, recent
advancements in the pathogenesis of these two conditions have highlighted several
therapeutic targets. These include novel anti-inflammatory agents, antioxidants,
macrolides, and antiageing molecules. New treatments targeting single mediators

have been mostly disappointing in clinical trials. Broad-spectrum anti-inflammatory treatments such as dual PDE3/PDE4 inhibitors and PI3K inhibitors have shown greater promise in preclinical development. The development of these new emerging classes of drugs in asthma and COPD is very exciting. However, adverse effects associated with systemic distribution need to be addressed to optimize therapy and patient compliance. Long-term studies will surely need to be conducted to determine whether these novel anti-inflammatory drugs reduce disease progression, exacerbations, and mortality in patients.

ACKNOWLEDGMENTS

Dr Omar S. Usmani is a recipient of a UK National Institute of Health Research (NIHR) Career Development Fellowship. This article was supported by the NIHR Respiratory Disease Biomedical Research Unit at the Royal Brompton and Harefield NHS Foundation Trust and Imperial College London.

REFERENCES

1. Barnes PJ. Chronic obstructive pulmonary disease: A growing but neglected global epidemic. *PLOS Med.* 2007 May;4(5):e112.
2. Akinbami LJ, Moorman JE, Bailey C, Zahran HS, King M, Johnson CA et al. Trends in asthma prevalence, health care use, and mortality in the United States, 2001–2010. *NCHS Data Brief.* 2012 May(94):1–8.
3. Barnes PJ. New anti-inflammatory targets for chronic obstructive pulmonary disease. *Nat Rev Drug Discov.* 2013 July;12(7):543–559.
4. Vestbo J, Hurd SS, Agusti AG, Jones PW, Vogelmeier C, Anzueto A et al. Global strategy for the diagnosis, management, and prevention of chronic obstructive pulmonary disease: GOLD executive summary. *Am J Respir Crit Care Med.* 2013 February 15; 187(4):347–365.
5. Hastie AT, Moore WC, Meyers DA, Vestal PL, Li H, Peters SP et al. Analyses of asthma severity phenotypes and inflammatory proteins in subjects stratified by sputum granulocytes. *J Allergy Clin Immunol.* 2010 May;125(5):1028–1036.e13.
6. Suissa S, Barnes PJ. Inhaled corticosteroids in COPD: The case against. *Eur Respir J.* 2009 July;34(1):13–16.
7. Moore WC, Meyers DA, Wenzel SE, Teague WG, Li H, Li X et al. Identification of asthma phenotypes using cluster analysis in the Severe Asthma Research Program. *Am J Respir Crit Care Med.* 2010 February 15;181(4):315–323.
8. Woodruff PG, Boushey HA, Dolganov GM, Barker CS, Yang YH, Donnelly S et al. Genome-wide profiling identifies epithelial cell genes associated with asthma and with treatment response to corticosteroids. *Proc Natl Acad Sci USA.* 2007 October 2; 104(40):15858–15863.
9. Mercado N, Hakim A, Kobayashi Y, Meah S, Usmani OS, Chung KF et al. Restoration of corticosteroid sensitivity by p38 mitogen activated protein kinase inhibition in peripheral blood mononuclear cells from severe asthma. *PLOS ONE.* 2012;7(7):e41582.
10. Martinez FD, Vercelli D. Asthma. *Lancet.* 2013 October 19;382(9901):1360–1372.
11. Bedouch P, Marra CA, FitzGerald JM, Lynd LD, Sadatsafavi M. Trends in asthma-related direct medical costs from 2002 to 2007 in British Columbia, Canada: A population based-cohort study. *PLOS ONE.* 2012;7(12):e50949.

12. Reddy AP, Gupta MR. Management of asthma: The current US and European guidelines. *Adv Exp Med Biol.* 2014;795:81–103.
13. Jarjour NN, Erzurum SC, Bleecker ER, Calhoun WJ, Castro M, Comhair SA et al. Severe asthma: Lessons learned from the National Heart, Lung, and Blood Institute Severe Asthma Research Program. *Am J Respir Crit Care Med.* 2012 February 15; 185(4):356–362.
14. Cohn L, Elias JA, Chupp GL. Asthma: Mechanisms of disease persistence and progression. *Annu Rev Immunol.* 2004;22:789–815.
15. Haldar P, Pavord ID, Shaw DE, Berry MA, Thomas M, Brightling CE et al. Cluster analysis and clinical asthma phenotypes. *Am J Respir Crit Care Med.* 2008 August 1;178(3):218–224.
16. Rabe KF, Hurd S, Anzueto A, Barnes PJ, Buist SA, Calverley P et al. Global strategy for the diagnosis, management, and prevention of chronic obstructive pulmonary disease: GOLD executive summary. *Am J Respir Crit Care Med.* 2007 September 15;176(6):532–555.
17. Mannino DM, Buist AS. Global burden of COPD: Risk factors, prevalence, and future trends. *Lancet.* 2007 September 1;370(9589):765–773.
18. Barnes PJ. Immunology of asthma and chronic obstructive pulmonary disease. *Nat Rev Immunol.* 2008 March;8(3):183–192.
19. Kirkham PA, Barnes PJ. Oxidative stress in COPD. *Chest.* 2013 July;144(1):266–273.
20. Usmani OS, Barnes PJ. Assessing and treating small airways disease in asthma and chronic obstructive pulmonary disease. *Ann Med.* 2012 March;44(2):146–156.
21. Lee EY, Lee ZH, Song YW. The interaction between CXCL10 and cytokines in chronic inflammatory arthritis. *Autoimmun Rev.* 2013 March;12(5):554–557.
22. Donnelly LE, Barnes PJ. Chemokine receptors as therapeutic targets in chronic obstructive pulmonary disease. *Trends Pharmacol Sci.* 2006 October;27(10):546–553.
23. Woodruff PG, Modrek B, Choy DF, Jia G, Abbas AR, Ellwanger A et al. T-helper type 2-driven inflammation defines major subphenotypes of asthma. *Am J Respir Crit Care Med.* 2009 September 1;180(5):388–395.
24. Nair P, Pizzichini MM, Kjarsgaard M, Inman MD, Efthimiadis A, Pizzichini E et al. Mepolizumab for prednisone-dependent asthma with sputum eosinophilia. *N Engl J Med.* 2009 March 5;360(10):985–993.
25. Barnes PJ. New therapies for chronic obstructive pulmonary disease. *Med Princ Pract.* 2010;19(5):330–338.
26. Holz O, Khalilieh S, Ludwig-Sengpiel A, Watz H, Stryszak P, Soni P et al. SCH527123, a novel CXCR2 antagonist, inhibits ozone-induced neutrophilia in healthy subjects. *Eur Respir J.* 2010 March;35(3):564–570.
27. Costa C, Rufino R, Traves SL, Lapa E SJR, Barnes PJ, Donnelly LE. CXCR3 and CCR5 chemokines in induced sputum from patients with COPD. *Chest.* 2008 January;133(1):26–33.
28. Mahler DA, Huang S, Tabrizi M, Bell GM. Efficacy and safety of a monoclonal antibody recognizing interleukin-8 in COPD: A pilot study. *Chest.* 2004 September;126(3):926–934.
29. Doe C, Bafadhel M, Siddiqui S, Desai D, Mistry V, Rugman P et al. Expression of the T helper 17-associated cytokines IL-17A and IL-17F in asthma and COPD. *Chest.* 2010 November;138(5):1140–1147.
30. Wenzel S, Ford L, Pearlman D, Spector S, Sher L, Skobieranda F et al. Dupilumab in persistent asthma with elevated eosinophil levels. *N Engl J Med.* 2013 June 27; 368(26):2455–1266.
31. Corren J, Lemanske RF, Hanania NA, Korenblat PE, Parsey MV, Arron JR et al. Lebrikizumab treatment in adults with asthma. *N Engl J Med.* 2011 September 22; 365(12):1088–1098.

32. Rennard SI, Fogarty C, Kelsen S, Long W, Ramsdell J, Allison J et al. The safety and efficacy of infliximab in moderate to severe chronic obstructive pulmonary disease. *Am J Respir Crit Care Med.* 2007 May 1;175(9):926–934.
33. Paul-Pletzer K. Tocilizumab: Blockade of interleukin-6 signaling pathway as a therapeutic strategy for inflammatory disorders. *Drugs Today (Barc).* 2006 September;42(9):559–576.
34. De Sanctis JB, Garmendia JV, Moreno D, Larocca N, Mijares M, Di Giulio C et al. Pharmacological modulation of Th17. *Recent Pat Inflamm Allergy Drug Discov.* 2009 June;3(2):149–156.
35. Abboud RT, Vimalanathan S. Pathogenesis of COPD. Part I. The role of protease-antiprotease imbalance in emphysema. *Int J Tuberc Lung Dis.* 2008 April; 12(4):361–367.
36. Gaggar A, Jackson PL, Noerager BD, O'Reilly PJ, McQuaid DB, Rowe SM et al. A novel proteolytic cascade generates an extracellular matrix-derived chemoattractant in chronic neutrophilic inflammation. *J Immunol.* 2008 April 15;180(8):5662–5669.
37. Churg A, Wang R, Wang X, Onnervik PO, Thim K, Wright JL. Effect of an MMP-9/MMP-12 inhibitor on smoke-induced emphysema and airway remodelling in guinea pigs. *Thorax.* 2007 August;62(8):706–713.
38. Magnussen H, Watz H, Kirsten A, Wang M, Wray H, Samuelsson V et al. Safety and tolerability of an oral MMP-9 and -12 inhibitor, AZD1236, in patients with moderate-to-severe COPD: A randomised controlled 6-week trial. *Pulm Pharmacol Ther.* 2011 October;24(5):563–570.
39. Tomita K, Barnes PJ, Adcock IM. The effect of oxidative stress on histone acetylation and IL-8 release. *Biochem Biophys Res Commun.* 2003 February 7;301(2):572–577.
40. Puente-Maestu L, Perez-Parra J, Godoy R, Moreno N, Tejedor A, Gonzalez-Aragoneses F et al. Abnormal mitochondrial function in locomotor and respiratory muscles of COPD patients. *Eur Respir J.* 2009 May;33(5):1045–1052.
41. Malhotra D, Thimmulappa R, Navas-Acien A, Sandford A, Elliott M, Singh A et al. Decline in NRF2-regulated antioxidants in chronic obstructive pulmonary disease lungs due to loss of its positive regulator, DJ-1. *Am J Respir Crit Care Med.* 2008 September 15;178(6):592–604.
42. Gold R, Kappos L, Arnold DL, Bar-Or A, Giovannoni G, Selmaj K et al. Placebo-controlled phase 3 study of oral BG-12 for relapsing multiple sclerosis. *N Engl J Med.* 2012 September 20;367(12):1098–1107.
43. Rossing P. Diabetic nephropathy: Could problems with bardoxolone methyl have been predicted? *Nat Rev Nephrol.* 2013 March;9(3):128–130.
44. Chatzopoulou M, Pegklidou K, Papastavrou N, Demopoulos VJ. Development of aldose reductase inhibitors for the treatment of inflammatory disorders. *Expert Opin Drug Discov.* 2013 November;8(11):1365–1380.
45. Giembycz MA. Can the anti-inflammatory potential of PDE4 inhibitors be realized: Guarded optimism or wishful thinking? *Br J Pharmacol.* 2008 October;155(3):288–290.
46. Grootendorst DC, Gauw SA, Verhoosel RM, Sterk PJ, Hospers JJ, Bredenbroeker D et al. Reduction in sputum neutrophil and eosinophil numbers by the PDE4 inhibitor roflumilast in patients with COPD. *Thorax.* 2007 December;62(12):1081–1087.
47. Calverley PM, Sanchez-Toril F, McIvor A, Teichmann P, Bredenbroeker D, Fabbri LM. Effect of 1-year treatment with roflumilast in severe chronic obstructive pulmonary disease. *Am J Respir Crit Care Med.* 2007 July 15;176(2):154–161.
48. Fabbri LM, Calverley PM, Izquierdo-Alonso JL, Bundschuh DS, Brose M, Martinez FJ et al. Roflumilast in moderate-to-severe chronic obstructive pulmonary disease treated with longacting bronchodilators: Two randomised clinical trials. *Lancet.* 2009 August 29;374(9691):695–703.

49. Watz H, Mistry SJ, Lazaar AL, for the IPC101939 investigators. Safety and tolerability of the inhaled phosphodiesterase 4 inhibitor GSK256066 in moderate COPD. *Pulm Pharmacol Ther.* 2013;26:588–595.
50. Giembycz MA. Phosphodiesterase-4: Selective and dual-specificity inhibitors for the therapy of chronic obstructive pulmonary disease. *Proc Am Thorac Soc.* 2005;2(4):326–333; discussion 40–41.
51. Banner KH, Press NJ. Dual PDE3/4 inhibitors as therapeutic agents for chronic obstructive pulmonary disease. *Br J Pharmacol.* 2009 July;157(6):892–906.
52. Boswell-Smith V, Spina D, Oxford AW, Comer MB, Seeds EA, Page CP. The pharmacology of two novel long-acting phosphodiesterase 3/4 inhibitors, RPL554 [9,10-dimethoxy-2(2,4,6-trimethylphenylimino)-3-(n-carbamoyl-2-aminoethyl)-3,4,6, 7-tetrahydro-2H-pyrimido[6,1-a]isoquinolin-4-one] and RPL565 [6,7-dihydro-2- (2,6-diisopropylphenoxy)-9,10-dimethoxy-4H-pyrimido[6,1-a]isoquino lin-4-one]. *J Pharmacol Exp Ther.* 2006 August;318(2):840–848.
53. Cazzola M, Page CP, Calzetta L, Matera MG. Emerging anti-inflammatory strategies for chronic obstructive pulmonary disease. *Eur Respir J.* 2012 April 10; 40(3):724–741.
54. Medina-Tato DA, Ward SG, Watson ML. Phosphoinositide 3-kinase signalling in lung disease: Leucocytes and beyond. *Immunology.* 2007 August;121(4):448–461.
55. Marwick JA, Caramori G, Stevenson CS, Casolari P, Jazrawi E, Barnes PJ et al. Inhibition of PI3Kdelta restores glucocorticoid function in smoking-induced airway inflammation in mice. *Am J Respir Crit Care Med.* 2009 April 1;179(7):542–548.
56. Doukas J, Eide L, Stebbins K, Racanelli-Layton A, Dellamary L, Martin M et al. Aerosolized phosphoinositide 3-kinase gamma/delta inhibitor TG100-115 [3-[2,4-diamino-6-(3-hydroxyphenyl)pteridin-7-yl]phenol] as a therapeutic candidate for asthma and chronic obstructive pulmonary disease. *J Pharmacol Exp Ther.* 2009 March;328(3):758–765.
57. Reutershan J, Saprito MS, Wu D, Ruckle T, Ley K. Phosphoinositide 3-kinase gamma required for lipopolysaccharide-induced transepithelial neutrophil trafficking in the lung. *Eur Respir J.* 2010 May;35(5):1137–1147.
58. Ward S, Sotsios Y, Dowden J, Bruce I, Finan P. Therapeutic potential of phosphoinositide 3-kinase inhibitors. *Chem Biol.* 2003 March;10(3):207–213.
59. Sturgeon SA, Jones C, Angus JA, Wright CE. Advantages of a selective beta-isoform phosphoinositide 3-kinase antagonist, an anti-thrombotic agent devoid of other cardiovascular actions in the rat. *Eur J Pharmacol.* 2008 June 10;587(1–3):209–215.
60. Renda T, Baraldo S, Pelaia G, Bazzan E, Turato G, Papi A et al. Increased activation of p38 MAPK in COPD. *Eur Respir J.* 2008 January;31(1):62–69.
61. Medicherla S, Fitzgerald MF, Spicer D, Woodman P, Ma JY, Kapoun AM et al. p38alpha-selective mitogen-activated protein kinase inhibitor SD-282 reduces inflammation in a subchronic model of tobacco smoke-induced airway inflammation. *J Pharmacol Exp Ther.* 2008 March;324(3):921–929.
62. Lomas DA, Lipson DA, Miller BE, Willits L, Keene O, Barnacle H et al. An oral inhibitor of p38 MAP kinase reduces plasma fibrinogen in patients with chronic obstructive pulmonary disease. *J Clin Pharmacol.* 2012 March;52(3):416–424.
63. Chung KF. p38 mitogen-activated protein kinase pathways in asthma and COPD. *Chest.* 2011 June;139(6):1470–1479.
64. Rajendrasozhan S, Yang SR, Kinnula VL, Rahman I. SIRT1, an antiinflammatory and antiaging protein, is decreased in lungs of patients with chronic obstructive pulmonary disease. *Am J Respir Crit Care Med.* 2008 April 15;177(8):861–870.
65. Birrell MA, Wong S, Hardaker EL, Catley MC, McCluskie K, Collins M et al. IkappaB kinase-2-independent and -dependent inflammation in airway disease models: Relevance of IKK-2 inhibition to the clinic. *Mol Pharmacol.* 2006 June;69(6):1791–1800.

66. Keslacy S, Tliba O, Baidouri H, Amrani Y. Inhibition of tumor necrosis factor-alpha-inducible inflammatory genes by interferon-gamma is associated with altered nuclear factor-kappaB transactivation and enhanced histone deacetylase activity. *Mol Pharmacol*. 2007 February;71(2):609–618.
67. Catley MC, Sukkar MB, Chung KF, Jaffee B, Liao SM, Coyle AJ et al. Validation of the anti-inflammatory properties of small-molecule IkappaB Kinase (IKK)-2 inhibitors by comparison with adenoviral-mediated delivery of dominant-negative IKK1 and IKK2 in human airways smooth muscle. *Mol Pharmacol*. 2006 August;70(2):697–705.
68. Courtine E, Pene F, Cagnard N, Toubiana J, Fitting C, Brocheton J et al. Critical role of cRel subunit of NF-kappaB in sepsis survival. *Infect Immun*. 2011 May;79(5):1848–1854.
69. Barnes PJ. Emerging pharmacotherapies for COPD. *Chest*. 2008 December; 134(6):1278–1286.
70. Sugawara A, Sueki A, Hirose T, Nagai K, Gouda H, Hirono S et al. Novel 12-membered non-antibiotic macrolides from erythromycin A; EM900 series as novel leads for anti-inflammatory and/or immunomodulatory agents. *Bioorg Med Chem Lett*. 2011 June 1; 21(11):3373–3376.
71. Nakamaru Y, Vuppusetty C, Wada H, Milne JC, Ito M, Rossios C et al. A protein deacetylase SIRT1 is a negative regulator of metalloproteinase-9. *FASEB J*. 2009 September;23(9):2810–2819.
72. Wilkinson JE, Burmeister L, Brooks SV, Chan CC, Friedline S, Harrison DE et al. Rapamycin slows aging in mice. *Aging Cell*. 2012 August;11(4):675–682.
73. Baur JA, Pearson KJ, Price NL, Jamieson HA, Lerin C, Kalra A et al. Resveratrol improves health and survival of mice on a high-calorie diet. *Nature*. 2006 November 16; 444(7117):337–342.
74. Donnelly LE, Newton R, Kennedy GE, Fenwick PS, Leung RH, Ito K et al. Anti-inflammatory effects of resveratrol in lung epithelial cells: Molecular mechanisms. *Am J Physiol Lung Cell Mol Physiol*. 2004 October;287(4):L774–L783.

5 Inhaled Anticancer Agents

Rajiv Dhand

CONTENTS

INTRODUCTION

The search for alternative therapies for patients with surgically unresectable lung cancer continues because currently available regimens of chemotherapy, radiation therapy, and other newer treatment modalities have not made a significant impact on their grim prognosis. Inhalation therapy has intuitive advantages over systemic routes of administration because it is possible to achieve high local concentrations of therapeutic agents with minimal systemic effects. Rapid progress has been made in the ability to target aerosols to specific lung regions and in formulating inhaled therapies with lower toxicity and prolonged effects. A variety of modalities, including inhalation of immunomodulators, chemotherapeutic agents, and gene therapies, have been tested in preclinical and early-phase clinical trials, but no breakthrough treatments for lung cancer have emerged as yet. Nevertheless, these novel and promising approaches are being vigorously pursued and have the potential to improve outcomes for patients with lung cancer.

Lung cancer accounts for 14% of all new cancers and is the most common cause of cancer death in both men and women in the United States. Despite significant advances in prevention, screening, and treatment, approximately 224,000 new cases and 158,000 deaths from lung cancer were expected to occur in 2016, accounting for about 25% of all cancer deaths, in the United States (American Cancer Society 2016). The majority of new cases of lung cancer are now arising in the developing and less developed regions of the world, which have large populations of individuals who smoke cigarettes and are therefore at risk of developing lung cancer. Thus, newer, cost-effective, and well-tolerated treatments that can prolong survival among patients with lung cancer are urgently needed.

Non–small cell lung cancer (NSCLC), small cell lung cancer (SCLC), and carcinoid tumors constitute the vast majority of primary lung cancers. In addition, the lungs become involved by metastatic spread of other common tumors, such as carcinomas of the breast, colon, and prostate, as well as sarcomas and melanoma. NSCLC is further broadly subclassified into adenocarcinoma, squamous cell carcinoma, large cell carcinoma, and NSCLC not otherwise specified. NSCLC accounts for the majority of patients (~75% of total cases), and most studies of inhaled anticancer treatments focus on patients with NSCLC because SCLC has often spread beyond the lungs at the time of diagnosis. Surgery, radiation therapy, and systemic chemotherapy are the primary modalities of treatment for NSCLC. The treatment of patients with early-stage disease (stages I and II by tumor-node-metastasis (TNM) classification) is primarily surgical, but the role for systemic chemotherapy has been gradually expanding, now playing an important role in the treatment of both early-stage (stage II disease with positive lymph nodes) and locally advanced NSCLC (stage III) (Leong et al. 2014). However, systemic treatment with cytotoxic chemotherapy has the potential to produce serious adverse effects, and a significant proportion of patients may not be candidates for such therapy because of comorbidities and poor performance status.

DELIVERY OF INHALED ANTICANCER AGENTS

AEROSOL DEPOSITION

Inhalation therapy provides a method for regional administration of anticancer agents to treat lung cancer. Other solid tumors have been successfully controlled with regional administration of immunotherapy, chemotherapy, and genetic manipulation. Inhalational delivery is a noninvasive method to achieve high pulmonary concentrations of the delivered agent, with low systemic toxicity, potential to target therapy, and avoid hepatic metabolism of drugs. The ability to achieve high concentrations of chemotherapeutic agents within lung tumors may be a critical factor in reducing treatment failures as well as emergence of resistance to treatment (Minchinton and Tannock 2006). With this approach, tumors that have become refractory to systemic chemotherapy could respond to inhalation treatment (Hershey et al. 1999; Chou et al. 2013). The development of novel, local administration of anticancer agents may help to better target the tumors and potentially reduce the occurrence of adverse effects due to systemically administered treatments. Inhalation therapy, therefore, has the potential to become an effective and safe treatment for patients with lung cancer.

Aerosol particle size, inspiratory flow rate, tidal volume, and airway geometry are among the several factors that influence aerosol deposition in the lungs (Dolovich and Dhand 2011). The optimal site for inhaled drug deposition may vary depending on the site of the tumor. Aerosols with larger mass median aerodynamic diameter (MMAD) of 4–5 μm target centrally located lung tumors, whereas slow inhalation of aerosols containing drug particles of 1–3 μm in diameter increases the likelihood of drug deposition in peripheral airways and alveoli and is more appropriate for targeting peripheral tumors (e.g., adenocarcinoma and pulmonary metastasis). Airway obstruction by the tumor or the presence of associated obstructive lung disease could influence aerosol deposition patterns. Likewise, the high humidity environment in the lung could alter the particle size of some drugs and change their deposition. Other physical properties of the aerosol particles, such as pH, electrostatic charge, and osmolarity, also play a role in drug deposition (Eschenbacher et al. 1984).

After deposition drugs undergo dissolution and are transported across the epithelial membranes for absorption into the circulation. In the conducting airways, the mucociliary clearance mechanisms transport particulate matter up to the oropharynx, whereas in the alveoli, the principal mechanism of clearance is by alveolar macrophage phagocytosis. In patients with lung cancer, drugs depositing on the conducting airways in the vicinity of tumors may not be rapidly removed by mucociliary clearance because tumor cells lack functioning cilia, allowing the drug more opportunities to reach the tumor by direct local penetration. Moreover, drugs depositing on the airways are distributed to other regions of the lung via a rich plexus of bronchial capillaries that have pre- and postcapillary connections with the pulmonary circulation (Deffebach et al. 1987). Due to these communications between the bronchial and pulmonary circulations, drugs administered by inhalation could achieve adequate drug concentrations even within small tumors that are located in the lung parenchyma and lack direct communication with a major airway.

The chemical characteristics and biological effects of drugs strongly influence their efficacy as anticancer agents. In addition, tumor size influences drug penetration. Drugs show variable penetration into tumors; drugs such as 5-fluorouracil (5-FU), which bind macromolecules minimally, readily penetrate and are uniformly cytotoxic throughout the tumor. In contrast, penetration of other drugs, such as paclitaxel, within tumors is influenced by tumor cellularity, density of the interstitium, and apoptotic activity of the drug. In normal tissues, the net outward flow of fluid from the blood vessels is balanced by reabsorption into the lymphatic circulation. The interstitial pressure within tumors may be higher because they lack functional lymphatics, and the elevated interstitial fluid pressure could limit the distribution of some inhaled anticancer agents within the tumor. Thus, inhalation has the potential to achieve higher drug concentrations in the vicinity of the tumor; however, several other factors have to be considered in determining the ability of these agents to eradicate cancer cells.

TARGETING AIRWAY DEPOSITION OF DRUGS

Many lung tumors are localized to one lobe or segment of the lung; therefore, selective targeting of tumors could exponentially enhance local concentrations within the tumor while avoiding exposure of uninvolved areas of the lung to potentially toxic agents. Both *passive* and *active* targeting approaches have been utilized in an attempt to localize inhaled agents to specific sites in the lung. In the *passive targeting* approach, modification of aerosol droplet size; breathing pattern, depth, and duration of breath-hold; timing of the aerosol bolus in relation to inspiratory airflow; and the density of the inhaled gas are employed to enhance deposition at specific sites (Kleinstreuer et al. 2008). However, variations in patient's lung volumes and airway geometry make it difficult to achieve precise regional targeting even with a specified breathing pattern and size of aerosol particles (Clark and Hartman 2012). Thus, it is not possible to define a single set of parameters to target specific lung regions that are applicable to all patients. Newer devices (e.g., the Akita system® or I-neb adaptive aerosol delivery system®) provide attractive options for delivery of inhaled anticancer agents because the ability to synchronize aerosol generation with the patient's breathing enhances aerosol delivery efficiency and allows more precise control over the delivered dose (Diaz et al. 2012). Enhanced condensational growth is another technique to bypass upper airway deposition and achieve optimal lower respiratory tract deposition (Longest et al. 2013). In this technique, a submicrometer aerosol is provided to one nostril at slightly subsaturated humidification, whereas a humidified airstream saturated with water vapor is delivered to the other nostril with a temperature a few degrees above *in vivo* wall conditions. The two airstreams are physically separated by the nasal septum; the submicrometer aerosol is able to retain its small size as it traverses the nose and nasal deposition is minimized. The two airstreams combine in the nasopharynx with condensational growth of the aerosol particles as the airstream moves downward into the lungs. Mean drug deposition in the nose, mouth, and throat model could be reduced from 72.6% to 14.8%, whereas aerosol size increased from an initial MMAD of 900 nm to approximately 2 µm at the exit of the model (Longest et al. 2011). This technique overcomes the barrier imposed to aerosol particles by the nasal passages and could be employed to enhance lung deposition of agents delivered by inhalation while breathing through the nose. In addition, tumors have a leaky vasculature and the size of drug particles could be modulated to promote selective uptake by tumors that have increased permeability of the vascular endothelium—the enhanced permeability and retention effect (Torchilin 2010).

In the *active targeting* approach, either the aerosol is directed to the diseased area of the lung or some molecular or biological recognition that allows the drug to bind to the target cells is employed. For this purpose, therapy with an intracorporeal nebulizing catheter (INC), target-specific receptor ligands (tyrosine kinase inhibitors or folate), target-specific anti–epidermal growth factor receptor antibodies coupled to drugs, or an external magnetic field that guides inert superparamagnetic iron oxide nanoparticles (NPs) to a desired lung region has been employed (Dolovich and Dhand 2011). These active targeting techniques offer promising and novel approaches to treatment of lung cancers; however, they have not as yet been employed in clinical practice.

FORMULATIONS

Solutions

Nebulizers have been most commonly employed to deliver solution formulations of inhaled anticancer agents. Solution formulations employed in nebulizers were not specifically prepared for inhalation and had the potential to produce local irritant effects. However, the active moiety in the solution retained efficacy after nebulization. Repeated inhalations of the intravenous (IV) formulations of cisplatinum and gemcitabine (GEM) were shown to be well tolerated in anesthetized, mechanically ventilated dogs (Selting et al. 2008, 2011). No signs of significant local or systemic toxicity were observed after administration of escalating doses of cisplatin (10, 15, 20, and 30 mg/m^2 given by INC every 2 weeks for 10 weeks; cumulative dose 75 mg/m^2) (Selting et al. 2008). In a follow-up study, administration of escalating doses of combination chemotherapy (GEM 1, 2, 3, or 6 mg/kg and cisplatin 10 mg/m^2 given by INC every 2 weeks for 10 weeks) also did not produce clinical or biochemical side effects (Selting et al. 2011). All the dogs developed focal pneumonitis radiologically limited to the treated lobe, which increased in severity over time following increasing doses of chemotherapy. At autopsy, these radiologic changes correlated with chronic pneumonitis with fibrosis. Other investigators employed a freeze-dried powder of GEM or carboplatin solution reconstituted with normal saline for inhalation (Lemarie et al. 2011; Zarogoulidis et al. 2012). Because of problems in maintaining stability of solution formulations, many newer inhaled anticancer agents are now being formulated as dry powders, especially in an NP form.

Dry Powders

Dry powders are more stable than solutions and powder formulations may be preferable to aqueous solutions for delivery of inhaled anticancer agents. Ideal formulations of dry powders have the majority of drug particles in the range of 1–5 μm in size, and they exhibit desirable flow properties, low agglomeration tendency, and good batch-to-batch uniformity. Carrier particles (e.g., lactose) are added as excipients to improve handling and dispensing of the active agent and to reduce cohesiveness between particles. Small particles of the active agent adhere to the surface of the larger carrier particles to form agglomerates. Dry powders may also be formulated without excipients as loose agglomerates, which disperse into small particles with the application of energy from a patient's breath or other active sources. Particles of the active agent in the desired size range are commonly produced either by micronization involving milling techniques, commonly air jet milling, or by *in situ* micronization by various forms of controlled precipitation (Weers et al. 2007; Chan and Kwok 2013). Spray-drying is a widely used technique to manufacture particles by forcing a solution (less commonly a suspension) under pressure into a drying chamber through a spray nozzle. The dried particles that remain after the solvent or liquid evaporates are collected through a cyclone separator. Spray-drying allows various compounds to be incorporated into a single particle and is also employed to produce porous particles that have a density <0.1 g/cm^3. Porous particles (e.g., PulmoSpheres, Nektar Therapeutics) have a larger particle size, but their aerodynamic diameter is smaller (because of their lower density), and their deposition in the respiratory tract is similar to smaller particles of unit density. The larger size and surface area of porous particles allows them to carry a higher drug payload. Alveolar macrophages are unable to rapidly ingest such particles, they have a prolonged residence time within the deep lung, and they could potentially release their payload over extended periods of time (Edwards et al. 1997).

Inhaled agents could also be incorporated into the matrix of biodegradable synthetic polymers (polylactic acid [PLA], polylactic-co-glycolic acid [PLGA], natural polymers such as albumin and gelatin, and poly(ether-anhydrides)). Supercritical fluid technology is another promising method for preparing dry powders for inhalation. Particles of uniform size and shape can also be prepared by particle replication in nonwetting templates technology, in which a silicon master template is fabricated with photolithography and a polymeric mold is made from this silicon master template that has cavities of the precise particle size and required shape. The drug or excipient is filled into the cavities through capillary forces; the particles are then solidified in the mold and extracted by using an adhesive layer. The adhesive layer is dissolved to recover the particles and they can be used as a suspension or they may be lyophilized or evaporated to obtain dry free-flowing powder (Garcia et al. 2012).

Liposomes

Encapsulation of an aqueous solution within a hydrophobic phospholipid membrane has been employed to prepare liposomes of a variety of drugs, with a wide range of lipophilicities, including small molecules, nucleotides, deoxyribonucleic acid (DNA) constructs, peptides, and proteins (Cipolla et al. 2013). Typically, liposomes are formed by natural or synthetic phospholipids that may be electrically neutral or carry a net positive or negative charge. Their site of deposition within the respiratory tract and rate of drug release depend on their composition, size, charge, drug/lipid ratio, and method of delivery. The advantages of liposomal formulations are that they have minimal toxicity and prolonged drug effect compared to aqueous solutions. For example, CsA liposomes prepared for pulmonary delivery had a prolonged drug release compared to the free drug (Arppe et al. 1998). Liposomes are selectively taken up by mononuclear phagocytes and are also absorbed into lymphatic vessels—a common route for spread of lung tumors—allowing targeting of cancer cells that have metastasized to the lymph nodes.

The uptake of liposomes by macrophages could be avoided, and their effect further prolonged, by coating their surface with polyethylene glycol (PEG). Attaching monoclonal antibodies or ligands to the liposome surface allows targeting to specific cell surface receptors ("stealth" liposomes), or liposomes may be designed to release the drug on encountering a specific environment, such as the lower pH within cancers ("pH-sensitive" liposomes). Inhaled liposomal cisplatin has been tested on humans with lung cancer (Chou et al. 2013).

Liposomal formulations can be delivered by microspray or instillation or by jet or ultrasonic nebulizers. Drugs may leak from liposomes due to high shear stresses during nebulization, and therapeutic responses could be altered depending on the magnitude of leakage. Leakage of drug from liposomes could be reduced by using vibrating mesh nebulizers compared to jet nebulizers. Several investigators have attempted to minimize drug leakage during liposome administration. To avoid leakage of encapsulated drug or active agent during rehydration of dry powders, liposomes may be created *in situ* in the airways from the individual dried components (lipids, drug, and a powder dispersing agent such as lactose). In this technique, phospholipid-based dry powder formulations are dispersed in saline and spontaneously form multilamellar vesicles with a higher efficiency of drug encapsulation compared to other techniques (Desai et al. 2002).

Microparticles

Microparticles (size range 0.1–500 μm), produced from naturally occurring or synthetic polymers, are physically and chemically more stable than liposomes and have the capability to carry a higher drug load. Natural synthetic biocompatible and biodegradable polymers (chitosan, PLGA, PLA, poly(butylcyanoacrylate), and poly(lactic-co-lysine graft lysine) are commonly employed in producing such particles (Smola et al. 2008; Kaur et al. 2012). These particles can be coated with PEG to enhance their sustained-release property. Other techniques, including addition of dipalmitoylphosphatidylcholine, chitosan, or hydroxypropylcellulose, also prolong residence of particles in the lung. Microparticles produced by these techniques have higher stability, are able to carry a higher drug load, release drug slowly, and have longer pharmacological activity than liposomal formulations (Feng et al. 2003). The morphology, size, and porosity of these particles could be modulated for specific pulmonary indications (Feng et al. 2003). Docetaxel-loaded microspheres demonstrate sustained drug release, increased lung bioavailability, and reduced systemic toxicity (Wang et al. 2014).

Nanoparticles

Carrier particles are used to enhance lung deposition of inhaled NPs (size range 10–100 nm). NPs deposit in the deep lung lining fluid and escape mucociliary clearance and they are not engulfed by alveolar macrophages so that they have a more prolonged residence time in the lung (Ehrhardt et al. 2002), therefore having the advantage of requiring once or twice daily dosing. However, particle accumulation within alveoli could occur after repeated dosing. Lipid-coated NPs have less local toxicity than microspheres. In experimental models, paclitaxel-loaded solid lipid NPs (SLNs) and doxorubicin-loaded NPs effectively reduced the number and size of tumors. Other investigators have employed PLGA-coated NPs for delivery of chemotherapeutic agents. Abraxane®, an injectable suspension of albumin NPs with bound paclitaxel, has been employed clinically for the past few years but is not available as an inhaled formulation.

Drug-loaded NPs have been encapsulated within microparticles (so-called "Trojan" particles) by spray-drying of NPs followed by assembly into hollow porous particles, which can be delivered into the deep lung and provide sustained drug release (Tsapis et al. 2002). Such techniques have been employed for pulmonary delivery of antibodies (Kaye et al. 2009).

NPs have the ability to concurrently deliver drugs and genes to the same cells, and they can be coated with a variety of targeting molecules. SLNs have a hydrophobic core and a monolayer phospholipid shell. Drug-loaded SLNs can be administered within microparticles to enhance bioavailability and increase therapeutic effectiveness (Weber et al. 2014).

Swellable Hydrogels

Another approach to delivery of inhaled anticancer agents is to employ 1–5 μm particles in the dry state that swell to form larger particles in the warm and humid environment of the lung, are able to evade being engulfed by alveolar macrophages, and could be employed as carriers for drug-loaded NPs (El-Sherbiny et al. 2010).

Micelles

Amphipathic surfactant molecules self-assemble to a core–shell nanostructure in aqueous solution at a certain concentration and temperature to form polymeric micelles. Micelles represent colloidal dispersions with particle size from 5 to 50–100 nm. At low concentrations, these amphiphilic molecules exist separately as unimers; however, at a critical micelle concentration, they aggregate to form micelles, which are close to spherical in shape. The hydrophobic fragments of amphiphilic molecules form the core of a micelle, and poorly soluble pharmaceuticals can be carried in the core. The structure of these micelles can be chemically altered to improve drug stability, provide controlled drug release, and provide targeted drug delivery (Lavsanifar et al. 2002).

AEROSOL DELIVERY DEVICES

Traditionally, pressurized metered-dose inhalers (pMDIs), dry powder inhalers (DPIs), and nebulizers have been employed as aerosol generators, but pMDIs and DPIs are rarely employed for delivery of anticancer agents. More modern technologies generate aerosols by passing a solution through a vibrating mesh (e.g., Aeroneb® or eFlow®), by producing a soft mist from a drug solution (e.g., Respimat® and AERx®), or by evaporative condensation of a drug powder (e.g., Staccato® inhaler) (Dolovich and Dhand 2011). Other DPIs utilize compressed air (e.g., Exubera®) or electrical vibration (e.g., Microdose®) to disperse powder formulations. Aerosols generated by the Microsprayer® could be targeted to specific intrapulmonary sites.

INHALED ANTICANCER AGENTS

IMMUNOLOGICS/CYTOKINES

Tumors have developed several systems to evade or overwhelm the host's immune system and exogenous stimulation of the immune system could be utilized to lyse tumor cells. Tumor-associated macrophages have a significant role in controlling the tumor microenvironment, and these cells could be activated by inhalation of granulocyte macrophage colony-stimulating factor (GM-CSF). In humans, inhaled GM-CSF (500 µg/day in 2 divided doses) has modest effects in patients with pulmonary metastasis (Anderson et al. 1999). In patients with metastatic melanoma, aerosol delivery of GM-CSF may induce melanoma-specific immunity, similar to an *in vivo* dendritic cell vaccination (Markovic et al. 2008). In experimental and human studies, alveolar macrophages can be induced to destroy tumor cells and prolong survival.

In experimental animals, the anticancer activity of inhaled interleukin 2 (IL-2) is enhanced by liposomal encapsulation compared to free IL-2. Two or three times a day inhalation of 1×10^6 units of IL-2 was found to be effective for the treatment of canine osteosarcoma lung metastases. In metastatic renal carcinoma in humans, high-dose inhaled IL-2 in combination with low-dose subcutaneous IL-2 and subcutaneous interferon (IFN)-α improved median survival. However, inhaled IL-2 alone did not achieve significant efficacy in the treatment of patients with renal cancer and NSCLC. Inhaled IL-2 also had only modest effects against human metastatic melanoma and sarcoma.

IFNs are important mediators of immunity against tumors, and at low doses, cIFNs stimulate the immune system against cancer cells. IFN-γ is the most potent, and its effects are augmented by coadministration of tumor necrosis factor-α. Inhaled IFN-γ could achieve high lung levels and stimulate the local immune system, but it had limited efficacy in treating diffuse or locally advanced bronchoalveolar carcinoma.

CHEMOTHERAPY

Systemic chemotherapy is the primary treatment option for patients with advanced-stage lung cancer. However, with systemic chemotherapy, less than 6% of the administered dose is distributed to the lungs, and this may limit the concentrations of chemotherapy that are achieved in the lung (Litterst et al. 1976). Inhalation of chemotherapeutic agents could greatly enhance the concentrations achieved in the lung (Tatsumura et al. 1993; Selting et al. 2008). Inhaled chemotherapeutic agents are rapidly absorbed into the systemic circulation because of the large surface area of the alveoli and rich vascular supply; however, the peak blood levels achieved after inhalation are much lower than those after IV administration (Litterst et al. 1976; Selting et al. 2008).

The efficacy, safety, and pharmacokinetics of several inhaled chemotherapeutic agents, including doxorubicin, cisplatin, GEM, and liposomal encapsulated forms of paclitaxel and 9-nitrocamptothecin (9-NC) have been demonstrated in proof-of-concept studies in animal models of primary and metastatic lung cancer (Gagnadoux et al. 2008; Carvalho et al. 2011; Zarogoulidis et al. 2012). In dogs with spontaneous primary and metastatic lung cancers, including sarcoma, carcinomas, and malignant melanoma, partial responses were observed to inhaled paclitaxel or doxorubicin administered every 2 weeks. Inhalation of liposomal camptothecin and 9-NC reduced the size of human breast, colon, and lung cancer cells implanted subcutaneously in mice. Likewise, liposomal 9-NC effectively reduced metastasis in a murine malignant melanoma model and in a nude mice model with pulmonary metastasis of human osteosarcoma cells (Koshkina et al. 2000). Inhalation of liposomal paclitaxel (3 days per week) was effective in reducing lung metastasis and prolonging survival in a murine renal cell carcinoma pulmonary metastasis model (Koshkina et al. 2001).

GEM aerosol (given twice or thrice a week) after osteosarcoma tumor cell inoculation in mice inhibited the growth of lung metastasis and reduced subcutaneous tumor growth, indicating a possible systemic effect of aerosolized GEM. Furthermore, in an orthotopic model of large cell undifferentiated primary lung cancer produced by implantation of NCI-H460 cancer cells in BALB/c nude mice, administration of GEM with an endotracheal sprayer completely inhibited tumor growth in about one-third of animals and partially inhibited growth in the remainder. Higher doses of inhaled GEM produced more profound tumor suppression; however, lower doses were better tolerated and were not associated with any observed clinical or histological signs of toxicity (Gagnadoux et al. 2005).

Concomitant systemic and inhaled therapy could enhance the efficacy of treatment without increasing overall toxicity.

Pharmacokinetics

Following aerosol administration of ^{14}C-labeled doxorubicin in dogs, levels of radioactivity achieved in the lungs with aerosol delivery were higher, seemed to persist for longer period of time, and produced significantly lower systemic radioactivity levels than those observed after IV administration (Sharma et al. 2001). Similarly, liquid chromatography identified higher concentrations and slower clearance of paclitaxel from lung tissue extracts in dogs treated with inhaled liposomal paclitaxel versus IV administration of the same drug (Koshkina et al. 2001).

Cisplatin administered by an INC to the right caudal lung lobe of healthy dogs produced high platinum concentrations in the lung parenchyma (Selting et al. 2008). Immediately following a single inhaled dose, mean platinum levels in the lung were 44 times greater than in most other tissues, and peak blood levels were 15.6 times lower than those observed after IV infusion of a comparable dose. Later studies with inhaled liposomal cisplatin corroborated these findings (Chou et al. 2013).

Kelsen et al. reported that serum levels of cisplatin 5 min after an IV dose of 100–120 mg/m^2, the dose commonly employed for treatment of osteosarcoma, ranged from 1600 to 9500 ng/mL (median 5500 ng/mL), (Kelsen et al. 1985). After 24 h of IV dosing, the serum cisplatin levels ranged from 400 to 3500 ng/mL (median 1400 ng/mL) (Kelsen et al. 1985). In contrast, following inhalation of cisplatin, serum levels after 30 min ranged from 43.6 to 157.4 ng/mL (median 84.6 ng/mL) and at 18–24 h postdose, the levels were 47.0–153.5 ng/mL (median 81.9 ng/mL) (Chou et al. 2013). As expected, cisplatin levels in the lung after inhalation were much higher than those achieved after IV administration of cisplatin. In 3 patients who had bronchoalveolar lavage (BAL) performed within 24 h of receiving inhaled lipid cisplatin, the levels in BAL (9.4, 2,951.9, and 11,201.6 ng/mL) tended to be variable but generally higher than the corresponding levels in serum (61.9, 50.2, and 80.4 ng/mL) (Chou et al. 2013). Similarly, 24 and 96 h after instillation of cisplatin conjugated with hyaluronan into the lungs of rats, platinum levels in the lung were 5.7 and 1.2-fold higher, respectively, compared to rats receiving IV cisplatin (Xie et al. 2010). The levels of platinum in the draining lymph nodes were higher and plasma platinum levels were more sustained with a reduced peak plasma concentration after instillation compared to IV administration; however, the animals developed patchy areas of moderate inflammation after instillation, suggesting that aerosolization may be preferable to instillation for delivering such cisplatin conjugates to the lung (Xie et al. 2010).

Preclinical Efficacy

The aerosolization process does not affect the cytotoxic effect of the chemotherapy as shown by similar levels of growth inhibition with nebulized and nonnebulized GEM in NCI-H460 and A549 NSCLC cell lines (Gagnadoux et al. 2006). *In vivo* efficacy of aerosol chemotherapy has been evaluated in mouse models for lung metastasis treated with inhaled liposomal 9-NC (Koshkina et al. 2000), inhaled GEM (Koshkina and Kleinerman 2005), or inhaled liposomal paclitaxel (Koshkina et al. 2001). Another murine model found that weekly inhalation of GEM achieved complete or partial inhibition of tumor growth after intrabronchial implantation of large cell undifferentiated primary lung cancer cells (NCI-H460) in BALB/c nude mice (Gagnadoux et al. 2005).

In dogs with primary lung cancer or lung metastases, inhaled paclitaxel and doxorubicin resulted in tumor shrinkage in 25% of the dogs, without producing adverse effects commonly seen with IV chemotherapy (Hershey et al. 1999). Aerosol administration of GEM to dogs who naturally developed lung metastases from osteosarcoma was well tolerated but did not produce any cures and did not prolong survival among the treated dogs (Rodriguez et al. 2010).

While earlier studies demonstrated the feasibility and relative safety of targeted direct local administration of chemotherapeutic agents to the lung, concerns about local toxicity could be reduced by employing formulations designed specifically for inhalation rather than the IV formulations of cisplatin and GEM that were employed in the previous investigations. Further investigations have been conducted to fulfill the need for formulations that are suitable for inhalation and do not cause local toxicity. For example, Feng and colleagues insufflated freeze-dried porous microspheres of PLGA loaded with doxorubicin and pacli-taxel into the lungs of C57BL/6J mice implanted with B16F10 melanoma cells (Feng et al. 2014). The combination of doxorubicin and paclitaxel had a synergis-tic effect in reducing the number of tumor lesions in the lungs of the mice without causing histological evidence of damage to healthy alveoli. Other novel formu-lations that could enhance the safety of inhaled chemotherapeutic agents while preserving their efficacy for treating lung cancers are under active investigation (Meenach et al. 2013, 2014).

Inhaled Chemotherapeutic Agents

Treatment with aerosolized 5-FU, doxorubicin, 9-NC, liposomal paclitaxel, and platinum agents has shown activity against lung cancer and metastasis to the lung in preclinical studies. Subsequent phase I/II clinical trials have assessed the safety and anticancer effect of several chemotherapeutic agents, including inhaled 5-FU, GEM, 9-NC, doxorubicin, and platinum agents (Table 5.1).

Nucleoside Analogs

5-FU is a fluoropyrimidine that acts as an antimetabolite inhibiting DNA and ribo-nucleic acid (RNA) synthesis. In the first study of inhaled chemotherapy in humans, Tatsumura and colleagues observed that 5-FU concentrations in the airways and regional lymph nodes were at therapeutic levels, whereas only a trace of the drug was detected in the serum (Tatsumura et al. 1993). Interestingly, the levels of 5-FU were significantly higher in the tumor tissue than in the normal lung tissue. Six of 10 patients with unresectable lung cancer who were previously untreated and received inhaled 5-FU responded to therapy with no significant adverse effects from these treatments (Tatsumura et al. 1993).

GEM belongs to the same class of drugs as 5-FU. Inhaled GEM administered once a week for 9 weeks to 11 patients with lung cancer resulted in a partial response in one patient and stable disease in four patients (Lemarie et al. 2011).

Doxorubicin

Inhaled doxorubicin has shown preclinical activity against both primary lung cancer and lung metastasis. A phase I trial evaluated the safety of increasing doses of inhaled doxorubicin in 53 patients with lung metastases (Otterson et al. 2007). Pulmonary toxicities were the most frequently reported adverse events, and five patients had severe adverse effects ($\geq$grade 3). Partial response was reported in one patient, and stable disease was reported in eight patients.

In a subsequent phase I/II study, patients with treatment-naive advanced-stage NSCLC were treated with the maximal tolerated dose (MTD) for inhaled doxorubi-cin (6 mg/m^2) along with IV cisplatin and docetaxel (Otterson et al. 2010). The inves-tigators reported a 29% response rate (7 responders out of 24 evaluable patients) and stable disease rate of 54%. Toxicities were primarily due to systemic chemotherapy, and pulmonary toxicities were generally mild (grade 1–2). In this study, the addition of inhaled doxorubicin to IV chemotherapy did not result in significant improvement in treatment outcomes, and the authors did not recommend further evaluation of this combination (Otterson et al. 2010).

TABLE 5.1

Clinical Studies of Inhaled Chemotherapy

First Author	Year	Chemotherapy Agent/ Delivery Device	Disease State	Evaluation	Outcome
Tatsumura, T	1993	5-FU nebulizer	Lung cancer	Bronchoscopy, HPLC, histopathology	Aerosolized 5-FU accumulated at therapeutic concentrations in airways and regional lymph nodes; partial responses in 60% of patients without significant pulmonary or systemic side effects.
Verschraegen, CF	2004	9-NC liposomal nebulizer	Primary lung cancer or metastases to the lung	HRCT, blood, BAL, urine analysis	Chemical pharyngitis was dose limiting. Other side effects included nausea, vomiting, cough, bronchial irritation, fatigue, and reversible fall in FEV_1. Partial remissions were observed in some patients.
Witgen, BP	2007	Cis liposomal nebulizer	Lung cancer	Blood, pulmonary function, chest x-ray, chest CT, PK, RECIST	Dose-escalating study in 17 patients with primary or metastatic lung cancer. There was no dose-limiting toxicity at maximum delivered dose. The side effects also include generally reversible fall in pulmonary function, nausea, and vomiting, but no other systemic toxicity was reported. Stability of disease was observed in 12 patients.
Otterson, GA	2007	DOX nebulizer	Metastases to the lung	CT, RECIST, HPLC, V/Q, blood	Phase I study of 53 patients with cancer metastatic to the lungs. Increasing doses of DOX ($0.4-9.4$ mg/m^2) were given every 3 weeks. Pulmonary toxicity was dose limiting. Partial responses were observed in some patients.

(Continued)

TABLE 5.1 (*Continued*)
Clinical Studies of Inhaled Chemotherapy

First Author	Year	Chemotherapy Agent/ Delivery Device	Disease State	Evaluation	Outcome
Otterson, GA	2010	DOX nebulizer	Advanced NSCLC	CT, RECIST; V/Q	Phase I/II dose escalation study of inhaled DOX in combination with IV docetaxel and Cis. Forty-three patients with metastatic NSCLC were treated, with partial responses in 6 patients and complete response in 1 patient; some patients developed late decreases in pulmonary function.
Lemarie E	2011	GEM vibrating mesh nebulizer with a vertical chamber spacer	NSCLC	Gamma scintigraphy, blood, chest x-ray, chest CT, head CT, pulmonary function tests, PK	Patients with NSCLC ($n =11$) unresponsive to chemotherapy were treated with inhaled GEM doses between 1 and 4 mg/kg body weight. A maximum dose of 3 mg/kg/week was safe. Side effects included cough, dyspnea, vomiting, and bronchospasm. Partial responses were observed in some patients.
Zarogoulidis, P	2011	CARBO nebulizer	NSCLC	HRCT, RECIST, blood	Sixty patients with untreated NSCLC received IV docetaxel and either inhaled CARBO, inhaled and IV CARBO, or IV CARBO. The combination of inhaled and IV CARBO prolonged survival. Fever and cough were the common side effects.
Chou, AJ	2013	Cis liposomal nebulizer	Recurrent osteosarcoma with metastases to the lungs	PFT, blood, urine, V/Q, CT scan	Nineteen children with high-grade metastatic osteosarcoma. Side effects include nausea, vomiting, dyspnea, wheezing, and cough.

Abbreviations: 5-FU, 5-fluorouracil; 9-NC, 9-nitro camptothecin; BAL, bronchoalveolar lavage; CARBO, carboplatin; Cis, cisplatin; CT, computer tomography; DOX, doxorubicin; FEV₁, forced expiratory volume in 1 s; GEM, gemcitabine; HPLC, high-performance liquid chromatography; HRCT, high resolution computer tomography; NSCLC, non-small cell lung cancer; PK, pharmacokinetics; RECIST, response evaluation criteria in solid tumors; V/Q, ventilation/perfusion scan.

Liposomal 9-Nitrocamptothecin

A phase I trial evaluated the feasibility and safety of inhaled 9-NC in the treatment of patients with primary or metastatic lung cancer (Verschraegen et al. 2004). 9-NC was administered on days 1–5 every week for a period of 6 weeks. The MTD was 20 µg/kg/day, but a lower-dose level of 13.3 µg/kg/day was well tolerated. Two patients with metastatic endometrial cancer had partial response to treatment, and the treatment benefit was not confined to the lung tumors (Verschraegen et al. 2004). Overall, inhaled 9-NC was found to be well tolerated with an acceptable safety profile; however, no further clinical development of this formulation has been reported.

Platinum Agents

Cisplatin and carboplatin are the primary treatment agents used in several combination chemotherapy regimens for systemic treatment of lung cancer. The safety of inhaled cisplatin encapsulated in microscopic phospholipid spheres or sustained-release lipid inhalation targeting (SLIT)™ was evaluated in a phase I study by Wittgen and colleagues (2007). The treatment was well tolerated, and the serum levels of cisplatin varied between low to undetectable in most cases. No treatment response was reported, but 12 of 17 patients were reported to have stable disease at the time of evaluation (Zarogoulidis et al. 2012). Cisplatin lipid complex was also evaluated in the treatment of 19 pediatric patients with pulmonary metastases from recurrent osteosarcoma in a phase I/II study (Chou et al. 2013). In the eight patients with nonbulky disease (size of lesions ≤2 cm), one had partial response and two patients had stable disease. Because dose-limiting toxicity was not reported in the clinical trials reported with SLIT™ (Wittgen et al. 2007; Chou et al. 2013), further studies would be needed to determine if the efficacy of treatment could be improved with higher doses or use of alternative formulations of cisplatin.

Carboplatin is frequently used in the frontline treatment of advanced-stage NSCLC. Inhaled carboplatin in the treatment of NSCLC was evaluated in a small trial (Zarogoulidis et al. 2012). In this trial, 60 patients with advanced-stage NSCLC were randomized into 3 groups. The first group received IV carboplatin and docetaxel (control arm), whereas the second group received IV docetaxel, two-thirds of the calculated carboplatin IV, and one-third carboplatin dose as an inhalant. The third group received the entire dose of carboplatin administered in the aerosol form along with IV docetaxel. Patients receiving both IV and inhaled carboplatin (group 2) had better survival outcomes compared to the control arm—275 days versus 211 days (Zarogoulidis et al. 2012). There was a trend toward improvement in the median overall survival for patients receiving inhaled carboplatin with IV docetaxel.

The development of resistance to chemotherapeutic agents is a frequent cause of treatment failure and tumor recurrence. Several approaches to reduce the development of resistance, such as adding pump and nonpump suppressors to inhaled chemotherapy (Hohenforsdt-Schmidt et al. 2014) or combining an active agent with an appropriate drug carrier that can specifically target sites in the respiratory tract where drug transporter genes are highly expressed or combining inhaled chemotherapy and gene therapy (Taratula et al. 2013), are currently under investigation.

GENE THERAPY

Specialized constructs of DNA are delivered to cells in order to correct specific abnormalities in mutated genes that are responsible for the development of cancer or those conferring resistance to chemotherapy. Other approaches have targeted genes that induce immune response to tumors or those that induce apoptosis in tumor cells. Liquid-suspended gene particles are difficult to nebulize at concentrations of DNA >5 mg/mL because of their viscosity. Shear stresses during nebulization cause fragmentation of naked DNA, and vector systems are needed as carriers to protect DNA from degradation. Both *ex vivo* and *in vivo* approaches have been employed for gene therapy, with the latter requiring direct transfer of genes to the patient's tissues with the help of vectors. These vectors are typically composed of viral capsid (Table 5.2), or they are packaged in nonviral systems, commonly involving the transfer of genes carried on plasmid DNA by cationic lipids, polymers, or peptides. The safety of viral delivery systems is enhanced by removing genes required for replication. Although these replication deficient viruses are efficient at transfection, their clinical use is challenging because they are inherently immunogenic. In phase I studies of patients with lung cancer, replacement of p53 tumor suppressor gene using an adenoviral vector did not yield promising results. However, in these investigations, the gene was not administered by inhalation.

Nonviral carriers are safer than viral carriers but their transfection efficiency is low. Among the several cationic polymers that have been employed, polyethylenimine achieves higher transfection efficiency both in tissue culture and *in vivo*. Several cationic lipids, such as dioleoyltrimethylammonium propane (DOTAP) and dioleoxipropyltrimethylammonium (DOTMA), have been employed as gene carriers, with DOTMA having higher transfection efficiency than DOTAP. Mixing cationic lipids with neutral lipids facilitates formation of liposomes and enhances their disassembly after uptake into the cell. Notably, a significant drawback of cationic lipoplexes is that high doses could trigger inflammatory responses in the lung. To avoid such toxicity, biodegradable polymer-based NPs, which have a prolonged residence time in the lung, have been investigated as gene carriers.

Several investigators have successfully delivered genes by inhalation using these nonviral carriers. Inhalation of p53 tumor suppressor gene in lipoplexes containing polylysine and protamine reduced lung metastasis in a murine model of malignant melanoma (Zou et al. 2007). Another approach involves transfection of tumors with a gene that codes for a specific enzyme that transforms a benign drug into a toxic metabolite that causes cell death ("suicide gene"). For example, transduction of herpes simplex virus 1 thymidine kinase (HSVtk) gene makes cells susceptible to ganciclovir, a nucleoside analog, which is normally poorly metabolized by mammalian cells. HSVtk converts ganciclovir to a metabolite that causes cell death by interfering with DNA replication. Clinical trials have employed an adenoviral vector to transduce HSVtk by intratumoral injection into mesothelioma with partial success (Sterman et al. 2008).

Various other physical techniques to facilitate DNA uptake into cells by transiently increasing membrane permeability involve application of electrical impulses (electroporation) or ultrasound energy (sonoporation).

TABLE 5.2
Viral Vectors for Gene Delivery

Viral Vector	Transduction Efficiency	Transduction of Nondividing Cells	Risk of Insertional Mutagenesis	Immune Response	Clinical Use
Adenovirus; non-enveloped DNA viruses, type 2 and type 5 are commonly employed for gene therapy.	Low to moderate; capable of packaging 8.5 kb of foreign DNA	Yes	Low	Occurrence of both antibody and cellular immune responses	Yes; transduced gene is expressed for short duration (1–6 weeks). Repeated dosing is needed.
Retrovirus; RNA virus that carry a gene for reverse transcriptase.	Very low; vector titers are low and particles are unstable	No	Moderate; viral genome is stably integrated into host genome and viral sequence is maintained during cell division; risk of toxicity if therapeutic gene is overexpressed	Inactivated by complement	Suitable for *ex-vivo* gene therapy and treatment of inherited and chronic diseases. Employed in several clinical trials.
Lentivirus (e.g., HIV-type 1; genetically modified virus is used).	Efficient transduction into lymphohematopoietic and central nervous system cells	Yes	Low	Low	Yes.

(Continued)

TABLE 5.2 (Continued)
Viral Vectors for Gene Delivery

Viral Vector	Transduction Efficiency	Transduction of Nondividing Cells	Risk of Insertional Mutagenesis	Immune Response	Clinical Use
Adeno-associated virus (AAV); parvovirus, most derived from AAV serotype 2. All internal coding sequences are removed and co-transfected with a helper virus (e.g., adenovirus, herpes simplex, vaccinia).	Low; only small amounts of DNA can be packaged (4–5 kb)	Latent infection; long-lasting expression of therapeutic gene	Low; higher level of safety	No	Yes; employed in clinical trials in cystic fibrosis, hemophilia B, and Parkinson's disease.
Herpes simplex virus; enveloped double-stranded DNA virus.	Natural human pathogen; replicates in dividing cells; able to stay latent in nondividing cells	Efficient for gene transfer; larger genes can be transferred (capacity 30–40 kb)	Low	No	In the latent state, most genes, including therapeutic gene, are turned off.
Pox viruses (e.g., vaccinia).	Yes	Efficient for gene transfer; potential to insert genes of ~10 kb	Low	Yes	Yes; attenuated virus enhances immunological rejection of tumors.
Alpha viruses (enveloped single stranded RNA viruses, e.g., Semliki forest virus)	Yes	Low	Low	Yes; induced cytotoxic T-cell responses	Useful for intratumoral gene therapy.

Despite recent advances, gene therapy for lung cancer needs to overcome several barriers to achieve meaningful success. Efficient delivery of the therapeutic gene to specific dysfunctional tumor cells is a significant hurdle. Carriers that target specific cells by utilizing receptor–ligand interactions must recognize receptors on the apical airway epithelial cell surface because receptors on the basal–lateral surface may not be accessible *in vivo*. Even after cellular uptake, the genetic material must overcome several intracellular barriers before protein translation occurs. Finally, effective suppression of tumors may require repeated dosing and vectors employed for gene delivery must be safe for both acute and chronic administration.

ANTISENSE THERAPY

In this approach, inhibition of gene expression is accomplished by administration of a targeted oligonucleotide that reduces transcription of complementary messenger ribonucleic acid. More recently, plasmid- or viral vector–mediated transfer of small interfering RNA or short hairpin RNA (shRNA) precursors has been employed in animal models. Inhibition of the Akt signaling pathway by aerosol delivery of a lung cancer cell–target shRNA has been reported to suppress lung tumorigenesis. However, it is difficult to achieve adequate concentrations of these molecules within tumors, and their efficacy is constrained by limited bystander effects on nontransduced cells within the tumor (Vachani et al. 2011).

BACTERIA

The innate ability of bacteria to invade cells has been employed to efficiently deliver DNA. Delivery of genetic material by bacteria is achieved by either of the two approaches: (1) specific replication of bacteria within tumors or (2) intracellular transfer of plasmids within cancer cells (bactofection) by various bacterial species, such as *Salmonella*, *Escherichia coli*, and *Listeria species*. Anaerobic and facultatively anaerobic bacteria are employed to specifically target the relative hypoxic environment within tumors. Bacteria also show chemotaxis to necrotic regions within tumors, and aberrant "leaky" vasculature and local immune suppression may also facilitate bacterial entry and colonization within tumors. Several bacterial species (*Bifidobacterium*, *Salmonella*, *E. coli*, *Vibrio cholerae* and *Listeria monocytogenes*) are capable of tumor-specific growth after IV administration, and they transport and amplify genes within tumors (Baban et al. 2010). However, the inhalation of bacteria has not been employed for DNA delivery and the potential for environmental spread of the vector will need to be carefully addressed if such a delivery mechanism is employed in clinical practice.

CLINICAL USE OF INHALED ANTICANCER AGENTS

IMMUNOLOGICS/CYTOKINES

Several attempts have been made to selectively activate local immunity in the lungs to control metastases. Inhaled IL-2 alone given for treatment of patients with renal cancer and NSCLC did not produce impressive results but was more effective when combined with systemic low-dose IL-2 and IFN-α, high-dose systemic IL-2, or chemotherapy (Huland et al. 2000). In patients with metastatic melanoma, aerosol delivery of GM-CSF has modest clinical effects, but it may induce melanoma-specific immunity. The use of inhaled monoclonal antibodies, such as cetuximab, merits further study because they retain activity after aerosolization and are able to penetrate into orthotopic lung tumors in BALB/c nude mice.

CHEMOTHERAPY

The efficacy of inhaled chemotherapy in a clinical setting has been reported by a few investigators (Table 5.1). Inhaled 5-FU achieved tumor tissue levels that were 5–15-fold higher than those in normal lung; the levels were higher than those needed for antineoplastic activity, and 5-FU alone or in combination with other chemotherapy agents was partially effective in patients with NSCLC (Tatsumura et al. 1993). Partial responses in lung tumors and liver metastasis were observed in patients with pulmonary metastasis from a variety of tumors who received inhaled liposomal 9-NC (Vershraegen et al. 2004). A liposomal formulation of cisplatin (SLIT) given over 1–4 consecutive days in 21-day treatment cycles to patients with lung cancer stabilized the disease in 12 out of 17 patients and was not associated with systemic side effects (Wittgen et al. 2007). In 11 patients with NSCLC (including 6 patients with diffuse bronchoalveolar carcinoma) who were unresponsive to previous chemotherapy, weekly inhalation of GEM (0.5 or 1 mg/kg) produced a minor response in one patient and stable disease in 4 patients (Lemarie et al. 2011). Likewise, survival benefit was shown in NSCLC patients after use of inhaled carboplatin in addition to systemic carboplatin in combination with IV docetaxel (Zarogoulidis et al. 2012). In early-stage (stage II) NSCLC patients who received inhaled cisplatin 2 h prior to surgery, the subcarinal lymph node had higher concentrations of cisplatin than those in the blood (Zarogoulidis et al. 2013). Thus, inhaled drugs could diffuse from the alveoli into the lymphatic circulation and regional lymph nodes. Whether inhaled drugs could achieve adequate concentration to lyse cancer cells within lymph nodes needs further evaluation.

In patients with metastatic osteosarcoma limited to the lungs, inhalation of liposomal cisplatin produced sustained benefit in some patients with less bulky disease without producing toxic effects that are commonly observed after IV cisplatin administration (Chou et al. 2013).

GENE THERAPY

There has been much progress in developing vectors for gene delivery and several experimental approaches have been employed, but these approaches have not yet been effectively applied in clinical practice. Replacement of a mutated or absent tumor suppressor gene should lead to suppression of tumor growth or tumor cell death. Several early-phase clinical trials have evaluated restoration of wild-type p53 in lung tumor cells. These approaches have employed direct intratumoral injection with adenoviral vectors and have shown partial responses, but the benefits over chemotherapy or radiotherapy alone have not been convincingly demonstrated in these trials. Promising gene therapy approaches involve stimulation of an endogenous immune response to the tumor and combining antisense therapy with chemotherapy (Taratula et al. 2013).

ADVERSE EFFECTS

Most adverse events of inhaled chemotherapy are due to direct local effects of the chemotherapeutic agents on the upper and lower respiratory tract. After IV administration, chemotherapeutic agents have the potential to produce a variety of pulmonary toxic effects, including some that are severe and life threatening. After inhaled chemotherapy, nonpulmonary side effects are infrequently reported. Metallic taste, cough, weight loss, neurotoxicity, and cardiotoxicity have been observed (Table 5.3).

Among a variety of agents given by inhalation, dose-limiting pulmonary toxicity was only observed with doxorubicin. Several symptoms such as cough, wheezing, shortness of breath, bronchospasm, and chest pain occur with varying frequency after inhalation of chemotherapy. An alveolar interstitial pattern is often seen radiologically and this is associated with histological findings of moderate fibrosis (Selting et al. 2008, 2011). Bilateral ground glass opacities and hypoxemia have been occasionally reported. Severe pulmonary toxicity has been observed with inhaled doxorubicin (Otterson et al. 2007), GEM (Lemarie et al. 2011), and liposomal cisplatin (Chou et al. 2013). Bronchoconstriction and a drop in pulmonary function observed after inhaled chemotherapy could be mitigated by prior administration of inhaled bronchodilators and corticosteroids (Otterson et al. 2007, 2010; Lemarie et al. 2011; Chou et al. 2013).

TABLE 5.3
Adverse Effects with Inhaled Chemotherapy

Type of Adverse Effect	Symptoms	Severity	Remarks
Respiratory	Cough, hoarseness, bronchoconstriction, dyspnea, fall in pulmonary function, acute lung injury	Dose-limiting lung toxicity can occur but is uncommon.	Pre-treatment with bronchodilators and corticosteroids is recommended.
Gastrointestinal (GI)	Glossitis, pharyngitis, nausea, vomiting	Glossitis and pharyngitis could be dose limiting.	GI side effects are common.
Hematological	Anemia, cytopenias	Hematological effects are uncommon.	Neutropenia may occur with repeated dosing.
Biochemical	No significant changes	Biochemical changes are rare.	Inhalation of chemotherapy is associated with very few biochemical derangements.
Miscellaneous	Metallic taste, fever, fatigue	These are usually not dose-limiting.	These side effects are more frequent. Other systemic side effects, e.g., ototoxicity, occur infrequently.

Adverse effects due to inhaled nonchemotherapeutic agents include reduction in forced vital capacity, bilateral infiltrates, pleural effusion, and bronchospasm with inhaled GM-CSF in patients with metastatic disease (Anderson et al. 1999; Markovic et al. 2008). In contrast, other investigators have reported only minor toxicity in patients who received inhaled GM-CSF. Inhalation of IL-2 is limited by the development of pulmonary vascular leakage, which is dose, route, and formulation dependent (Huland et al. 2003). Adenoviral vectors tend to create neutralizing antibodies and can be associated with significant local and systemic inflammation involving neutralizing antibodies and cytotoxic lymphocytes. In contrast, adenoassociated virus has not been associated with any significant toxicity. Nonviral vectors and polymers exhibit cytotoxicity, which is mainly due to their strong electrostatic charge. The molecular weight of the polymers plays an important role, with higher-molecular-weight polymers producing higher incidence of adverse respiratory effects.

LIMITATIONS OF INHALED ANTICANCER AGENTS

ENVIRONMENTAL CONTAMINATION

To minimize occupational exposure of healthcare workers or others who are administering inhaled chemotherapeutic agents, a well-ventilated room with a HEPA filter air cleaning system for aerosol administration is mandatory. However, Verschraegen and colleagues allowed patients to take their inhaled chemotherapy at home (Verschraegen et al. 2004). Establishing the safety of domiciliary chemotherapy could have enormous implications for convenience and cost of treatment.

UNANSWERED QUESTIONS

Further investigations are ongoing to establish the optimal drug regimens, formulations, and methods of inhaled drug delivery. When inhaled agents are used as adjuncts, whether they should be given before (neoadjuvant), concurrently with, or after (adjuvant) other forms of treatment have not been established. Future investigations will need to clarify if inhalation targeted only to the tumor site is more effective and less toxic compared to drug deposition in both lungs. Focused investigations could elucidate which tumor types (primary/secondary) respond best to inhalational treatment, whether such therapy is more effective at an early or late stage of the disease, and if inhaled therapy effectively treats micrometastases in the lungs and at other sites following lymphatic or vascular spread of the tumor. Successfully addressing these questions with well-designed clinical trials will aid in clarifying the role of inhalational anticancer therapy in clinical practice.

SUMMARY

- A variety of agents, including immunologics/cytokines, chemotherapy, gene therapy, antisense therapy, or gene transfer by bacterial infection, alone, or in combination, have been employed for treatment of primary or metastatic cancer in the lung.

- Aerosolized chemotherapy could target centrally located tumors with limited invasion or tumors that have relapsed after surgery as an adjunct to other well-established methods of treating lung malignancies.
- Inhaled chemotherapy also appears to be an attractive option for the treatment of bronchoalveolar carcinoma, a peripheral tumor that can be multifocal and spreads along alveolar walls, or multiple pulmonary metastases.
- Challenges to using inhaled anticancer formulations include the need for relatively large doses that lead to long administration times; delivering aerosol to the site of the tumor, especially past areas of airway obstruction; achieving adequate drug release within or in close proximity to the tumor; and adequate drug penetration into larger tumors. If the drug is rapidly absorbed into the systemic circulation, frequent administration may be required or formulations that have a prolonged effect are needed.
- Many oncology trials are performed in patients who have failed other treatments and have a poor outcome. Although this is appropriate from a safety viewpoint, efficacy may be better demonstrated in patients with an early disease (TNM stage I or stage II). However, surgical resection is the preferred treatment for early-stage lung cancer; other treatment modalities are the exception rather than the rule, generally being considered only for patients who are not surgical candidates.
- The effects of inhaled drugs in combination have not been tested in human studies even though doublet therapy is the cornerstone of systemic therapy for lung cancer. Targeted inhalation therapy of lung tumors could improve the duration and quality of life, even if the patient ultimately succumbs to the disease.
- Outcomes for patients with primary or metastatic lung cancer could be improved by future innovations in inhaled formulations of anticancer agents and their clinical application.

REFERENCES

American Cancer Society. 2016. Key statistics for lung cancer. http://www.cancer.org/cancer/lung cancer-non-small cell/detailedguide/non-small-cell-lung-cancer-key-statistics (accessed March 14, 2016).

Anderson PM, Markovic SN, Sloan JA et al. Aerosol granulocyte macrophage-colony stimulating factor: A low toxicity, lung-specific biologic therapy in patients with lung metastasis. *Clin Cancer Res* 1999;5:2316–2323.

Arppe J, Vidgren M, Waldrep J. Pulmonary pharmacokinetics of cyclosporine A liposomes. *Int J Pharm* 1998;161:205–214.

Baban CK, Cronin M, O'Hanlon D et al. Bacteria as vectors for gene therapy of cancer. *Bioengineered Bugs* 2010;1:385–394.

Carvalho TC, Carvalho SR, McConville JT. Formulations for pulmonary administration of anticancer agents to treat lung malignancies. *J Aerosol Med Pulm Drug Deliv* 2011;24:61–80.

Chan HK, Kwok PCL. Novel particle production technologies for inhalation products. Colombo P, Traini D, Buttini F, eds. *Inhalation Drug Delivery: Techniques and Products*. John Wiley and Sons, Ltd, Chichester, UK. Wiley-Blackwell; 2013, pp. 47–62.

Chou AJ, Gupta, R, Bell MD, Riewe KO, Meyers PA, Gorlick R. Inhaled lipid cisplatin (ILC) in the treatment of patients with relapsed/progressive osteosarcoma metastatic to the lung. *Pediatr Blood Cancer* 2013;60:580–586.

Cipolla D, Gonda I, Chan HK. Liposomal formulations for inhalation. *Ther Deliv* 2013;4:1047–1072.

Clark AR, Hartman MS. Regional lung deposition: Can it be controlled and have an impact on safety and efficacy? *Respir Drug Deliv* 2012;1:89–100.

Deffebach ME, Charan NB, Lakshminarayan S, Butler J. The bronchial circulation: Small, but a vital attribute of the lung. *Am Rev Respir Dis* 1987;135:463–481.

Desai TR, Wong JP, Hancock REW et al. A novel approach to the pulmonary delivery of liposomes in dry powder form to eliminate the deleterious effects of milling. *J Pharm Sci* 2002;9:482–491.

Diaz KT, Skaria S, Harris K et al. Delivery and safety of inhaled interferon-gamma in idiopathic pulmonary fibrosis. *J Aerosol Med Pulm Drug Deliv* 2012;25:79–87.

Dolovich MB, Dhand R. Aerosol drug delivery: Developments in device design and clinical use. *Lancet* 2011;377(9770):1032–1045.

Edwards DA, Hanes J, Caponetti G et al. Large porous particles for pulmonary drug delivery. *Science* 1997;276:1868–1872.

Ehrhardt C, Fiegel L, Fuchs S et al. Drug absorption by the respiratory mucosa: Cell culture models and particulate drug carriers. *J Aerosol Med* 2002;15:131–139.

El-Sherbiny IM, McGill S, Smyth HD. Swellable microparticles as carriers for sustained pulmonary drug delivery. *J Pharm Sci* 2010;99:2343–2356.

Eschenbacher WL, Boushey HA, Sheppard D. Alteration in osmolarity of inhaled aerosols cause bronchoconstriction and cough, but absence of a permeant anion causes cough alone. *Am Rev Respir Dis* 1984;129:211–215.

Feng SS, Chien S. Chemotherapeutic engineering: Application and further development of chemical engineering principles for chemotherapy of cancer and other diseases. *Chem Eng Sci* 2003;58:4087–4114.

Feng T, Tian H, Xu C et al. Synergistic co-delivery of doxorubicin and paclitaxel by porous PLGA microspheres for pulmonary inhalation treatment. *Eur J Pharm Biopharm* 2014;88:1086–1093.

Gagnadoux F, Hureaux J, Vecellio L et al. Aerosolized chemotherapy. *J Aerosol Med Pulm Drug Deliv* 2008;21:61–69.

Gagnadoux F, Leblond V, Vecellio L et al. Gemcitabine aerosol: *In vitro* antitumor activity and deposition imaging for preclinical safety assessment in baboons. *Cancer Chemother Pharmacol* 2006;58:237–244.

Gagnadoux F, Pape AL, Lemarié E, Lerondel S, Valo I, Leblond V, Racineux J-L, Urban T. Aerosol delivery of chemotherapy in an orthotopic model of lung cancer. *Eur Respir J* 2005;26:657–661.

Garcia A, Mack P, Williams S et al. Microfabricated engineered particle systems for respiratory drug delivery and other pharmaceutical applications. *J Drug Deliv* 2012;9:941243.

Hershey AE, Kurzman ID, Forrest LJ, Bohling CA, Stonerook M, Placke ME, Imondi AR, Vail DM. Inhalation chemotherapy for macroscopic primary or metastatic lung tumors: Proof of principle using dogs with spontaneously occurring tumors as a model. *Clin Cancer Res* 1999;5:2653–2659.

Hohenforst-Schmidt W, Zarogoulidis P, Linsmeier B et al. Enhancement of aerosol cisplatin chemotherapy with gene therapy expressing ABC10 protein in respiratory system. *J Cancer* 2014;5:344–350.

Huland E, Heinzer H, Huland H et al. Overview of interleukin-2 inhalation therapy. *Cancer J Sci Am* 2000;6(Suppl. 1):S104–S112.

Huland E, Burger A, Fleischer J, et al. Efficacy and safety of inhaled recombinant inter-leukin-2 in high risk renal cancer patients compared with systemic interleukin-2: an outcome study. *Folia Biologica (Praha)* 2003;49:183–190.

Kaur G, Narang RK, Rath G, Goyal AK. Advances in pulmonary delivery of nanoparticles. *Artif Cells Blood Substit Immobil Biotechnol* 2012;40:75–96.

Kaye RS, Purewal TS, Alpar HO. Simultaneously manufactured nano-in-micro (SIMANIM) particles for dry-powder modified-release delivery of antibodies. *J Pharm Sci* 2009;98:4055–4068.

Kelsen DP, Alcock N, Young CW. Cisplatin nephrotoxicity: correlation with plasma platinum concentrations. *Am J Clin Oncol* 1985;8:77–80.

Kleinstreuer C, Zhang Z, Donohue JF. Targeted drug-aerosol delivery in the human respira-tory system. *Ann Rev Biomed Eng* 2008;10:195–220.

Koshkina NV, Kleinerman ES. Aerosol gemcitabine inhibits the growth of primary osteosar-coma and osteosarcoma lung metastases. *Int J Cancer* 2005;116:458–463.

Koshkina NV, Kleinerman ES, Waldrep JC, Jia S-F, Worth LL, Gilbert BE, Knight V. 9-Nitrocamptothecin liposome aerosol treatment of melanoma and osteosarcoma lung metastases in mice. *Clin Cancer Res* 2000;6:2876–2880.

Koshkina NV, Waldrep JC, Roberts LE, Golunski E, Melton S, Knight V. Paclitaxel liposome aerosol treatment induces inhibition of pulmonary metastases in murine renal carci-noma model. *Clin Cancer Res* 2001;10:3258–3262.

Lavasanifar A, Samuel J, Kwon GS. Poly (ethylene oxide)-block-poly(l-amino acid) micelles for drug delivery. *Adv Drug Deliv Rev* 2002;54:169–190.

Lemarie E, Vecellio L, Hureaux J et al. Aerosolized gemcitabine in patients with car-cinoma of the lung: Feasibility and safety study. *J Aerosol Med Pulm Drug Deliv* 2011;24:261–270.

Leong D, Rai R, Nguyen B, Lee A, Yip D. Advances in adjuvant systemic therapy for non-small-cell lung cancer. *World J Clin Oncol* 2014;5:633–645.

Litterst CL, Gram TE, Dedrick RL, Leroy AF, Guarino AM. Distribution and disposition of platinum following intravenous administration of cis-diamminedichloroplatinum(II) (NSC 119875) to dogs. *Cancer Res* 1976;36:2340–2344.

Longest PW, Tian G, Hindle M. Improving the lung delivery of nasally administered aerosols during noninvasive ventilation—An application of enhanced condensational growth (ECG). *J Aerosol Med Pulm Drug Deliv* 2011;24:103–118.

Longest PW, Walenga RL, Son YJ et al. High-efficiency generation and delivery of aerosols through nasal cannula during noninvasive ventilation. *J Aerosol Med Pulm Drug Deliv* 2013;26:266–279.

Markovic SN, Suman VJ, Nevala WK et al. A dose-escalation study of aerosolized sar-gramostim in the treatment of metastatic melanoma: An NCTG study. *Am J Clin Oncol* 2008;31:573–579.

Meenach SA, Anderson KW, Hilt JZ, McGarry RC, Mansour HM. Characterization and aerosol dispersion performance of advanced spray-dried chemotherapeutic PEGylated phospholipid particles for dry powder inhalation delivery in lung cancer. *Eur J Pharm Sci* 2013;49;699–711.

Meenach SA, Anderson KW, Hilt JZ, McGarry RC, Mansour HM. High-performing dry powder inhalers of paclitaxel DPPC/DPPG lung surfactant-mimic multifunctional par-ticles in lung cancer: Physicochemical characterization, *in vitro* aerosol dispersion, and cellular studies. *AAPS PharmSciTech* 2014;15:1574–1587.

Minchinton AI, Tannock IF. Drug penetration in solid tumors. *Nat Rev Cancer* 2006;6:583–592.

Otterson GA, Villalona-Calero MA, Hicks W et al. Phase I/II study of inhaled doxorubicin combined with platinum-based therapy for advanced non-small cell lung cancer. *Clin Cancer Res* 2010;16:2466–2473.

Otterson GA, Villalona-Calero MA, Sharma S et al. Phase I study of inhaled doxorubicin for patients with metastatic tumors to the lungs. *Clin Cancer Res* 2007;13:1246–1252.

Rodriguez CO Jr, Crabbs TA, Wilson DW et al. Aerosol gemcitabine: Preclinical safety and *in vivo* antitumor activity in osteosarcoma-bearing dogs. *J Aerosol Med Pulm Drug Deliv* 2010;23:197–206.

Selting K, Waldrep J, Essman S et al. Targeted combined aerosol chemotherapy in dogs and radiologic toxicity grading. *J Aerosol Med Pulm Drug Deliv* 2011;24:43–48.

Selting K, Waldrep JC, Reinero C et al. Feasibility and safety of targeted cisplatin delivery to a select lung lobe in dogs via the AeroProbe intracorporeal nebulization catheter. *J Aerosol Med Pulm Drug Deliv* 2008;21:255–268.

Sharma S, White D, Imondi AR, Placke ME, Vail DM, Kris MG. Development of inhalational agents for oncologic use. *J Clin Oncol* 2001;19:1839–1847.

Smola M, Vandamme T, Sokolowski A. Nanocarriers as pulmonary drug delivery systems to treat and diagnose respiratory and non respiratory diseases. *Int J Nanomed* 2008;3:1–19.

Sterman DH, Treat J, Litzky LA et al. Adenovirus-mediated herpes simplex virus thymidine kinase/ganciclovir gene therapy in patients with localized malignancy: Results of a Phase I clinical trial in malignant mesothelioma. *Hum Gene Ther* 2008;9:1083–1092.

Taratula O, Kuzmov A, Shah M, Garbuzenko OB, Minko T. Nanostructured lipid carriers as multifunctional nanomedicine platform for pulmonary co-delivery of anticancer drugs and siRNA. *J Control Release* 2013;171:349–357.

Tatsumura T, Koyama S, Tsujimoto M et al. Further study of nebulization chemotherapy, a new chemotherapeutic method in the treatment of lung carcinomas: Fundamental and clinical. *Br J Cancer* 1993;68:1146–1149.

Torchilin VP. Passive and active drug targeting: Drug delivery to tumors as an example. *Handb Exp Pharmacol* 2010;197:3–53.

Tsapis N, Bennett D, Jackson B, Weitz DA, Edwards D. Trojan particles: Large porous carriers of nanoparticles for drug delivery. *Proc Nat Acad Sci* 2002;99:12001–12005.

Vachani A, Moon E, Wakeam E, Haas AR, Sterman DH, Albelda SM. Gene therapy for lung neoplasms. *Clin Chest Med* 2011;32:865–885.

Verschraegen CF, Gilbert BE, Loyer E et al. Clinical evaluation of the delivery and safety of aerosolized liposomal 9-nitro-20(s)-camptothecin in patients with advanced pulmonary malignancies. *Clin Cancer Res* 2004;10:2319–2326.

Wang H, Xu Y, Zhou X. Docetaxel-loaded chitosan microspheres as a lung targeted delivery system: *In vitro* and *in vivo* evaluation. *Int J Mol Sci* 2014;15:3519–3532.

Weber S, Zimmer A, Pardeike J. Solid lipid nanoparticles (SLN) and nanostructured lipid carriers (NLC) for pulmonary application: A review of the state of the art. *Eur J Pharm Biopharm* 2014;86:7–22.

Weers JG, Tarara TE, Clark AR. Design of fine particles for pulmonary drug delivery. *Expert Opin Drug Deliv* 2007;4(3):297–313.

Wittgen BP, Kunst PW, van der Born K et al. Phase I study of aerosolized SLIT cisplatin in the treatment of patients with carcinoma of the lung. *Clin Cancer Res* 2007;13:2414–2421.

Xie Y, Aillon KL, Cai S, Christian JM, Davies NM, Berkland CJ, Forrest ML. Pulmonary delivery of cisplatin-hyaluronan conjugates via endotracheal instillation for the treatment of lung cancer. *Int J Pharm* 2010;392:156–163.

Zarogoulidis P, Chatzaki E, Porpodis K et al. Inhaled chemotherapy in lung cancer. *Int J Nanomedicine* 2012;7:1551–1572.

Zarogoulidis P, Darwiche K, Krauss L et al. Inhaled cisplatin deposition and distribution in lymph nodes in stage II lung cancer patients. *Future Oncol* 2013;9:1307–1313.

Zarogoulidis P, Eleftheriadou E, Sapardanis I et al. Feasibility and effectiveness of inhaled carboplatin in NSCLC patients. *Invest New Drugs* 2012;30:1628–1640.

Zou Y, Tornos C, Qiu X, Lia M, Perez-Soler R. p 53 aerosol formulation with low toxicity and high efficiency for early lung cancer treatment. *Clin Cancer Res* 2007;13:4900–4908.

6 Inhaled Countermeasures for Respiratory Tract Viruses

Ralph A. Tripp and Jarod M. Hanson

CONTENTS

AEROSOL BIOLOGY

Aerosol biology (aerobiology) as it relates to respiratory viral diseases is an understudied area considering the vast microbiome in the nasopharynx and related upper respiratory tract (URT) airways [1–3]. Despite the abundance of microbes that coexist at mucosal surfaces, comparatively few of these microorganisms are pathogenic with most occupying commensal or opportunistic niches in the URT microbiome. However, several pathogens have evolved airborne transmission as a primary route of infection in part to gain direct access to the respiratory system in order to facilitate host-to-host transmission. One example is influenza virus, which can be considered an obligate airborne pathogen. Influenza infection induces host generation of large quantities of virus-laden aerosols via coughs and sneezes that typically serve as a means for virus transmission via the respiratory system. Infectious aerosols produced by the affected host typically range in size from 0.1 to 20 μm [3]. Aerosol generation induced by a pathogen is one way to efficiently enable multiple passages through several hosts, an effect that may ultimately lead to a general increase in relative virulence via virus modifications induced by passaging in successive hosts. Aerosols generated during infection vary in both droplet size and virus content; that is, those larger than 5 μm in diameter are classified as droplets (and have a relatively low virus content), while those smaller than 5 μm are classified as particles and typically have increased virus content [4,5].

Experimentally, intranasal inoculation is a surrogate method used to emulate aerosol infection and involves putting an inoculum directly into the nasal passage(s). It should be noted that the aerosol dispersion patterns and droplet sizes in the respiratory tract change when surrogate methods are used compared to natural aerosol inhalation of respiratory droplets. Typically, intratracheal instillation is used in animal models to provide better control of the inoculation process, although this surrogate method often does not adequately reproduce the full spectrum of clinical disease typically seen following natural infection via inhalation using the same virus concentration [3]. Importantly, the aerosolized particulates include variable numbers of viral particles that can also affect infection and disease outcome [3]. Others have shown direct links between aerosol particle size and the quantity of influenza A virus (IAV) carried in the particle during natural infection with fine particles (<5 μm) containing significantly more viral copies than coarse particles (>5 μm), which indicates potential particle size effects on the spatial dynamics of IAV infection in the respiratory tract [5].

The respiratory tract consists of a large mucosal surface and is second only to the digestive system in terms of mucosal surface area [6]. Thorough knowledge of mucosal immunity is necessary not only for the conceptualization and actualization of the next-generation vaccines but also for the advancement of other prevention and treatment strategies targeting infectious respiratory diseases, particularly those involving viruses [6,7]. Mucosal immunity influences aerobiology in the large airways found in the respiratory tract as well as in the microenvironments found within the small airways and alveoli [8].

The mammalian respiratory tract is often referred to as the upper (trachea) and lower (lung) respiratory tracts based in part on anatomical differences between the regions [6]. The URT can be further subdivided into the nasopharynx (from nose to trachea) and oropharynx (from oral cavity to trachea). Historically, in healthy individuals, the lower respiratory tract was presumed to be largely sterile; therefore, once infection occurred in this area, subsequent host inflammatory responses then led to the development of pneumonia [9]. However, that paradigm has begun to shift with the identification of various airway microbiota in the lower respiratory tract identified via PCR-based methods, many of which are implicated as having significant roles in disease prevention especially in those with preexisting airway complications such as smokers and asthmatics [10]. The URT is colonized not only by resident microbes but also by opportunistic and pathogenic microorganisms, for example, influenza virus and various bacteria, and other foreign substances such as particulates including pollen, smoke, and dust [6]. Interestingly, there is evidence that aerobiology and susceptibility to respiratory infection can be programmed by signals from the gut microbiome [11], which is not unexpected given the multisystemic nature of mucosal immunity [12]. Several studies have elucidated the enhanced susceptibility of germ-free mice to respiratory pathogens including influenza virus, Coxsackievirus, and Friend leukemia virus [1,13,14]. However, resistance to infection is generally attributed to facets of the innate immune response mediated by cells lining the respiratory tract, including the respiratory epithelium's role as a physical barrier as well as its associated mucociliary clearance mechanisms [3,15–17].

The respiratory epithelium serves as the initial, and highly critical, line of defense against viral infections of the respiratory tract [16]. The physical barrier function of the epithelia is augmented by innate immune cell-like macrophages that traverse the respiratory tract in part to destroy pathogenic organisms including viruses and bacteria [3,18]. There are adaptive immune cells that also affect aerobiology via contributions made to respiratory tract immunity as well as epithelia cells contributing further to innate defense via mucin production, mucociliary clearance, etc. Type I epithelial cells have been shown to internalize particles in the respiratory tract directly, while type II cells are unable to do so, implicating cell targeting as a crucial mechanism for drug or particle-based vaccine uptake, with at least one study indicating pulmonary surfactants are also involved in uptake by epithelial cells [19]. Additionally, the relative size of a particle determines its ability to successfully penetrate the respiratory epithelium as ~50 nm particles can enter epithelial cell cytoplasm via passive diffusion, while ~100 nm particles rely on clathrin- or caveolin-mediated endocytosis, and yet neither particle can cross cellular tight junctions, which demonstrates the added importance of particle size in drug and/or particle-based vaccine uptake [19]. Also of note is the potential for particle size to directly influence drug uptake as was shown with ciprofloxacin delivered to the respiratory tract via successively increasing diameter liposomes with direct implications for drug concentrations relative to the diameter of the delivery particle [20]. The size and cellular specificity afforded by the respiratory epithelium likely includes additional screening interactions facilitated by transmembrane mucins, pattern recognition receptors (PRRs), PAMPs, etc. that directly affects the uptake of a given particle based on a multitude of host and particle factors.

Mucins can have somewhat contradictory roles during viral infection in the airways in that they can not only potentially induce innate immunity and act as a physical barrier to virus entry to host cells but may also enable viral penetration to host cells depending on specific viral properties such as the neuraminidase (NA) associated with influenza. Mucins can be split into two groups based on which layer they partition to *in vivo*: the transporting mucous layer (TML) on the apical cell surface and the periciliary layer (PCL) located above the TML and spanning the distance between the TML and the apical portion of the cilia. Two polymeric mucins, MUC5AC and MUC5B, are enriched in the TML (as well as many additional globular proteins), while the PCL is rich in keratin sulfate as well as the tethered mucins MUC1, MUC4, and MUC16, but it has relatively few proteoglycans compared to the TML [21]. While these mucins may be enriched in their respective layers, they are not solely found there.

With respect to innate immunity and viral infections, MUC1 in particular has been implicated in T cell responses as well as being a modulator of the airway during inflammation and infection [22]. This would imply a potential immunomodulatory effect of mucins themselves (in the absence of any viral or inflammatory initiator). Additionally, the mucins mentioned earlier have associated alpha-2,6-linked sialic acids (but not alpha-2,3-) with them, which has been postulated to help neutralize influenza virus. However, this effect is probably transient at best in that NA has been shown to aid mucous penetration via the cleavage of sialic acid molecules although at least one study showed greater than 80% neutralization of influenza virus *in vitro* by cellular subunit preparations containing MUC1.

If penetration of the initial mucin barrier is achieved, actual infection of respiratory epithelial cells by pathogenic viruses and live-attenuated vaccines results in the production of antiviral cytokines and other defensive compounds such as type I and III interferons (INFs) and nitric oxides [23]. This stimulates the release of various chemokines involved in the recruitment of inflammatory and immune cells that influence adaptive immunity [23]. The respiratory tract's adaptive immune response includes B and T cells, immunoglobulins, and antigen-presenting cells that are typically diffusely associated with the epithelium. Alternately, they can be found within the lungs, airways, and nasal passages in specific locations defined as mucosal-associated lymphoid tissues (MALTs) [24] consisting of aggregated lymphoid tissues and immune cells [3]. Additionally, bronchial-associated lymphoid tissues (BALTs) and nasal-associated lymphoid tissues (NALTs) have been described in mice [25–27] to have a similar functional role as MALTs in humans. The MALT, NALT, and BALT appear to be sites of antibody production within the respiratory tract [3].

T cells subsist in MALTs and are broadly classified by their receptors. The alpha–beta T cells found in the respiratory tract may be either effector or effector memory T cells, while those located in associated lymphatic tissues, such as lymph nodes, may be of the effector or central memory phenotypes [3,28–32]. CD8 T cells are primarily cytotoxic T lymphocytes involved in the destruction of host cells infected with viruses, while CD4 T cells are primarily of the Th1 variety and are involved in the initiation of cell-mediated immunity [3,23,33,34]. Gamma–delta T cells can be found in various mucosal tissues, including those lining the respiratory tract [3,35]. This T cell type is predominately an innate immune cell type, but pulmonary gamma–delta T lymphocytes can produce IL-17, which functions in host adaptive immune-mediated responses [3,36]. B cells produce immunoglobulins that can directly, or with the addition of complement, bind to and destroy pathogens such as viruses [3,37,38]. Plasma cells capable of secreting antibodies make up the majority of B cells, or memory B lymphocytes (these are present in germinal centers [lymph nodes] and follicle-associated epithelium) [3,39]. Plasma cells lining the respiratory tract can produce immunoglobulin, which is expressed as IgG and IgA [40–42]. IgA is the predominant antibody type present in mucous secretions. It is also present in the alveolar spaces although IgG is the primary immunoglobulin isotype in this locale [3,43].

Mucosally induced S-IgA antibodies are an essential arm of adaptive immunity for protecting the host from infection, but take several days to generate at the site(s) of infection and replication. During that generation time, the innate immune response, which is antigen nonspecific, can respond and confront the pathogen by producing inflammatory cytokines, IFNs, and IFN-stimulated cytokines [44].

The proinflammatory cytokines include IL-6, IL-12, and TNFα [38] that are needed for the induction of antigen-specific T and B cell responses to pathogens; thus, the innate immune response is needed to induce, activate, and expand adaptive immune responses [45].

Influenza virus infection serves as a useful example of a prominent respiratory tract pathogen as the virus affects aerosol biology when it first attaches to respiratory mucosal epithelial cells and then invades the cell cytoplasm by endocytosis [45]. This event signals PRRs and Toll-like receptors (TLRs), particularly when the viral single-strand RNA (ssRNA) is released into the cytoplasmic region of the epithelial cell [46]. ssRNA viruses like influenza virus are recognized by TLR7 in humans located on the inside of the endosome [47]. Also, retinoic-acid inducible gene I (RIG-I) is a prominent PRR during the innate immune response [48,49].

RIG-I, a cytoplasmic RNA helicase, is especially important because it is capable of binding virus-specific RNA structures [49]. RIG-I recognizes genomic RNA released into the cytoplasmic region of infected cells [49]. TLR7 and RIG-I activated by ssRNA trigger intracellular signal transductions, hence leading to the expression and production of IFNs, IFN-stimulated genes, and proinflammatory cytokines. A better understanding of host aerobiology features as they relate to respiratory tract pathogens is important for developing infection countermeasures utilizing aerosol or pulmonary methods of delivery for vaccines or therapeutics.

SMALL ANIMAL MODELS AND AEROSOL TRANSMISSION

The use of guinea pigs as laboratory models to evaluate influenza transmission dynamics was a substantial step forward in understanding influenza virus aerosol transmission [50–52]. Guinea pigs have been shown to be readily susceptible to human strains of IAV without first adapting the virus to the host, capable of replicating IAV in the upper and lower respiratory tracts, and able to easily spread IAV via aerosols among themselves if housed in the same air space [50,51,53,54]. Influenza virus pathogenicity in guinea pigs varies considerably with the Hartley strain of guinea pigs that are often asymptomatic [55], while strain 13 animals may exhibit both loss of body condition and disease [56].

Studies utilizing guinea pigs as models for influenza transmission were performed using a single infected source animal with the sentinel, naive guinea pigs housed in separate cages [51,57]. Transmission between the cages is highly indicative of aerosol transmission among guinea pigs. Importantly, influenza spread via aerosols depends largely on environmental factors such as humidity level and ambient temperature [38]. Extrapolating from this finding, the intermediate sized droplets that left the infected guinea pig likely partially desiccated in ambient air depending on size and relative humidity in the room, while smaller droplets that remained in the air were likely responsible for transmission to cohort naïve guinea pigs. This is reinforced by the previously mentioned clinical study that showed smaller particles (<5 μm) had higher numbers of viral copies, thus indicating greater viral load compared to the large diameter particles [5].

Several caveats from these studies require further elucidation since influenza-infected guinea pigs do not typically exhibit respiratory signs such as sneezing or coughing [55]. More conclusive studies pinpointing why certain guinea pig strains appear to differ in their ability to effectively transmit viruses via aerosols are also needed [51,55,58,59]. The guinea pig model of aerosol transmission has also been used in IAV coinfection studies where a naïve guinea pig was exposed to two cage mates; one infected with wild-type influenza virus and the other with a variant influenza virus [60]. This exposure method was able to produce coinfection as well as reassortment, although the percentage of isolates with reassortant genomes varied from 50% to 100% depending on the time point that was observed [60]. This finding led to the conclusion that coinfection achieved through some degree of direct and/or aerosol transmission is capable of producing large numbers of reassortant viruses. The main advantages of using guinea pigs as influenza models include the overall susceptibility of the model to infection with human influenza virus strains, the transmission efficiency of influenza among cohoused guinea pigs as well as between the guinea pig and other species, and the commercial availability of the model [55]. The primary disadvantages include the relative lack of visible clinical signs of influenza depending on the variety of guinea pig used and a paucity of immunological reagents that severely limits comparison of immunological parameters in the model with those seen in other models, clinical infections, etc. [51,58].

Beyond guinea pigs, mice, ferrets, cotton rats, and macaques have all been evaluated as laboratory models to study aerosol biology, although each species presents its own set of distinct advantages and disadvantages [52,61]. A significant advantage is that current animal models, that is, ferrets and guinea pigs, are naturally hosts for many human influenza strains, while a significant disadvantage is that mice typically require adaptation of a given influenza virus prior to regular use in the species [52,55]. However, inbred mice may yield more severe clinical signs and outcomes if infected intranasally with some IAV strains, including A/Puerto Rico/8/1934 (H1N1, PR8), whereas wild-type, noninbred mice exhibit much greater resistance to viral infection with the identical strain [61]. This apparent difference in disease severity is postulated to be due in part to the failure of the inbred mice to express a functional Mx1 protein, which is important for host antiviral activity [62].

Ferrets are naturally infected with a number of influenza A and B subtypes and are another commonly used animal model to investigate aerosol transmission [52,53,63,64]. Historically, in the early 1930s, they were demonstrated to be the first species infected with human influenza isolates [65–67]. A primary factor for influenza virus studies in this animal model is their susceptibility to many human isolates (without first adapting the virus to ferrets), allowing for the growth and evaluation of human clinical isolates with minimal risk of adaptation-related antigenic or phenotypic changes in the virus due to the adaptation process. During IAV infections, ferrets emulate many aspects of human influenza illness, including URT infection profiles and similar clinical symptoms to those observed in humans [52,68]. However, the specific influenza strain utilized for challenge, as well as the route the virus inoculum is administered, affects the overall clinical disease picture and the relative severity of the observed symptoms [69].

As animal models are required for efficacy studies and preclinical evaluations of drug or vaccine candidates, the ability to better understand the mechanisms affecting aerosol transmission or aerosol vaccination in these small animal models is critical. Guinea pig and ferret models have been tailored to these types of studies although both models possess distinct advantages and disadvantages. In summary, the primary advantages of the ferret model are its relative ease of infection with field influenza virus strains that have not been adapted after being isolated from human patients, ready dissemination of the virus among cohoused ferrets, and similar clinical disease profile to that seen in human influenza patients. The ferret model's primary limitations are the relative lack of commercial availability (compared to mice), paucity of inbred strains, greater expense relative to other aerosol animal models making statistical power more costly to achieve, and a deficiency of commercially available ferret-specific immunological reagents. Finally, there is only a draft sequence of the ferret genome currently available, hence preventing definitive studies involving virus and host genome interplay [70].

RESPIRATORY VIRUS INFECTION

Respiratory infection is the most common route of transmission for most viral diseases. Viruses commonly spread via aerosols from the respiratory track include well-known pathogens such as respiratory syncytial virus (RSV) and IAV. In addition to respiratory transmission, these viruses as well as many others can also be transmitted by fomites, often in conjunction with a direct inoculation event whereby the host touches an infected surface and then touches the face, nose, etc., directly introducing the virus to a mucosal surface. Direct inoculation of a host can also occur between individuals via direct contact such as handshaking and kissing.

There are several parameters related to the aerosolized droplets that help predict whether an airborne virus successfully infects a naïve host, including the size of the aerosol droplets following sneezing or coughing, the velocity of the aerosol, the season, and the relative humidity of the environment in which the droplet is generated [3,71–76]. The time an aerosol remains in the air depends on particle size and the time required for the desiccation of the particles outside the host [77]. Particles <10 μm have a longer aerosolization time compared to larger particles. Importantly, particles greater than 10 μm in diameter are readily filtered in the nasal and nasopharyngeal passages, where they are also more easily expelled prior to the virus actually infecting the epithelial cells lining the large airways [77]. Small diameter particles (0.5–5 μm) easily pass through to the trachea and large airways where they then attach to the host epithelial cells; particles smaller than 0.5 μm in diameter easily transit to the most distal alveolar spaces where they too can generate patent infection. However, aerosolized particles reaching portions of the airway capable of hosting an infection may not actually contact cells susceptible to that pathogen; thus, cell tropism is an essential factor in determining whether a person is infected by an aerosolized virus (like influenza virus) [78].

The potential size(s) of aerosolized particles containing a respiratory pathogen that a person may be exposed to is unpredictable because aerosols from coughs, sneezes, and other sources comprise a plume of a particle size distribution that varies with exposure time as well as distance from the source due to environmental conditions including temperature and humidity [78]. Thus, inhalational infection progresses as a continuum of airway deposition events following a cough or sneeze. A range of URT tissues and cell types are susceptible postinhalation with the site of particle deposition impacting disease kinetics and pathogenesis.

In the late 1960s, aerosol transmission of respiratory viral diseases was investigated in a joint study by the U.S. Army Biological Laboratories and the Laboratory of Clinical Investigations, National Institute of Allergy and Infectious Diseases [79]. Prior studies had demonstrated successful aerosol inoculation and infection of volunteers with Coxsackievirus [80,81]. In the later studies, natural contact and airborne transmission was evaluated using nasal drops and aerosols containing the rhinovirus strain Coxsackievirus A type 21. Recovery from infection was evaluated, and specifically, virus transmission was determined from the natural aerosols produced by coughing and sneezing, as well as from air in rooms contaminated by coughing and sneezing patients. The inoculation procedures involved volunteers who received aerosol inoculums containing either 0.2–3.0 μm particles or ~15 μm particles. Nasopharyngeal inoculations were performed by the instillation of 0.25 mL of virus inoculum into each nostril of the volunteer. Some volunteers received 0.5 mL of inoculum deposited into each nostril and an additional 0.5 mL sprayed into each nostril [79].

Nasopharyngeal inoculation, as well as small particle (0.2–3.0 μm) or large droplet (15 μm) aerosols, efficiently infected individuals. However, the type of administration (based primarily on the generation of small particles over larger droplets) affected the prevalence of pathological disease in the various locales within the respiratory tract. Importantly, this was the first direct evidence for aerosol spread of virus via the detection of virus in aerosols produced by coughing, sneezing, or normal respiration. Virus titrations were performed for 61 cough and 58 sneeze samples collected from volunteers infected with Coxsackievirus A type 21. Interestingly, 39% of cough specimens and 50% of sneeze specimens were positive for virus, and 30% of air samples were strongly positive for virus implicating the potential for aerosol transmission and infection [79]. Similar results were found for other viruses tested, including adenovirus. This was the first study to show that airborne transmission was a potential route of infection for respiratory viruses. Today, many related studies have been completed in animal models, field studies, and clinical settings, with similar findings relative to aerosol transmission. However, viral infections are not limited to aerosol transmission alone.

Infectious respiratory disease is propagated via three routes of transmission: airborne, contact, and droplet. Contact transmission is either direct or indirect, with the former involving transfer of the pathogen from an infected individual to a naïve one. Indirect transmission involves movement of the pathogen from a susceptible person via a fomite, a contaminated surface, or other object [82]. Droplet transmission, also a type of direct contact, refers to respiratory droplets with diameters 5 μm or greater from an infected individual that are capable of direct contact with the respiratory and/or facial mucosal tissues of a naïve person [82]. The transmission of a respiratory virus requires the infected individual to release the agent into the environment where it is subsequently acquired by a naïve, susceptible host [82]. Since not all biological transmission routes are plausible for person-to-person transmission, aerosol transmission of a given pathogen usually only occurs if the following conditions are met: infectious aerosols are generated from a host, the agent can maintain viability in the environment for the period of time necessary to encounter a susceptible host, and the pathogen's susceptible tissues are accessible to the agent in its aerosol form [82]. For example, influenza virus must be released via aerosols from an infected patient, stay viable in the environment (whether as an aerosol or on a surface), and then contact respiratory epithelial cells in an uninfected patient via inhalation or direct inoculation from a fomite to the patient as would occur if the uninfected patient touches his or her nose after contacting a contaminated surface.

Notably, respiratory barriers (such as N95 respirators) are the only reliable means of filtering out infectious aerosol particles prior to inhalation although handwashing can reduce or eliminate indirect infection [82]. As such, the first step to minimize transmission events is frequent handwashing using proper techniques. Second, personal protective equipment (PPE) is recommended such as appropriate respirators that can effectively filter respiratory particles that have diameters 5 µm or less. PPE is appropriate for health-care workers and susceptible people who may become infected through airborne transmission. Latex gloves are another PPE item that should be worn and can help to control infection provided the gloves are changed between patients. Failure to do so can result in the gloves serving as a fomite for infectious agent transfer.

COUNTERMEASURES FOR RESPIRATORY TRACT INFECTIONS

A basic strategy for controlling the spread of an infectious disease is to interrupt the transmission cycle. This strategy relies on having a fundamental understanding of the virus, host(s), and environmental factors contributing to virus spread. Countermeasures for controlling a pathogen typically rely on inhibiting infection or replication, but a variety of chemicals (soaps, sanitizers, disinfectants, and/or detergents) can also be used to minimize or eliminate potential environmental exposure. Effective prevention can also be achieved through interventions such as preventing contact through isolation or wearing PPE. Unfortunately, transmission often occurs before infection control measures are put in place due to vague (or no) symptoms initially present with many respiratory diseases and as such, transmission may still occur despite adequate infection control strategies once a putative diagnosis is made. This delay between initial onset of pathogen shedding and diagnosis then necessitates further prophylactic countermeasures directed to those exposed, but not yet showing disease, or as therapeutics to those with symptoms of the disease (either pre- or postlaboratory confirmation, if confirmation is possible depending on the agent involved).

There are a number of therapeutic countermeasures available where antimicrobial agents target susceptible stages in the replicative cycle of the pathogen. Unfortunately, there are very few antiviral drugs that are broadly effective for respiratory viruses. However, many new candidate drugs that target host genes and pathways used by the virus for replication are being identified on a regular basis [83–86]. Many of these drugs can be rapidly repurposed with their safety having been previously established [84,85]. These host-targeted drugs may provide means to target multiple viruses with a single drug, but the efficacy of this type of broad-spectrum approach has yet to be established. With many respiratory infections, and specifically viral ones, lack of effective therapeutic interventions often leads to increased disease severity due to the host immune response, secondary or opportunistic pathogen involvement, etc. For example, bronchiolitis is a common sequela of uncontrolled viral replication in the lower reaches of the respiratory tract, especially in newborns, and often causes considerable morbidity and occasional mortality. RSV is one of the several agents capable of inducing bronchiolitis (often referred to as croup) in newborn children, as well as being the primary cause for hospitalization due to respiratory diseases in early childhood [87,88]. The treatment of infants with bronchiolitis is largely supportive as there are no truly efficacious therapies for bronchiolitis relative to reducing clinical endpoints such as duration of ICU or hospital stay.

Beyond antiviral drugs, vaccines have been used to help mitigate the transmission of respiratory viruses where possible. Key to aerosol vaccination efficacy is that the vaccine must generate humoral and/or mucosal immune correlates of protection that are biologically capable of preventing the initial infection, preventing reinfection, and/or reducing clinical disease in the vaccinee. The vaccine should provide robust, long-term protection and result in few or no side effects or adverse reactions, induction of clinical disease, enhanced virulence of endemic strains, etc. Ideally, administration should require a simple regimen in a form acceptable to the target population [89].

There are several categories of vaccines including live-attenuated, killed/inactivated, subunit, vectored, and DNA, and these have all been tested for pulmonary delivery in the respiratory tract. Vaccine design, application, and actual field use vary among target pathogens. Influenza virus vaccines are a good example as seasonal vaccines include virus strains projected to circulate in the target region during the next flu season [90]. Historically, influenza vaccines were formulated as a trivalent mixture to provide protection against influenza A H3N2, H1N1, and an influenza B strain. However, continued circulation of two distinct clusters of influenza B led to the development and implementation of quadrivalent vaccines that include both the circulating influenza B lineages [90].

Vaccine delivery to the airways became feasible with the advent of commercially available pressurized metered-dose inhalers (MDIs) that were initially developed to treat asthma and chronic obstructive pulmonary disease (COPD) patients. However, MDIs suffered from difficulties due to the propellant used in the device to deliver vaccines and drugs [91]. Depending on the formulation of the preparation to be administered, that is, solution or suspension, issues arose regarding solubility and/or stability. Additionally, the devices had a low efficiency of drug targeting to the small airways and reformulation of the compound(s) to be aerosolized was required.

Approaches to overcome these limitations led to the development of dry powder inhalers (DPIs) [91]. The DPIs were designed to reproducibly deliver the vaccine to the lower respiratory tract and alveoli, typically via a mass median aerodynamic diameter of 1–5 μm. However, the extent and depth deposition within the airways was largely due to the patient's inspiratory flow rate and volume, either of which can drastically affect the actual dosage received at a given region in the lower airways [92].

As a major issue with aqueous vaccines is loss of efficacy due to degradation many are instead prepared as a dry powder to enhance stability [93]. This method has the added benefit of limiting hydrolysis, which can further compromise the efficacy of the final product, and dry powder formulations are typically more cost effective and can reduce or eliminate cold chain requirements compared with aqueous products [93]. Several dry powder formulations are available for use with protein subunit vaccines, whole virus vaccines, and DNA vaccines, while several techniques can be utilized for the actual generation of the powder including spray-drying, freeze-drying (lyophilization), and spray-freeze-drying [93,94]. There are additional factors that affect vaccine stability and efficacy that become critically important for the stability of powdered formulations. The particle size distribution is just one of these critical factors that impact dry powder vaccine efficacy [93]. Dry powder vaccines targeting mucosal surfaces have shown promising stability and antigenicity in several preclinical and clinical studies, suggesting an expanded role for this route of administration in the future [93,95–97].

There is increasing interest in the pulmonary route for delivering both drugs and vaccines. DPIs are a promising option for the delivery of vaccines to certain patient populations, and the recent introduction of disposable devices will expand the range of DPI vaccine applications. Currently, there is a demand for needleless, shelf-stable/cold chain–independent vaccines—two inherent features of DPI-based vaccines [93]. Dry powder vaccines against respiratory pathogens have been shown to induce protective immunity in several animal models [96–98]. Most effort has been focused on influenza, with respect to the variations in the generation of the antigenic component of the vaccine such as whole inactivated virus, split virus, subunit, and virosomal vaccines. The rationale is that there is a yearly demand for influenza vaccines produced by lyophilization, spray-drying, freeze-drying, spray-freeze-drying, and/or vacuum drying due to their enhanced shelf stability [93,98,99], and effective dry powder influenza vaccines can be accurately and efficiently delivered to a variety of target populations with minimal cold chain and equipment requirements. With respect to drug delivery via a DPI system, other technologies exist for drug isolation/purification, including supercritical fluid technology, solvent precipitation (using ultrasonic waves), double emulsion/solvent evaporation, and particle replication in nonwetting templates [100]. While DPI remains a promising technology, the agent being delivered and its ability to be purified or concentrated into a powder formulation, and that powder's specific structural characteristics, plays a large role in the success or failure of administration using a specific DPI device and powder formulation.

INFLUENZA VIRUS, A PROTOTYPICAL RESPIRATORY TRACT VIRUS

Influenza virus is a respiratory pathogen transmitted via aerosol and fomite, which variably infects both the upper and lower respiratory tracts [101,102]. Annual epidemics of influenza A and influenza B viruses often generate significant morbidity and mortality in susceptible populations. The elderly and very young comprise the most serious disease, hospitalization, and mortality, out of the 5%–20% of the total population affected [103,104]. Vaccination is considered the most efficacious method to prevent disease, hospitalization, and mortality associated with influenza or complications from influenza virus infection [105,106]. Both parenteral and inhaled vaccines are licensed for use to prevent influenza virus infection. Similarly, oral and inhaled antiviral drugs are approved for therapeutic use against influenza virus infection. In this section, pulmonary delivery of influenza vaccines and anti-influenza drugs will be discussed as influenza provides model case studies for the employment of multiple respiratory virus countermeasures.

Influenza virus is an enveloped, single-strand, negative-sense RNA virus of the Orthomyxoviridae family [101,102]. Three influenza genera, A, B, and C, make up the causative agents of influenza illness, with a fourth version, influenza D, which is proposed as a distinct quasi-species (initially classified as influenza C) found in cattle and pigs with unknown significance in humans [107,108]. The genome of influenza A virus is composed of eight negative-sense RNA segments that encode 10–13 proteins. Two major viral glycoproteins are located on the surface of the viral envelope, that is, hemagglutinin (HA) and NA. HA binds to sialic acids that serve as the virus receptor, while NA enzymatically cleaves these receptors to mediate virus exit. Influenza virus primarily infects the respiratory tract in humans eliciting responses that result in exacerbated pulmonary inflammation of the respiratory tract, which in some cases leads to life-threatening pneumonia, respiratory failure, and death generally in the young, old, and immune compromised [101]. Influenza B virus is similar to influenza A, having an eight-segment, negative-sense RNA genome encoding 10 proteins, including the HA and NA surface glycoproteins [102].

Influenza A viruses circulate on a nearly constant basis in several species, including waterfowl, poultry, swine, and horses [109], although they are also found less commonly in dogs, cats, and several other mammalian species [110]. Influenza A viruses are further subtyped based on the antigenicity of their two viral surface glycoproteins, HA and NA. Currently, 18 HA and 11 NA subtypes are known although only viruses of three HA subtypes (H1, H2, and H3) and two NA subtypes (N1 and N2) have circulated regularly (over the last two centuries) in humans, hence leading to annual epidemics and more rarely large-scale pandemics [109]. Current influenza vaccines rely primarily on antibody-based immunity to the HA epitope and, to a lesser extent, NA proteins [111]. Virus mutations in response to immune pressure leading to enhanced virus adaptation in a given host and natural changes in the viral genome due to the intrinsic errors induced by the viral RNA-dependent RNA polymerase are both referred to as antigenic drift [112]. These changes, which occur primarily within the HA and NA, help the virus evade the immune response and are the antigenic basis for continuous influenza circulation in a population as well as annual influenza epidemics.

Persistent antigenic drift of influenza viruses requires that influenza vaccines be regularly reformulated to compensate for newly drifted viruses that often emerge and overtake less well-adapted viruses in circulation [113]. Antigenic drift, though problematic, is of less concern than antigenic shift, where influenza virus gene reassortment occurs between influenza viruses from different species (e.g., avian, swine), which can lead to a completely novel virus that is unrecognized by the population [101]. Only three subtypes of influenza A virus currently circulate on a regular basis in humans, that is, H1, H2, and H3 [112], and thus embody the greatest menace for antigenic shift events; while influenza B virus does transmit between humans, it primarily infects humans minimizing the reassortment potential between viruses adapted to different species and thus does not represent a significant pandemic threat.

CONTROLLING INFLUENZA VIRUS DISEASE BURDEN

The primary control of seasonal influenza epidemics is achieved through a comprehensive vaccination program [111]. There are two competing influenza vaccine moieties currently licensed for use in the United States: killed or inactivated and live-attenuated vaccines (Table 6.1). Trivalent inactivated influenza vaccines (TIVs or IIV3s) consist of three viruses that are propagated independent of one another in embryonated chicken eggs, detergent inactivated, and then combined together to be administered as a single inactivated vaccine preparation [111]. Historically,

TABLE 6.1
Current Licensed Influenza Vaccines Available in the United States

Vaccine Type	Brand Name/Manufacturer	Delivery	ACIP Indication for Use[a]
Inactivated, egg grown			
Trivalent (IIV3)	Afluria/CSL Limited	Intramuscular	≥9 years
	Fluarix/GSK	Intramuscular	≥3 years
	FluLaval /ID Biomedical	Intramuscular	≥3 years
	Fluvirin/Novartis	Intramuscular	≥4 years
	Fluzone/Sanofi Pasteur	Intramuscular	6–35 months[b]
			≥36 months
			≥6 months
	Fluzone Intradermal/Sanofi Pasteur	Intradermal	18–64 years
Trivalent (IIV3), high dose	Fluzone High-Dose/Sanofi Pasteur	Intramuscular	≥65 years
Quadrivalent (IIV4)	Fluarix Quadrivalent/GSK	Intramuscular	≥3 years
	FluLaval Quadrivalent/ID Biomedical	Intramuscular	≥3 years
	Fluzone Quadrivalent/Sanofi Pasteur	Intramuscular	6–35 months[b]
			≥36 months
Inactivated, cell culture grown			
Trivalent (ccIIV3)	Flucelvax/Novartis	Intramuscular	≥18 years
Recombinant			
trivalent (RIV3)	FluBlok/Protein Sciences	Intramuscular	18–49 years
Live attenuated			
Quadrivalent (LAIV4)	FluMist Quadrivalent/MedImmune	Intranasal	2–49 years

[a] Prevention and Control of Seasonal Influenza with Vaccines: Recommendations of the Advisory Committee on Immunization Practices—United States, 2013–2014 [103].
[b] Multiple formulations.

TIVs contained H3N2 and H1N1 influenza A viruses and one influenza B virus. These viruses were mixed to improve the breadth of coverage against circulating influenza strains and administered intramuscularly [112]. In 2012, quadrivalent inactivated influenza vaccines (IIVs) containing viruses of the H3N2 and H1N1 influenza A lineages and two influenza B lineages were approved for use to improve vaccine coverage against influenza B viruses. Production, approval, and administration of these vaccines are essentially the same. These new quadrivalent vaccines, in conjunction with the development of live-attenuated vaccines, have resulted in a modification of the nomenclature from TIV to IIV3 and IIV4 for IIVs [103].

Two new, cell culture–generated influenza vaccines were approved in 2012. The first is similar to the classical inactivated vaccines, but the vaccine viruses are grown in Madin–Darby canine kidney (MDCK) cells instead of the more traditional embryonated chicken eggs. This MDCK cell–based vaccine is available as a trivalent vaccine and referred to as ccIIV3 (cell culture–inactivated influenza). More recently, a recombinant HA vaccine consisting of purified recombinant HA proteins generated using insect cells was also approved for use and is referred to as RIV3 (recombinant influenza vaccine) [103]. Strictly speaking, this is not an inactivated vaccine but falls under the umbrella of HA antigen–based vaccines due to its primary antigenic component. Both of these new vaccines avoid reliance on egg availability and potential contraindications due to egg allergies. However, all of these new vaccines are incremental improvements, still administered via injection, and rely upon induction of HA-specific antibody responses.

Live-attenuated, cold-adapted, temperature-sensitive influenza vaccines (LAIV) are also available. These are weakened strains of influenza that only replicate at temperatures present in the upper airways and are reassorted in order to generate expression of HA and NA proteins from influenza A and B viruses expected to circulate during the upcoming influenza season. Live-attenuated influenza vaccines (LAIVs) are typically administered via a nasal spray device and are particularly effective in preventing influenza disease in young children but also are effective in the elderly [114]. Interestingly, the age range for which LAIVs are approved varies significantly by region with Europe allowing use in those 2–18 years of age, the United States from 2–49 years or age, and Canada from 2–59 years of age [90]. These vaccines are trivalent or quadrivalent (LAIV3 and LAIV4, respectively), although only the LAIV4 was utilized in the United States during the 2013–2014 influenza season [103,115].

BRIEF HISTORY OF INFLUENZA VACCINES

Influenza vaccines were introduced in the late 1930s, but the first large-scale programs were supported by the United States military in the early 1940s through the Commission on Influenza. In 1942, the commission developed a trivalent vaccine containing two influenza A strains (A/Puerto Rico/8/1934 and A/Weiss/1943) and one influenza B strain (B/Lee/1940), which was formalin inactivated and commercially produced. A trial in 1943 that involved 12,500 students demonstrated efficacy [116]. The trivalent vaccine was approved for use in the military in 1945 and subsequently approved for public use in 1946 [116]. Two decades later, inactivated split and subunit vaccines were introduced to reduce the reactogenicity observed with whole virus vaccines [117]. At the same time, the first LAIVs were being developed, but it would be decades before they were approved for use in part because of issues with attenuating the virus without significantly impacting replication in the vaccinee in order to maximize the response against the vaccine [118].

The backbone for the current licensed LAIV, A/Ann Arbor/6/60-ca, was developed in 1967 [119]. A/Ann Arbor/6/60 was attenuated through serial passage, in conjunction with sequentially lower incubation temperatures, in primary chicken kidney tissue cultures [119]. The genetic basis of this and other similarly attenuated cold-adapted, temperature-sensitive influenza viruses was explored into the 1980s, as well as other approaches for the generation of reassortants from the cold-adapted seed strain [120]. Later, an influenza B cold-adapted strain (B/Ann Arbor/1/86-ca) was developed [121]. Interestingly, cold-adapted influenza vaccines were developed about the same time in Russia; however, these vaccines were in use by the late 1970s as monovalent formulations and, more recently, as trivalent, live-attenuated vaccines [121].

LIVE-ATTENUATED INFLUENZA VACCINES

LAIVs are often viewed as immunologically superior to traditional killed vaccines due to the perception that they induce immunity in a similar manner to a natural influenza infection [122]. LAIVs typically undergo at least one round of replication that aids in the induction of several adaptive immune responses such as the production of serum and mucosal antibodies as well as the generation of stronger memory responses. In addition, several variations on the existing LAIV paradigm are being tested in clinical trials [122]. There has been substantial evolution of the LAIV field with regard to their safety, immunogenicity, and recommendations for use in human patients [122].

Cold-adapted Ann Arbor–based LAIV was first used in 2003 in the United States and has demonstrated efficacy against multiple influenza strains. Additionally, LAIV was the first intranasally administered influenza vaccine in the United States, and the first new vaccine to market since trivalent influenza vaccines (TIVs) were developed and utilized clinically in the 1940s [123]. In addition to the cold-adapted A/Ann Arbor/6/60 (H2N2) virus, B/Ann Arbor/1/66 virus was also added for additional coverage against influenza B. Both viruses donate their phenotype to a 6:2 reassortant cold-adapted vaccine virus containing six internal protein gene segments of the A or B donor strains as well as the HA and NA proteins present on the wild-type virus. Current LAIV variants are produced in specific-pathogen-free embryonated chicken eggs in the same manner as viruses grown for traditional inactivated vaccines, which remains one of its primary drawbacks.

Beneficial features of LAIV include the ability to mass vaccinate a population easily, broader coverage against heterologous strains, and some measure of herd immunity in the general vaccinee population [123]. Seasonal LAIV consists of three or four viruses including influenza A H1N1 and H3N2, influenza B Victoria, and/or Yamagata strains depending on which LAIV is used [123]. The 2009 pandemic included the use of LAIV, and they have also been evaluated clinically for use in future pandemics involving the more nontraditional influenza H2, H5, H6, H7, and H9 subtypes [123].

One drawback is that LAIVs utilize small volume intranasal (0.25 mL per nostril) administration that limits vaccine spread to the nasopharynx and URT only due in part to the size of the aerosol particles generated [111]. The dose of LAIV necessary to achieve an effective immune response varies based on age, previous influenza infection history, and existing immunity against influenza, which decreases with age [124]. However, a typical dose contains approximately 10^7 TCID$_{50}$ (50% tissue culture infectious dose) of each of the three or four vaccine strains [124]. LAIVs have demonstrated satisfactory safety profiles, minimal horizontal spread from vaccine recipients to nonrecipients, and have proven efficacious in the face of viral challenge while still maintaining their desired attenuation and replication characteristics in seasonal vaccine programs [111,124–126].

As noted previously, the lateral spread of LAIV is minimal since the initial round of replication leads to few, if any, clinical signs, thus minimizing the potential for aerosol transmission events via a cough or sneeze. Additionally, the single round of virus replication produces very little virus compared to a natural infection making transmission very inefficient due primarily to the lack of a sufficient dose of virus to achieve a patent infection. However, a controlled study performed in a daycare setting has previously shown that LAIV component viruses can in fact be shed from the vaccinee and infect a nonvaccinee indicating that while rare, vaccine virus infecting nonvaccinees is still possible under the right conditions [126]. This could be due to environmental conditions, route of infection, existing immunity of both the vaccinee and the subsequently infected contact, etc.

Immune correlates of protection for LAIV are not absolute, as serum hemagglutination inhibition antibody from LAIVs varies. Seasonal LAIVs are capable of inducing not only serum antibody responses but also mucosal and cell-mediated immunity, which are known to be involved in protection [123]. While largely considered efficacious, recent LAIV formulations have shown reduced efficacy in eliciting immunity to the H1N1 component of the vaccine [106,127]. While the reasons for the poor efficacy have not been determined, stability of the HA antigen in the live-attenuated vaccine is under investigation. The pandemic H1N1 vaccine strain may have an unpredicted susceptibility to heat, thus reducing vaccine efficacy [128]. While overall efficacy is established and LAIV formulations continue to have improvements in cold chain requirements, this and other issues could reduce use of live-attenuated inhaled influenza vaccines due to real or perceived efficacy concerns.

PULMONARY DELIVERY

Pulmonary delivery of countermeasures for viral respiratory diseases has several advantages and disadvantages. One such advantage is that pulmonary administration improves the overall bioavailability of several antiviral drugs, which typically suffer from poor absorption if given orally and may lead to increased concentrations of the drug in alveolar macrophages targeting the specific pathogen [20,129]. Additionally, nasal vaccine administration offers enhanced safety since no needles are required, and it also offers durable immunity compared to the traditional inactivated vaccines given via intramuscular injection. Importantly, administration of antiviral drugs or vaccines at the site of infection may offer another approach to better address respiratory viruses [130].

Furthermore, aerosol administration minimizes the loss of the drug due to first pass metabolism and/or excretion as the drug initially passes from the stomach into the bloodstream and circulates through the major metabolic and excretory organs (liver and kidney) while potentially overcoming solubility and bioavailability issues commonly encountered with oral drug administration [131]. However, this also limits aerosol delivery to those drugs not requiring systemic metabolic processes to generate the biologically active metabolite of the drug in the host. For instance, oseltamivir uses hepatic carboxylesterase I in the liver to generate the active metabolite, which then disseminates throughout the body [132]. However, a pulmonary-delivered drug such as laninamivir requires activation by hydrolysis that readily occurs in the pulmonary tissues indicating that if the drug is not metabolically active upon administration, it must be designed to utilize localized lung metabolic machinery to achieve activation [133,134]. In contrast to intramuscular administration, aerosol inhalation treatment is not painful and has been shown to improve patient compliance, thus leading to improved outcomes [135].

Since the mucosa is the site of infection and replication for influenza virus, mucosally delivered vaccines such as LAIV can improve immunity through the induction of IgM, IgG, IgA, and sIgA antibodies. However, the contribution of mucosal antibody responses toward protection in humans is not well understood because of the lack of mucosal samples, relative to serum specimens, in part because of the invasiveness of procedures required to collect mucosal tissue specimens [136]. This is also true for experimental animal models such as ferrets and mice; thus, clinical correlates of mucosal immunity are not always available or relevant, hence making comparison of vaccine efficacy difficult for licensed LAIVs against more traditional vaccine preparations [136].

Prior to the licensure of IIVs, a HA inhibition (HI) titer was shown to correlate with protection in clinical trials [136]. The HI assay uses the agglutination of red blood cells as a measure of virus binding and potential for infection. Inhibition of agglutinating capacity by influenza-specific serum is understood to be associated with a reduction in infectivity. The measure of immunity used for licensure of IIVs is seroconversion as measured by a $\geq$1:40 serum HI titer or a $\geq$4-fold increase in titer from baseline. Vaccination with LAIV can induce serum antibody HI titers, but seroconversion rates are variable and can be as low as 1%–4% in seropositive adults. However, despite the poor serum antibody response to LAIV, vaccination generally induces similar or better efficacy compared to inactivated vaccines [137]. In a study designed to test delivery of a LAIV in ferrets, a piezoelectric vibrating mesh system was used to generate aerosols with defined particle sizes; ferrets receiving the LAIV aerosol exhibited diminished viral titers during either a homologous or a heterologous challenge [71]. The study showed low-dose LAIV aerosol vaccination, followed by heterologous challenge, was able to decrease the duration and magnitude of viral shedding as well.

Despite the lack of a correlate of efficacy, LAIVs have repeatedly been shown to be more efficacious than inactivated vaccines, particularly in children [137]. While recent failures have been reported for H1N1 antigens, the lack of efficacy in these cases has not been associated with the vaccine mechanism of action, but rather vaccine strain stability [106,128]. Achieving site-specific immunity remains a critical requirement for any new influenza vaccine technology [138]. It has been recognized that tradition injectable vaccinations fail to generate adequate immunogenicity in many cases [138,139]. Development of new or improved influenza vaccines that target mucosal immunity will likely require new definitions of specific correlates of protection.

A limited set of alternatives to the HI assay exist to measure influenza-specific antibody responses. Microneutralization (MN) assays detect antibodies that neutralize influenza virus replication in cell culture [136]. This is a more sensitive assay than the HI titer and is likely a better correlate of protection than HI. However, there are no human infection data demonstrating a 50% protective MN titer, and thus it is not used as a correlate of protection. Enzyme-linked immunosorbent assays (ELISAs) can quantitatively measure antigen-specific antibodies (e.g., HA or virus specific) and can further determine the antibody isotype inferring function. The ELISA additionally provides information regarding the nature of the immune response as well as potential mucosal (IgA) immunity [136]. Cellular immune responses, CD8+ T cells in particular, have also been associated with protection against influenza infection. T cells can recognize conserved peptide epitopes from the virus and potentially provide heterosubtypic immunity. Epitope specificity, cytokine production, and effector function (e.g., killing of target cells) can all be assessed using established flow cytometry-based assays [136]. Importantly, serum antibody responses, mucosal antibody responses, and T cell responses have all been associated with protection in LAIV (mucosally)-vaccinated individuals [125,137,140].

The LAIV licensed in the United States is not the only inhaled influenza vaccine. As previously noted, a LAIV has been in use in Russia since the 1970s [141]. More recently, an inactivated virosomal-subunit vaccine was approved for administration in Switzerland. Virosomes are made by extracting the HA from influenza virus and then reconstituting the antigen in synthetic phosphatidylcholine and phosphatidylethanolamine liposomes. These liposomes were immunogenic in animals and humans, but interestingly the vaccine was still used in conjunction with either endotoxins or heat-labile toxin (LT) as a mucosal adjuvant [142]. The vaccine was shown to induce both serum HI and mucosal antibody responses and have efficacy rates of ≥89% in adults in protection from clinically diagnosed influenza-like illness [142]. Clinical trials showed the vaccine to be safe and effective, and the vaccine was approved and used in Switzerland beginning in 2000. However, postlicensure monitoring identified an increase in the rate of Bell's palsy among vaccines and the vaccine was discontinued in 2001 [143].

PULMONARY DRUG DELIVERY

The detection of viral pathogens by laboratory methods including PCR, cell culture, and/or serologic tests is often too complicated to provide timely information during the initial cases of an outbreak but is ultimately useful for elucidating the underlying cause of the outbreak. There are several point-of-care diagnostic tests available for influenza, RSV, and several other common respiratory viruses, but the overall usefulness of these rapid tests is not clearly defined given the wide variations in sensitivity and specificity of any one testing modality. Management of pulmonary disease is based on clinical presentation, patient vital signs, and laboratory data, and as such treatment for viral respiratory tract viruses is generally limited to supportive care. Antibacterial drugs (often referred to more generally as antibiotics) are ineffective against viruses but often are used as prophylaxis against secondary bacterial infections, a practice that has been implicated in the exacerbation of drug resistance and is thus generally not recommended without definitive clinical evidence of bacterial involvement. However, in patients with chronic lung disease, antibiotics are generally administered to mitigate risk given the underlying pathology and propensity for the patient to develop more severe lung disease, develop more or enhanced complications, etc.

Inhaled antiviral drugs have been studied for a variety of viruses, including influenza virus, Coxsackievirus, echovirus, adenovirus, RSV, rhinovirus, parainfluenza virus, corona virus, human metapneumovirus, hantavirus, human bocavirus, polyomaviruses, and polyomaviruses [144]. The most common etiology of respiratory tract disorders due to viral infection is the "common cold" (coryza). This is most commonly due to rhinovirus infection (over ~150 rhinovirus serotypes are currently known) [145]. Twenty percent of colds are due to coronavirues, but many symptoms overlap with those caused by influenza viruses, parainfluenza viruses, adenoviruses, RSV, and/or enteroviruses (EVs) [146]. Infection with many of these viruses induces a descending infection of the respiratory tract although adenoviruses may also cause a viral pharyngitis [146]. Croup is primarily due to parainfluenza virus infection although RSV is capable of inducing croup-like illness as well [147]. All the viruses mentioned often induce acute bronchitis (even in healthy populations) and may worsen symptoms in patients suffering from COPD [148].

Rhinoviruses primarily adhere to the cell surface glycoprotein intercellular adhesion molecule-1 (ICAM-1) [149]. There are two specific antivirals that are available to treat rhinovirus via pulmonary delivery. They are a soluble form of ICAM-1 that will adhere to rhinovirus binding domains, thereby inhibiting virus binding and attachment to the cell surface receptors and preventing replication [150]. They have been demonstrated to have inhibited human rhinovirus *in vitro*, and in phase II clinical trials, when given intranasally, decreased overall symptoms of experimentally induced rhinoviral disease even if the drug was given after viral challenge [150,151]. However, research in this area is limited due to the short dwell time of the drug in the nasal passages. Mucociliary clearance, in combination with subsequent sneezing and nose blowing, remains the primary issue associated with pulmonary drug delivery.

The limited dwell time of these medications in the nasopharynx combined with problems associated with achieving necessary concentrations of the drug in the target locations likely explains why compounds that initially had positive results in trials failed to advance in larger scale studies. In a lethal coronavirus model in rats, 7-thia-8-oxoguanosine demonstrated excellent efficacy but failed to advance due to the problems noted previously [152,153]. In contrast, the anti-influenza drug zanamivir is very efficacious when administered intranasally [154] with approximately 50% of the drug remaining in the nasopharynx for at least 1.5 h. Why this drug did not suffer the same fate as the first remains unknown, but IAV infection can reduce mucociliary clearance and may explain the prolonged dwell time relatively to the coronavirus model mentioned previously [155,156]. Thus, it appears that prolonging the intranasal dwell time of inhaled drugs will be a critical prognostic feature when developing and assessing new drug formulations.

Amantadine, rimantadine, oseltamivir, and zanamivir are antiviral drugs with variable efficacy often used for influenza therapy. For influenza A and B viruses, the NA inhibitors oseltamivir and zanamivir are approved for use in adults, but not pediatric patients. Another NA inhibitor, Rapivab (peramivir), has also been approved for use in adults [157]. These drugs can be administered for either postinfluenza exposure prophylaxis or treatment of influenza infection if given within 48 h after exposure [158,159]. NA inhibitors (except peramivir) are recommended only for children with protracted morbidity and who are at an elevated risk of enhanced disease [159].

There are currently two classes of drugs utilized to treat influenza infections. Amantadine and rimantadine both block the M2 proton channel that inhibits virus uncoating. Oseltamivir, peramivir, and zanamivir are NA inhibitors that prevent virus egress [158,160]. There are other long-acting NA inhibitors and the polymerase inhibitor (favipiravir), as well as several experimental drugs that target virus features such as the HA inhibitors, cyanovirin-N, and thiazolides or those that target the host (DAS181) [160,161]. The development of drug-resistant influenza strains has grown rapidly in the past few years, and influenza strains resistant to both classes of drugs have been described [29,36,37,158]. The usefulness of M2 inhibitors is particularly limited, not only due to drug resistance but also because of their specificity for influenza A viruses only; they are ineffective against influenza B since it does not have an M2 membrane protein. NA inhibitors are not immune to the development of drug-resistant strains. Moreover, both classes of anti-influenza drugs are associated with the occurrence of neuropsychiatric side effects. Importantly, these inhibitors do little for an established influenza infection and do not improve severe LRTI.

The powder-based pulmonary inhalant, laninamivir, is a long-acting antiviral drug against influenza that requires only one dose for treatment [162]. This makes it a viable alternative to other multidose NA inhibitors. Laninamivir (licensed only in Japan) is given as the prodrug laninamivir octanoate (LO) and is administered as a dry powder at a dosage of 40 mg for adults and 20 mg for children [162,163]. Clinical trials in humans have shown a reduction in the duration of clinical signs [133,162]. More importantly, metabolic degradation of the drug is limited initially as the activating hydrolysis reaction that occurs in the pulmonary tissue itself as noted previously [134].

Ribavirin (Virazole) is a broad-spectrum antiviral guanosine analog that inhibits replication of many RNA and DNA viruses. It has seen sporadic use in severely immunocompromised patients with lower respiratory tract disease due to RSV [34], although ribavirin has also been considered for use during pandemic influenza infection [35]. It is approved for the treatment of RSV in high-risk infants as well as for Lassa fever virus and hepatitis C virus [144]. Ribavirin is also a prodrug (like laninamivir) and is metabolized to its active 5′-monophosphate form that resembles guanosine; due to the structural similarity, it interferes with viral replication via the incorporation of the analog into the viral transcripts during replication in

RNA viruses [144]. Inhaled ribavirin has been used in influenza challenge models in several animal species and demonstrated protection against a lethal influenza A challenge [144,164].

A promising antiviral is pleconaril, a drug targeting EV-induced diseases including the common cold, meningitis, encephalitis, pneumonia, and myocarditis [165–168]. This drug is classified as a pyrazolopyrimidine, is well tolerated, and is a potent EV inhibitor with good bioavailability, attaining robust drug levels in nasal epithelium [165,169]. Rupintrivir (AG-7088), a specific 3C protease inhibitor, demonstrated similar antiviral activity to pleconaril when administered intranasally [170–172]. In phase II clinical trials, healthy volunteers challenged via experimental infection exhibited a reduction in symptoms, nasal secretions, and viral titers.

AEROSOL INHALERS

There are three aerosol inhalers designed for pulmonary delivery: the small volume nebulizer, the MDI, and the DPI [173–176]. And "aerosol device" refers to a nebulizer, while "inhaler" most often refers to an MDI; generally, all are classified as aerosol inhalers [117]. Additionally, *aerosol* refers to a suspension of liquid or solid particles in a carrier gas, not necessarily a liquid spray. Microspray devices have also been developed, which use room air or mechanical force to create pulmonary mists or clouds without another carrier gas or propellant, but these devices have not seen widespread adoption outside controlled research settings due to cost and availability [177].

Each of the commonly encountered aerosol devices has distinctive performance characteristics, making the choice of the system used dependent not only on the solution to be aerosolized but also on the intended target, particle size, etc. Since there is substantial drug loss in the oropharynx, holding chambers and spacers are utilized on many MDIs, which results in a large amount of wastage of the active drug. Also, there are several generalizable advantages and disadvantages of the inhalation route.

The main advantage of aerosol administration over systemic administration is that aerosol doses are usually lower than systemic doses to achieve the same efficacy resulting in considerably less wastage of drug and/or lower drug costs. Also, the drug is carried directly to the desired location limiting the time to onset for the patient primarily due to limiting transit time from the GI tract to the blood stream, that is, the onset of action for inhaled agents is much quicker than an oral dosage regimen (albuterol takes 30 min or less to take effect if taken orally while inhaled albuterol takes 5 min to achieve therapeutic effect in the lung) [178,179]. Some disadvantages are that lung deposition is a relatively low fraction of the total aerosol dose, so there is typically some amount of drug/vaccine loss, and many variables such as breathing pattern among individuals and mucous viscosity and thickness can affect lung deposition and dose reproducibility.

Particle size, particle velocity, and settling times are important in aerosol deposition in the airways [20,78,175,180,181]. Particle deposition in the oropharyngeal cavity increases with large diameter particles (those above 5 µm), while expiration removes particles 1 µm or less; particles 1–5 µm can readily spread in the lung with those 5–10 µm in diameter mostly ending up in larger airways [180,182].

Many aerosolization devices utilize compressed air to disperse dry powders to deliver drugs or vaccines into a spacer before inhalation [183]. The location of deposition of aerosol particles varies with the particle size where particles <10 μm have an increased likelihood of reaching the lower airways [184]. Vaccine deposition in the lungs or lower airways is neither required nor advantageous (and actually may be contraindicated for optimal vaccine efficacy) as most LAIV and related vaccines are not designed to replicate outside of the nasopharynx [103]. Large particle size reduces the likelihood of delivery to the lower lungs, which is a safety benefit.

Notably, there are three major limitations of DPIs: exposure to moisture, chemical/electrostatic interactions between the drug molecules themselves as well as to the administration device, and a dependence on the person's inspiratory volume that is often limited in both acute and chronic lung disease conditions [185,186]. Further, DPIs are extremely susceptible to moisture accumulation on the unit during exhalation, which means users have to consciously remember to exhale away from the mouthpiece of the DPI unit in order to minimize drug loss due to wetting of the surfaces by previous exhalation. Last, DPIs depend on reasonable inspiration volume, so there is a legitimate question as to whether the very young and very old can generate the tidal volume necessary to achieve optimal dosing with these devices [185].

Nebulization is one of the earliest techniques used to deliver liquid formulations as aerosols. Nebulizers are distinctly different from inhalers in that they typically use battery or mechanical power to convert a liquid solution into a fine mist (in some cases via the generation and incorporation of a compressed gas) and deliver it via a mouthpiece or face mask, instead of a pressurized carrier gas as with most inhalers. Multiple types of nebulizers are commercially available including jet, ultrasonic wave, vibrating mesh, and human powered, as well as several relying on mechanical force [100,187]. However, significant disparities exist in the overall size distribution of droplets and/or particles that an individual nebulizer can generate based mainly on the method used to generate the aerosol [187]. As such, picking a nebulizer suited not only to the liquid being aerosolized but also to the downstream host requirements relative to target area in the respiratory tract, optimum particle size for effective uptake, and potential interactions with host defense mechanisms is critically important to ensure maximal drug or vaccine efficacy. Historically, nebulization was used as a first step in many clinical trials followed quickly by the development of specific inhalers for the drug of interest, due primarily to the lack of portability of many nebulization units as well as their cost and ease of use relative to handheld inhalers. However, nebulizers based on more recent technology may supplant the need for a transition to MDIs as well as allow for a larger array of drugs and vaccines to be delivered via nebulization, including many that are not readily amenable to conversion to an inhaler-based delivery system due to solubility, viscosity, etc.

SAFETY OF AEROSOL VACCINES

Aerosol vaccination paradigms currently employ delivery of the vaccine directly into the nasal cavity, especially in infants that only breathe through their nasal passages. However, this strategy is not without risk as the proximity of the nasal passages to the olfactory region in the nasal turbinates could result in inadvertent CNS exposure especially if preexisting inflammation is already present in this region. In the case of an LAIV, vaccine could be absorbed from the olfactory mucosa and pass onto the neuronal cells and then onto other parts of the CNS [188]. The possibility for this to occur was studied in adults inhaling aerosols delivered via nasal spray pumps or nebulizers [188]. The study showed the spray pump could not deliver aerosols to the nasal cavity, but a nebulizer was able to do so in part because of the small particle size it could generate, which suggests that small aerosol particles could be deposited in the mucosa of the olfactory region. With the experience gathered from studies done using the inhaled virosomal influenza vaccine, incorporation of adjuvants for inhalation is moving forward with caution. Adjuvants such as *Escherichia coli* heat-labile toxin (LT) and cholera toxin (CT), while being effective mucosal adjuvants, are believed to target olfactory nerves [189]. Despite the numerous advantages that are associated with aerosol immunization for live-attenuated vaccines, hazards remain regarding potential for transmission of the aerosols generated by the administration device or patient to the vaccine administrators, as well as to the vaccinees' contacts [126,190]. Several studies with measles, mumps, and rubella vaccines have indicated this potential, and there are documented seropositive responses to measles vaccine (presumably from the aerosol dispenser directly to vaccinators) as well as the previously mentioned LAIV transmission event documented in a daycare setting [126,191].

Host biological processes in response to vaccination may contribute to vaccine-enhanced disease. There are a variety of host responses that help limit infections, mediate vaccine-enhanced disease, or aid in overall disease progression in the patient [192]. For RSV, enhanced respiratory disease (ERD) linked to formalin-inactivated alum-precipitated RSV (FI-RSV) vaccine has forever changed how inactivated RSV vaccines are considered for use in terms of their safety [193]. In the late 1960s, children immunized intramuscularly using the FI-RSV vaccine showed enhanced disease after natural exposure to RSV, with one study noting that 69% of children receiving the immunization had pneumonia compared to just 9% of nonimmunized children in the control group [193,194].

FI-RSV vaccine-enhanced disease was subsequently classified as a severe RSV infection including bronchiolitis and pneumonia, but the majority of the severe and/or fatal vaccinees showed profound mononuclear cell infiltrates as well as pulmonary eosinophilia [193,194]. It is now well substantiated that FI-RSV-enhanced disease includes pulmonary eosinophilia with a substantial inflammatory response [195–197]. The lack of the G protein or G protein CX3C motif during FI-RSV vaccination or RSV challenge of FI-RSV-vaccinated mice or treatment with antisubstance P or anti-CX3CR1 antibodies has been shown to reduce the enhanced pulmonary disease typically observed [195,197]. Therefore, aerosol delivery of FI-RSV or related inactivated RSV vaccines is expected to induce ERD; however, there are no data currently available to confirm this outcome for aerosol-delivered RSV vaccine. It is important to understand the host response to vaccination to avoid unintended biological complications.

Although there are no effective vaccines or drugs for the prevention or treatment of dengue virus, it is an example of a pathogen capable of causing immune-mediated disease [192]. Dengue induces alterations in vascular permeability, hence leading to the translocation of microbial products from the intestinal lumen into the systemic circulation without a concurrent bacteremia [192]. Like RSV, supportive care is the only available treatment. A few live-attenuated vaccine candidates have been tested including intertypic dengue chimeric strains, yellow fever 17D vaccine–dengue chimeras, and flavivirus–nonflavivirus recombinant vaccine vectors [192,198,199]. Passive immunization using antibodies appears to be a viable option relative to the utter lack of effective antiviral treatment options [200]. Presently, there are several vaccine candidates in various stages of testing. The chimeric tetravalent vaccine based on the yellow fever 17D vector may be available in the near future, hence pending the successful outcome of ongoing clinical trials [192,201,202].

BENEFITS AND DRAWBACKS OF INHALED AGENTS

From the perspective of vaccinology, it is important to understand that respiratory viruses preferentially induce mucosal infections and that these viruses utilize mucosal tissues in order to enter the systemic compartment. Several viruses with mucosal tissue tropisms indicate that mucosal immunity by itself is necessary to prevent or clear viral infection demonstrating the need to include mucosal-associated lymphoid tissues as well [203]. "Integrated mucosal immune system" indicates that mucosal immune sites are linked, but mucosal immunity is not a single system in which all sites are integrated with one another although animal models have helped identify some key features in overall mucosal immune function [138]. MALT, NALT, and BALT are all critical to mucosal immune induction. As an example, the priming of the immune response in MALT may induce CD4 and CD8 T cell responses as well as B cell responses and SIgA [138].

Drug or dry particle vaccine administration via aerosols confers several distinct advantages over alternate methods of delivery, as typically the lung is the target organ relative to respiratory disease. Aerosol delivery can more rapidly achieve higher concentrations of drugs at the site of infection while minimizing systemic side effects, potentially allowing for a more rapid onset of drug action and elimination of oral or intravenous delivery, both of which have their own drawbacks [204]. It should be noted that aerosol delivery may alter the pharmacokinetics of the drugs and perhaps the robustness of the vaccine given the enormous surface area of the respiratory tract and its relatively permeable epithelial lining allowing for efficient transport from the lung into the systemic circulation [204]. Therefore, pulmonary delivery also offers a promising alternative approach to systemic drug delivery, particularly for drugs with poor bioavailability or those that are significantly degraded during first pass metabolism in the GI tract and liver.

Several studies have shown that the alveolar region is the preferred location for administration of vaccines or therapeutics. This is largely due to the fact that the alveolar spaces form a large surface area to absorb the components of the vaccine or therapeutic and mucociliary clearance in this area is minimal [205]. These characteristics prolong the dwell time of the agent in the alveolar space, which further enhances the absorption efficiency. In addition, the alveolar region and associated parenchyma is rich with antigen-presenting cells, such as dendritic cells and macrophages that are critical for initiating immunity.

LAIV does not target the alveolar region, instead relying on sustained replication in the nasopharynx. Several experimental inhaled influenza vaccines have been tested for dose, delivery, and efficacy (including split virus vaccines that are inactivated through detergent disruption then administered intranasally). Animal models have shown adequate protection is achievable with a single intranasal administration of adjuvanted influenza vaccine as long as the vaccine can reach sites in the lower respiratory tract capable of stimulating adequate induction of the immune system [206]. Importantly, the inclusion of adjuvants also improves the duration and breadth of the overall immune response to influenza vaccines. While concerns exist over the use of the heat-labile enterotoxins/CTs known as LT, both LT and CT have new mutant derivatives that have shown promise as safe and potent adjuvants [207].

CONSIDERATIONS

Administration of respiratory drugs at the site of infection offers key benefits of the patient, including the minimization of drug doses reducing systemic toxicity and exposure concerns [208]. Delivery via the respiratory route offers a more rapid response than traditional oral dosing techniques as well as the ability to bypass metabolism of the drugs in the GI tract as well as other shortfalls including poor absorption and degradation of the drug in the acidic environment of the stomach. [209]. Delivery via this route offers similar or enhanced drug concentrations to be achieved at the desired location at a fraction of the oral or systemic dose as well as the potential to minimize or eliminate hematogenous uptake and subsequent systemic spread, thus leading to not only higher initial concentrations but significantly prolonged drug activity as well [129,208].

There are three basic pulmonary delivery methods used, specifically MDIs, mist inhalers, nebulizers, and DPIs. Respiratory administration of relatively large drug doses is possible through nebulization of many liquid drug preparations [209]. However, drawbacks such as the limited portability of many nebulizers, power source requirements, and noise associated with the compressor for jet nebulizers must also be considered. Many of these obstacles are being overcome using portable battery-powered vibrating mesh nebulizers [71–73] as well as mechanical nebulizers using spring power to induce mist formation.

Drug delivery to the respiratory tract is currently being enhanced through the use of particle engineering studies in order to optimize not only particle size but also other parameters including surface charge, morphology, and structure [208]. Novel formulations may eliminate the need for carrier molecules to facilitate or improve aerosolization and for powders the increased dispersibility of the powder itself [208]. Optimized size, morphology, structure, and shape can substantially improve lung and respiratory delivery as well as tailor delivery to a specific location via careful selection of particle parameters. All these properties can contribute to more efficacious delivery of the compound, thus leading to enhanced and/or prolonged drug concentrations (often using lower total doses) at the desired location in the respiratory tract often with minimal spillover to the bloodstream or adjacent tissues.

High vaccination rates are critical for preventing morbidity and mortality due to infection by respiratory viruses like influenza and measles. As measles vaccine is administered via a traditional intramuscular injection, many challenges to achieving target levels of vaccine coverage in the population remain such as the need for trained personnel to give the vaccines, expensive handling and storage requirements, wastage and contamination concerns inherent to the use of multidose vials, as well as ongoing issues associated with needle usage including disposal and accessibility concerns [210,211]. Dry powder pulmonary vaccine delivery could overcome many of these issues given that aerosol administration of a dry powder live-attenuated measles vaccine was able to induce protective immunity in rhesus macaques challenged with wild-type measles of a comparable duration to existing measles vaccines [210].

Vaccine technology has dramatically advanced and dry powder formulation of live-attenuated vaccines is progressing. These thermostable, powdered vaccines eliminate issues associated with shipping liquids as well as issues surrounding proper reconstitution techniques (to preserve sterility) if they are administered as dry powders. This has already been demonstrated via the generation of small particle dry powder live-attenuated vaccine formulations. Accumulating pulmonary vaccination data in animal models confirms that live-attenuated vaccines when administered to the nasopharynx by spray or aerosol can not only be delivered to the nasal mucosa but can also actively replicate there. Additionally, virus-specific serum and mucosal antibodies, CD4 and CD8 T cells, and antiviral cytokine responses have all been induced via this technique, all of which are critical components for a successful response to a vaccination event. The relative breadth of immune responses induced by these vaccines suggests durable and broad protection is possible with many of these new technologies.

SUMMARY

- Achieving predictable, repeatable, and site-specific immunity is a major milestone for future influenza vaccine candidates.
- Intranasal vaccination shows great promise for respiratory pathogens since it generates both IgM- and IgG-mediated immune responses in the alveolar tissue while also generating IgA capable of protecting the mucosal surfaces lining the URT.
- Evidence supporting a nasal route for vaccine delivery comes from influenza virus aerosol vaccination that has been used in large populations, thus indicating it is a feasible and efficacious method for mass vaccinations across a diverse population.
- The benefits of aerosol vaccination outweigh the minor risks associated with them, as they are inherently no more dangerous than injectable vaccines, while minimizing the risk of blood-borne pathogens associated with traditional intramuscular vaccination.
- Improvements in therapeutic and vaccine delivery to newborns, including shelf-stable vaccines unaffected by wide variations in ambient temperature

and humidity, are desperately needed to further improve therapeutic options at a patient level as well as vaccine coverage across the developing world where shelf stability is a critical component for any vaccination campaign.

REFERENCES

1. Zhang N, He QS. Commensal microbiome promotes resistance to local and systemic infections. *Chinese Medical Journal*, 128(16), 2250–2255 (2015).
2. Hoffmann AR, Proctor LM, Surette MG, Suchodolski JS. The microbiome: The trillions of microorganisms that maintain health and cause disease in humans and companion animals. *Veterinary Pathology*, 53(1), 10–21 (2015).
3. Roy CJ, Reed DS, Hutt JA. Aerobiology and inhalation exposure to biological select agents and toxins. *Veterinary Pathology*, 47(5), 779–789 (2010).
4. Gralton J, Tovey ER, McLaws ML, Rawlinson WD. Respiratory virus RNA is detectable in airborne and droplet particles. *Journal of Medical Virology*, 85(12), 2151–2159 (2013).
5. Milton DK, Fabian MP, Cowling BJ, Grantham ML, McDevitt JJ. Influenza virus aerosols in human exhaled breath: Particle size, culturability, and effect of surgical masks. *PLOS Pathogens*, 9(3), e1003205 (2013).
6. Sato S, Kiyono H. The mucosal immune system of the respiratory tract. *Current Opinion in Virology*, 2(3), 225–232 (2012).
7. Kang H, Yan M, Yu Q, Yang Q. Characterization of nasal cavity-associated lymphoid tissue in ducks. *Anatomical Record*, 297(5), 916–924 (2014).
8. Yang W, Marr LC. Dynamics of airborne influenza A viruses indoors and dependence on humidity. *PLOS ONE*, 6(6), e21481 (2011).
9. Luke CJ, Subbarao K. The role of animal models in influenza vaccine research. In: *Influenza Vaccines for the Future*, Rappuoli, R, Del Giudice, G (eds.) (Springer, Basel, Switzerland, 2011) pp. 223–272.
10. Martin C, Burgel PR, Lepage P et al. Host-microbe interactions in distal airways: Relevance to chronic airway diseases. *European Respiratory Review: An Official Journal of the European Respiratory Society*, 24(135), 78–91 (2015).
11. Ichinohe T, Pang IK, Kumamoto Y et al. Microbiota regulates immune defense against respiratory tract influenza A virus infection. *Proceedings of the National Academy of Sciences of the United States of America*, 108(13), 5354–5359 (2011).
12. Macpherson AJ, McCoy KD, Johansen FE, Brandtzaeg P. The immune geography of IgA induction and function. *Mucosal Immunology*, 1(1), 11–22 (2008).
13. Smith K, McCoy KD, Macpherson AJ. Use of axenic animals in studying the adaptation of mammals to their commensal intestinal microbiota. *Seminars in Immunology*, 19(2), 59–69 (2007).
14. Pang IK, Iwasaki A. Control of antiviral immunity by pattern recognition and the microbiome. *Immunological Reviews*, 245(1), 209–226 (2012).
15. Gilley SK, Stenbit AE, Pasek RC et al. Deletion of airway cilia results in noninflammatory bronchiectasis and hyperreactive airways. *American Journal of Physiology: Lung Cellular and Molecular Physiology*, 306(2), L162–L169 (2014).
16. Vareille M, Kieninger E, Edwards MR, Regamey N. The airway epithelium: Soldier in the fight against respiratory viruses. *Clinical Microbiology Reviews*, 24(1), 210–229 (2011).
17. Blanco EE, Pinge MC, Andrade Neto OA, Pessoa NG. Effects of nitric oxide in mucociliary transport. *Brazilian Journal of Otorhinolaryngology*, 75(6), 866–871 (2009).

18. Evans SE, Xu Y, Tuvim MJ, Dickey BF. Inducible innate resistance of lung epithelium to infection. *Annual Review of Physiology*, 72, 413–435 (2010).
19. Thorley AJ, Ruenraroengsak P, Potter TE, Tetley TD. Critical determinants of uptake and translocation of nanoparticles by the human pulmonary alveolar epithelium. *ACS Nano*, 8(11), 11778–11789 (2014).
20. Chono S, Tanino T, Seki T, Morimoto K. Influence of particle size on drug delivery to rat alveolar macrophages following pulmonary administration of ciprofloxacin incorporated into liposomes. *Journal of Drug Targeting*, 14(8), 557–566 (2006).
21. Kesimer M, Ehre C, Burns KA, Davis CW, Sheehan JK, Pickles RJ. Molecular organization of the mucins and glycocalyx underlying mucus transport over mucosal surfaces of the airways. *Mucosal Immunology*, 6(2), 379–392 (2013).
22. Kesimer M, Scull M, Brighton B et al. Characterization of exosome-like vesicles released from human tracheobronchial ciliated epithelium: A possible role in innate defense. *FASEB Journal: Official Publication of the Federation of American Societies for Experimental Biology*, 23(6), 1858–1868 (2009).
23. Yoo JK, Kim TS, Hufford MM, Braciale TJ. Viral infection of the lung: Host response and sequelae. *The Journal of Allergy and Clinical Immunology*, 132(6), 1263–1276; quiz 1277 (2013).
24. Lamichhane A, Azegamia T, Kiyonoa H. The mucosal immune system for vaccine development. *Vaccine*, 32(49), 6711–6723 (2014).
25. Randall TD. Bronchus-associated lymphoid tissue (BALT) structure and function. *Advances in Immunology*, 107, 187–241 (2010).
26. Liang B, Hyland L, Hou S. Nasal-associated lymphoid tissue is a site of long-term virus-specific antibody production following respiratory virus infection of mice. *Journal of Virology*, 75(11), 5416–5420 (2001).
27. Wu HY, Nguyen HH, Russell MW. Nasal lymphoid tissue (NALT) as a mucosal immune inductive site. *Scandinavian Journal of Immunology*, 46(5), 506–513 (1997).
28. Doherty PC, Topham DJ, Tripp RA, Cardin RD, Brooks JW, Stevenson PG. Effector CD4+ and CD8+ T-cell mechanisms in the control of respiratory virus infections. *Immunological Reviews*, 159, 105–117 (1997).
29. Zens KD, Farber DL. Memory CD4 T cells in influenza. *Current Topics in Microbiology and Immunology*, 386, 399–421 (2015).
30. Hufford MM, Kim TS, Sun J, Braciale TJ. The effector T cell response to influenza infection. *Current Topics in Microbiology and Immunology*, 386, 423–455 (2015).
31. Chiu C, Openshaw PJ. Antiviral B cell and T cell immunity in the lungs. *Nature Immunology*, 16(1), 18–26 (2015).
32. Rossey I, Sedeyn K, De Baets S, Schepens B, Saelens X. CD8+ T cell immunity against human respiratory syncytial virus. *Vaccine*, 32(46), 6130–6137 (2014).
33. Shin H, Iwasaki A. Tissue-resident memory T cells. *Immunological Reviews*, 255(1), 165–181 (2013).
34. Hillaire ML, Rimmelzwaan GF, Kreijtz JH. Clearance of influenza virus infections by T cells: Risk of collateral damage? *Current Opinion in Virology*, 3(4), 430–437 (2013).
35. Werner JL, Steele C. Innate receptors and cellular defense against pulmonary infections. *Journal of Immunology*, 193(8), 3842–3850 (2014).
36. Moser EK, Sun J, Kim TS, Braciale TJ. IL-21R signaling suppresses IL-17+ gamma delta T cell responses and production of IL-17 related cytokines in the lung at steady state and after Influenza A virus infection. *PLOS ONE*, 10(4), e0120169 (2015).
37. Chiu C, Ellebedy AH, Wrammert J, Ahmed R. B cell responses to influenza infection and vaccination. *Current topics in Microbiology and Immunology*, 386, 381–398 (2015).

38. Boyden AW, Frickman AM, Legge KL, Waldschmidt TJ. Primary and long-term B-cell responses in the upper airway and lung after influenza A virus infection. *Immunologic Research*, 59(1–3), 73–80 (2014).
39. Keren DF. Antigen processing in the mucosal immune system. *Seminars in Immunology*, 4(4), 217–226 (1992).
40. Brandtzaeg P. Mucosal immunity: Induction, dissemination, and effector functions. *Scandinavian Journal of Immunology*, 70(6), 505–515 (2009).
41. Brandtzaeg P, Johansen FE. Mucosal B cells: Phenotypic characteristics, transcriptional regulation, and homing properties. *Immunological Reviews*, 206, 32–63 (2005).
42. Gourley TS, Wherry EJ, Masopust D, Ahmed R. Generation and maintenance of immunological memory. *Seminars in Immunology*, 16(5), 323–333 (2004).
43. Reynolds HY. Immunoglobulin G and its function in the human respiratory tract. *Mayo Clinic Proceedings*, 63(2), 161–174 (1988).
44. Hallstrand TS, Hackett TL, Altemeier WA, Matute-Bello G, Hansbro PM, Knight DA. Airway epithelial regulation of pulmonary immune homeostasis and inflammation. *Clinical Immunology*, 151(1), 1–15 (2014).
45. Ramos I, Fernandez-Sesma A. Modulating the innate immune response to influenza A virus: potential therapeutic use of anti-inflammatory drugs. *Frontiers in Immunology*, 6, 361 (2015).
46. Blasius AL, Beutler B. Intracellular toll-like receptors. *Immunity*, 32(3), 305–315 (2010).
47. Lund JM, Alexopoulou L, Sato A et al. Recognition of single-stranded RNA viruses by Toll-like receptor 7. *Proceedings of the National Academy of Sciences of the United States of America*, 101(15), 5598–5603 (2004).
48. Ramos I, Fernandez-Sesma A. Cell receptors for influenza a viruses and the innate immune response. *Frontiers in Microbiology*, 3, 117 (2012).
49. Weber F. The catcher in the RIG-I. *Cytokine*, 76(1), 38–41 (2015).
50. Lowen AC, Mubareka S, Steel J, Palese P. Influenza virus transmission is dependent on relative humidity and temperature. *PLOS Pathogens*, 3(10), 1470–1476 (2007).
51. Lowen AC, Mubareka S, Tumpey TM, Garcia-Sastre A, Palese P. The guinea pig as a transmission model for human influenza viruses. *Proceedings of the National Academy of Sciences of the United States of America*, 103(26), 9988–9992 (2006).
52. Tripp RA, Tompkins SM. Animal models for evaluation of influenza vaccines. *Current Topics in Microbiology and Immunology*, 333, 397–412 (2009).
53. Tellier R. Aerosol transmission of influenza A virus: A review of new studies. *Journal of the Royal Society, Interface/the Royal Society*, 6(Suppl. 6), S783–S790 (2009).
54. Lowen AC, Steel J, Mubareka S, Palese P. High temperature (30 degrees C) blocks aerosol but not contact transmission of influenza virus. *Journal of Virology*, 82(11), 5650–5652 (2008).
55. Thangavel RR, Bouvier NM. Animal models for influenza virus pathogenesis, transmission, and immunology. *Journal of Immunological Methods*, 410, 60–79 (2014).
56. Gabbard JD, Dlugolenski D, Van Riel D et al. Novel H7N9 influenza virus shows low infectious dose, high growth rate, and efficient contact transmission in the guinea pig model. *Journal of Virology*, 88(3), 1502–1512 (2014).
57. Pica N, Bouvier NM. Environmental factors affecting the transmission of respiratory viruses. *Current Opinion in Virology*, 2(1), 90–95 (2012).
58. Lowen AC, Bouvier NM, Steel J. Transmission in the guinea pig model. *Current Topics in Microbiology and Immunology*, 385, 157–183 (2014).
59. Lowen A, Palese P. Transmission of influenza virus in temperate zones is predominantly by aerosol, in the tropics by contact: A hypothesis. *PLOS Currents*, 1, RRN1002 (2009).

60. Tao H, Li L, White MC, Steel J, Lowen AC. Influenza A virus coinfection through transmission can support high levels of reassortment. *Journal of Virology*, 89(16), 8453–8461 (2015).

61. Bouvier NM, Lowen AC. Animal models for influenza virus pathogenesis and transmission. *Viruses*, 2(8), 1530–1563 (2010).

62. Staeheli P, Grob R, Meier E, Sutcliffe JG, Haller O. Influenza virus-susceptible mice carry Mx genes with a large deletion or a nonsense mutation. *Molecular and Cellular Biology*, 8(10), 4518–4523 (1988).

63. Herfst S, Schrauwen EJ, Linster M et al. Airborne transmission of influenza A/H5N1 virus between ferrets. *Science*, 336(6088), 1534–1541 (2012).

64. McLaren C, Potter CW, Jennings R. Immunity to influenza in ferrets. X. Intranasal immunization of ferrets with inactivated influenza A virus vaccines. *Infection and Immunology*, 9(6), 985–990 (1974).

65. Shope RE. Immunization experiments with swine influenza virus. *The Journal of Experimental Medicine*, 64(1), 47–61 (1936).

66. Francis T, Magill TP. Immunological studies with the virus of influenza. *The Journal of Experimental Medicine*, 62(4), 505–516 (1935).

67. Shope RE. The infection of ferrets with swine influenza virus. *The Journal of Experimental Medicine*, 60(1), 49–61 (1934).

68. Toms GL, Sweet C, Smith H. Behaviour in ferrets of swine influenza virus isolated from man. *Lancet*, 1(8002), 68–71 (1977).

69. Enkirch T, von Messling V. Ferret models of viral pathogenesis. *Virology*, 479–480, 259–270 (2015).

70. Peng X, Alfoldi J, Gori K et al. The draft genome sequence of the ferret (Mustela putorius furo) facilitates study of human respiratory disease. *Nature Biotechnology*, 32(12), 1250–1255 (2014).

71. Smith JH, Papania M, Knaus D et al. Nebulized live-attenuated influenza vaccine provides protection in ferrets at a reduced dose. *Vaccine*, 30(19), 3026–3033 (2012).

72. Smith JH, Nagy T, Barber J, Brooks P, Tompkins SM, Tripp RA. Aerosol inoculation with a sub-lethal influenza virus leads to exacerbated morbidity and pulmonary disease pathogenesis. *Viral Immunology*, 24(2), 131–142 (2011).

73. Smith JH, Brooks P, Johnson S et al. Aerosol vaccination induces robust protective immunity to homologous and heterologous influenza infection in mice. *Vaccine*, 29(14), 2568–2575 (2011).

74. Bohannon JK, Lackemeyer MG, Kuhn JH et al. Generation and characterization of large-particle aerosols using a center flow tangential aerosol generator with a non-human-primate, head-only aerosol chamber. *Inhalation Toxicology*, 27(5), 247–253 (2015).

75. Cowling BJ, Ip DK, Fang VJ et al. Aerosol transmission is an important mode of influenza A virus spread. *Nature Communications*, 4, 1935 (2013).

76. Yang W, Elankumaran S, Marr LC. Relationship between humidity and influenza A viability in droplets and implications for influenza's seasonality. *PLOS ONE*, 7(10), e46789 (2012).

77. Henning A, Schneider M, Nafee N et al. Influence of particle size and material properties on mucociliary clearance from the airways. *Journal of Aerosol Medicine and Pulmonary Drug Delivery*, 23(4), 233–241 (2010).

78. Thomas RJ. Particle size and pathogenicity in the respiratory tract. *Virulence*, 4(8), 847–858 (2013).

79. Couch RB, Cate TR, Douglas RG, Jr., Gerone PJ, Knight V. Effect of route of inoculation on experimental respiratory viral disease in volunteers and evidence for airborne transmission. *Bacteriological Reviews*, 30(3), 517–529 (1966).

80. Couch RB, Cate TR, Gerone PJ et al. Production of illness with a small-particle aerosol of coxsackie A21*. *The Journal of Clinical Investigation*, 44(4), 535–542 (1965).

81. Knight V, Gerone PJ, Griffith WR et al. Studies in volunteers with respiratory viral agents. *American Review of Respiratory Disease*, 88(3P2), 135–147 (1963).
82. Jones RM, Brosseau LM. Aerosol transmission of infectious disease. *Journal of Occupational and Environmental Medicine/American College of Occupational and Environmental Medicine*, 57(5), 501–508 (2015).
83. Perwitasari O, Yan X, Johnson S et al. Targeting organic anion transporter 3 with probenecid as a novel anti-influenza a virus strategy. *Antimicrobial Agents and Chemotherapy*, 57(1), 475–483 (2013).
84. Perwitasari O, Johnson S, Yan X et al. Verdinexor, a novel selective inhibitor of nuclear export, reduces influenza a virus replication *in vitro* and *in vivo*. *Journal of Virology*, 88(17), 10228–10243 (2014).
85. Perwitasari O, Yan X, O'Donnell J, Johnson S, Tripp RA. Repurposing kinase inhibitors as antiviral agents to control influenza A virus replication. *Assay and Drug Development Technologies*, Dec; 13(10), 638–49 (2015).
86. Tripp RA, Mark Tompkins S. Antiviral effects of inhibiting host gene expression. *Current Topics in Microbiology and Immunology*, 386, 459–477 (2015).
87. Chu HY, Englund JA. Respiratory syncytial virus disease: Prevention and treatment. *Current topics in Microbiology and Immunology*, 372, 235–258 (2013).
88. Lindeman RD. Successful aging. *Experimental Lung Research*, 31(Suppl. 1), 3–86 (2005).
89. Treanor JJ. Prospects for broadly protective influenza vaccines. *Vaccine*, 33, D39–D45 (2015).
90. Sridhar S, Brokstad KA, Cox RJ. Influenza vaccination strategies: Comparing inactivated and live attenuated influenza vaccines. *Vaccines*, 3(2), 373–389 (2015).
91. Berkenfeld K, Lamprecht A, McConville JT. Devices for dry powder drug delivery to the lung. *AAPS PharmSciTech*, 16(3), 479–490 (2015).
92. Feddah MR, Brown KF, Gipps EM, Davies NM. In-vitro characterisation of metered dose inhaler versus dry powder inhaler glucocorticoid products: Influence of inspiratory flow rates. *Journal of Pharmacy & Pharmaceutical Sciences: A Publication of the Canadian Society for Pharmaceutical Sciences, Societe Canadienne des Sciences Pharmaceutiques*, 3(3), 318–324 (2000).
93. Wang SH, Thompson AL, Hickey AJ, Staats HF. Dry powder vaccines for mucosal administration: Critical factors in manufacture and delivery. *Current Topics in Microbiology and Immunology*, 354, 121–156 (2012).
94. Saluja V, Hinrichs WL, Frijlink HW. Dried influenza vaccines: Over the counter vaccines. *Human vaccines*, 6(10), 854–856 (2010).
95. Sou T, Morton DA, Williamson M, Meeusen EN, Kaminskas LM, McIntosh MP. Spray-dried influenza antigen with trehalose and leucine produces an aerosolizable powder vaccine formulation that induces strong systemic and mucosal immunity after pulmonary administration. *Journal of Aerosol Medicine and Pulmonary Drug Delivery*, 28(5), 361–371 (2015).
96. Murugappan S, Patil HP, Kanojia G et al. Physical and immunogenic stability of spray freeze-dried influenza vaccine powder for pulmonary delivery: Comparison of inulin, dextran, or a mixture of dextran and trehalose as protectants. *European Journal of Pharmaceutics and Biopharmaceutics: Official Journal of Arbeitsgemeinschaft fur Pharmazeutische Verfahrenstechnik e.V*, 85(3 Pt A), 716–725 (2013).
97. Patil HP, Murugappan S, ter Veer W et al. Evaluation of monophosphoryl lipid A as adjuvant for pulmonary delivered influenza vaccine. *Journal of Controlled Release: Official Journal of the Controlled Release Society*, 174, 51–62 (2014).
98. Audouy SA, van der Schaaf G, Hinrichs WL, Frijlink HW, Wilschut J, Huckriede A. Development of a dried influenza whole inactivated virus vaccine for pulmonary immunization. *Vaccine*, 29(26), 4345–4352 (2011).

99. Amorij JP, Huckriede A, Wilschut J, Frijlink HW, Hinrichs WL. Development of stable influenza vaccine powder formulations: Challenges and possibilities. *Pharmaceutical Research*, 25(6), 1256–1273 (2008).
100. Patil JS, Sarasija S. Pulmonary drug delivery strategies: A concise, systematic review. *Lung India: Official Organ of Indian Chest Society*, 29(1), 44–49 (2012).
101. Wright PF, Neumann G, Kawaoka Y. Orthomyxoviruses. In: *Fields Virology*, Knipe, DM, Howley, PM et al. (eds.) (Lippincott Williams & Wilkins, Philadelphia, PA, 2013).
102. Shaw ML, Palese P. Orthomyxoviridae. In: *Fields Virology*, Knipe, DM, Howley, PM et al. (eds.) (Lippincott Williams & Wilkins, Philadelphia, PA, 2013).
103. Centers for Disease Control and Prevention. Prevention and control of seasonal influenza with vaccines. Recommendations of the Advisory Committee on Immunization Practices—United States, 2013–2014. *MMWR: Morbidity and Mortality Weekly Report*, 62(RR-07), 1–43 (2013).
104. Molinari NA, Ortega-Sanchez IR, Messonnier ML et al. The annual impact of seasonal influenza in the US: Measuring disease burden and costs. *Vaccine*, 25(27), 5086–5096 (2007).
105. Grohskopf LA, Olsen SJ, Sokolow LZ et al. Prevention and control of seasonal influenza with vaccines: Recommendations of the Advisory Committee on Immunization Practices (ACIP)—United States, 2014–2015 influenza season. *MMWR: Morbidity and Mortality Weekly Report*, 63(32), 691–697 (2014).
106. Grohskopf LA, Sokolow LZ, Olsen SJ, Bresee JS, Broder KR, Karron RA. Prevention and Control of Influenza with Vaccines: Recommendations of the Advisory Committee on Immunization Practices—United States, 2015–2016 influenza season. *MMWR: Morbidity and Mortality Weekly Report*, 64(30), 818–825 (2015).
107. Hause BM, Ducatez M, Collin EA et al. Isolation of a novel swine influenza virus from oklahoma in 2011 which is distantly related to human influenza C viruses. *PLOS Pathogens*, 9(2), e1003176 (2013).
108. Hause BM, Collin EA, Liu R et al. Characterization of a novel influenza virus in cattle and Swine: Proposal for a new genus in the Orthomyxoviridae family. *mBio*, 5(2), e00031-14 (2014).
109. Watanabe T, Watanabe S, Maher EA, Neumann G, Kawaoka Y. Pandemic potential of avian influenza A (H7N9) viruses. *Trends in Microbiology*, 22(11), 623–631 (2014).
110. Tanner WD, Toth DJ, Gundlapalli AV. The pandemic potential of avian influenza A(H7N9) virus: A review. *Epidemiology and Infection*, 143, 3359–3374, (2015).
111. Fiore AE, Bridges CB, Cox NJ. Seasonal influenza vaccines. *Current Topics in Microbiology and Immunology*, 333, 43–82 (2009).
112. Schultz-Cherry S, Jones JC. Chapter 3: Influenza vaccines: The good, the bad, and the eggs. In: *Advances in Virus Research*, Karl Maramorosch, AJS, Frederick, AM (eds.) (Academic Press, London, U.K., 2010) pp. 63–84.
113. Grebe KM, Yewdell JW, Bennink JR. Heterosubtypic immunity to influenza A virus: Where do we stand? *Microbes and Infection/Institut Pasteur*, 10(9), 1024–1029 (2008).
114. Peter MP. Engineering better influenza vaccines. In: *Medicinal Protein Engineering*, Khudyakov YE (ed.) (CRC Press, Boca Raton, FL, 2008).
115. Dhere R, Yeolekar L, Kulkarni P et al. A pandemic influenza vaccine in India: From strain to sale within 12 months. *Vaccine*, 29(Suppl. 1), A16–A21 (2011).
116. Eyler JM. De Kruif's boast: Vaccine trials and the construction of a virus. *Bulletin of the History of Medicine*, 80(3), 409–438 (2006).
117. Hampson AW. Vaccines for pandemic influenza. The history of our current vaccines, their limitations and the requirements to deal with a pandemic threat. *Annals of the Academy of Medicine*, 37(6), 510–517 (2008).

118. Jang YH, Seong B-L. Principles underlying rational design of live attenuated influenza vaccines. *Clinical and Experimental Vaccine Research*, 1(1), 35–49 (2012).
119. Maassab HF. Adaptation and growth characteristics of influenza virus at 25°C. *Nature*, 213(5076), 612–614 (1967).
120. Beare AS, Hall TS. Recombinant influenza-A viruses as live vaccines for man. Report to the Medical Research Council's Committee on Influenza and other Respiratory Virus Vaccines. *Lancet*, 2(7737), 1271–1273 (1971).
121. Alexandrova GI, Maassab HF, Kendal AP et al. Laboratory properties of cold-adapted influenza B live vaccine strains developed in the US and USSR, and their B/Ann Arbor/1/86 cold-adapted reassortant vaccine candidates. *Vaccine*, 8(1), 61–64 (1990).
122. Isakova-Sivak I, Rudenko L. Safety, immunogenicity and infectivity of new live attenuated influenza vaccines. *Expert Review of Vaccines*, 14(10), 1313–1329 (2015).
123. Jin H, Subbarao K. Live attenuated influenza vaccine. *Current Topics in Microbiology and Immunology*, 386, 181–204 (2015).
124. Cox RJ, Brokstad KA, Ogra P. Influenza virus: Immunity and vaccination strategies. Comparison of the immune response to inactivated and live, attenuated influenza vaccines. *Scandinavian Journal of Immunology*, 59(1), 1–15 (2004).
125. MedImmune. FluMist® Quadrivalent (Influenza vaccine live, intranasal). FDA, (2013) http://www.fda.gov/downloads/BiologicsBloodVaccines/Vaccines/ApprovedProducts/ucm294307.pdf.
126. Vesikari T, Karvonen A, Korhonen T et al. A randomized, double-blind study of the safety, transmissibility and phenotypic and genotypic stability of cold-adapted influenza virus vaccine. *The Pediatric Infectious Disease Journal*, 25(7), 590–595 (2006).
127. AAP. LAIV not effective against influenza A H1N1 viruses in children 2 through 8 years during the 2013–2014 influenza season. *AAP News*, (November 6, 2014).
128. Coelingh K. Update on live attenuated influenza vaccine (LAIV). CDC, Atlanta, GA (2015).
129. Chono S, Tanino T, Seki T, Morimoto K. Pharmacokinetic and pharmacodynamic efficacy of intrapulmonary administration of ciprofloxacin for the treatment of respiratory infections. *Drug metabolism and Pharmacokinetics*, 22(2), 88–95 (2007).
130. Wong JP, Christopher ME, Viswanathan S et al. Aerosol and nasal delivery of vaccines and antiviral drugs against seasonal and pandemic influenza. *Expert review of Respiratory Medicine*, 4(2), 171–177 (2010).
131. Pond SM, Tozer TN. First-pass elimination. Basic concepts and clinical consequences. *Clinical pharmacokinetics*, 9(1), 1–25 (1984).
132. Gibiansky L, Giraudon M, Rayner CR et al. Population pharmacokinetic analysis of oseltamivir and oseltamivir carboxylate following intravenous and oral administration to patients with and without renal impairment. *Journal of Pharmacokinetics and Pharmacodynamics*, 42(3), 225–236 (2015).
133. Kashiwagi S, Watanabe A, Ikematsu H et al. Laninamivir octanoate for post-exposure prophylaxis of influenza in household contacts: A randomized double blind placebo controlled trial. *Journal of Infection and Chemotherapy: Official Journal of the Japan Society of Chemotherapy*, 19(4), 740–749 (2013).
134. Koyama K, Ogura Y, Nakai D et al. Identification of bioactivating enzymes involved in the hydrolysis of laninamivir octanoate, a long-acting neuraminidase inhibitor, in human pulmonary tissue. *Drug Metabolism and Disposition: The Biological Fate of Chemicals*, 42(6), 1031–1038 (2014).
135. Giudice EL, Campbell JD. Needle-free vaccine delivery. *Advanced Drug Delivery Reviews*, 58(1), 68–89 (2006).
136. McCullers JA, Huber VC. Correlates of vaccine protection from influenza and its complications. *Human Vaccines & Immunotherapeutics*, 8(1), 34–44 (2012).

137. Carter NJ, Curran MP. Live attenuated influenza vaccine (FluMist(R); Fluenz): A review of its use in the prevention of seasonal influenza in children and adults. *Drugs*, 71(12), 1591–1622 (2011).

138. Vujanic A, Sutton P, Snibson KJ, Yen H-H, Scheerlinck J-PY. Mucosal vaccination: Lung versus nose. *Veterinary Immunology and Immunopathology*, 148(1–2), 172–177 (2012).

139. Pedersen G, Cox RJ. The mucosal vaccine quandary: Intranasal vs. sublingual immunization against influenza. *Human Vaccines & Immunotherapeutics*, 8(5), 689–693 (2012).

140. Esposito S, Montinaro V, Groppali E, Tenconi R, Semino M, Principi N. Live attenuated intranasal influenza vaccine. *Human Vaccines & Immunotherapeutics*, 8(1), 76–80 (2012).

141. Kendal AP, Maassab HF, Alexandrova GI, Ghendon YZ. Development of cold-adapted recombinant live, attenuated influenza A vaccines in the U.S.A. and U.S.S.R. *Antiviral Research*, 1(6), 339–365 (1982).

142. Glueck R. Review of intranasal influenza vaccine. *Advanced Drug Delivery Reviews*, 51(1–3), 203–211 (2001).

143. Mutsch M, Zhou W, Rhodes P et al. Use of the inactivated intranasal influenza vaccine and the risk of bell's palsy in Switzerland. *New England Journal of Medicine*, 350(9), 896–903 (2004).

144. Velkov T, Abdul Rahim N, Zhou QT, Chan HK, Li J. Inhaled anti-infective chemotherapy for respiratory tract infections: Successes, challenges and the road ahead. *Advanced Drug Delivery Reviews*, 85, 65–82 (2015).

145. Glanville N, Johnston SL. Challenges in developing a cross-serotype rhinovirus vaccine. *Current opinion in Virology*, 11, 83–88 (2015).

146. Turner RB. Epidemiology, pathogenesis, and treatment of the common cold. *Annals of Allergy, Asthma & Immunology: Official Publication of the American College of Allergy, Asthma, & Immunology*, 78(6), 531–539; quiz 539–540 (1997).

147. Marx A, Torok TJ, Holman RC, Clarke MJ, Anderson LJ. Pediatric hospitalizations for croup (laryngotracheobronchitis): Biennial increases associated with human parainfluenza virus 1 epidemics. *The Journal of Infectious Diseases*, 176(6), 1423–1427 (1997).

148. Greenberg SB, Allen M, Wilson J, Atmar RL. Respiratory viral infections in adults with and without chronic obstructive pulmonary disease. *American Journal of Respiratory and Critical Care Medicine*, 162(1), 167–173 (2000).

149. Palmenberg AC, Gern JE. Classification and evolution of human rhinoviruses. *Methods in Molecular Biology*, 1221, 1–10 (2015).

150. Turner RB, Wecker MT, Pohl G et al. Efficacy of tremacamra, a soluble intercellular adhesion molecule 1, for experimental rhinovirus infection: A randomized clinical trial. *Journal of the American Medical Association*, 281(19), 1797–1804 (1999).

151. Mediratta PK, Sharma KK, Verma V. A review on recent development of common cold therapeutic agents. *Indian Journal of Medical Sciences*, 54(11), 485–490 (2000).

152. Smee DF, Alaghamandan HA, Ramasamy K, Revankar GR. Broad-spectrum activity of 8-chloro-7-deazaguanosine against RNA virus infections in mice and rats. *Antiviral Research*, 26(2), 203–209 (1995).

153. Smee DF, Alaghamandan HA, Cottam HB, Jolley WB, Robins RK. Antiviral activity of the novel immune modulator 7-thia-8-oxoguanosine. *Journal of Biological Response Modifiers*, 9(1), 24–32 (1990).

154. Randomised trial of efficacy and safety of inhaled zanamivir in treatment of influenza A and B virus infections. The MIST (Management of Influenza in the Southern Hemisphere Trialists) Study Group. *Lancet*, 352(9144), 1877–1881 (1998).

155. Ishibashi Y, Inouye Y, Taniguchi A. Expression and role of sugar chains on airway mucus during the exacerbation of airway inflammation. *Yakugaku zasshi: Journal of the Pharmaceutical Society of Japan*, 132(6), 699–704 (2012).

156. Leophonte P. Infections in chronic obstructive pulmonary disease. *Bulletin de l'Academie nationale de medecine*, 188(1), 47–64; discussion 64–66 (2004).
157. BioCryst Pharmaceuticals I. Peramivr Package Label. FDA, (2014). http://www. accessdata.fda.gov/drugsatfda_docs/label/2014/206426lbl.pdf.
158. Li F, Ma C, Wang J. Inhibitors targeting the influenza virus hemagglutinin. *Current Medicinal Chemistry*, 22(11), 1361–1382 (2015).
159. Spanakis N, Pitiriga V, Gennimata V, Tsakris A. A review of neuraminidase inhibitor susceptibility in influenza strains. *Expert Review of Anti-Infective Therapy*, 12(11), 1325–1336 (2014).
160. Boltz DA, Aldridge JR, Jr., Webster RG, Govorkova EA. Drugs in development for influenza. *Drugs*, 70(11), 1349–1362 (2010).
161. Moorthy NS, Poongavanam V, Pratheepa V. Viral M2 ion channel protein: A promising target for anti-influenza drug discovery. *Mini Reviews in Medicinal Chemistry*, 14(10), 819–830 (2014).
162. Panozzo J, Oh DY, Margo K et al. Evaluation of a dry powder delivery system for laninamivir in a ferret model of influenza infection. *Antiviral Research*, 120, 66–71 (2015).
163. Yoshihara K, Ishizuka H, Kubo Y. Population pharmacokinetics of laninamivir and its prodrug laninamivir octanoate in healthy subjects and in adult and pediatric patients with influenza virus infection. *Drug Metabolism and Pharmacokinetics*, 28(5), 416–426 (2013).
164. Stephen EL, Walker JS, Dominik JW, Young HW, Berendt RF. Aerosol therapy of influenza infections of mice and primates with rimantadine, ribavirin, and related compounds. *Annals of the New York Academy of Sciences*, 284, 264–271 (1977).
165. Makarov VA, Braun H, Richter M et al. Pyrazolopyrimidines: Potent inhibitors targeting the capsid of rhino- and enteroviruses. *ChemMedChem*, 10, 1629–1634, (2015).
166. Bernard A, Lacroix C, Cabiddu MG, Neyts J, Leyssen P, Pompei R. Exploration of the anti-enterovirus activity of a series of pleconaril/pirodavir-like compounds. *Antiviral Chemistry & Chemotherapy*, 24(2), 56–61, (2015).
167. De Clercq E. Highlights in antiviral drug research: Antivirals at the horizon. *Medicinal Research Reviews*, 33(6), 1215–1248 (2013).
168. Fechner H, Pinkert S, Geisler A, Poller W, Kurreck J. Pharmacological and biological antiviral therapeutics for cardiac coxsackievirus infections. *Molecules*, 16(10), 8475–8503 (2011).
169. Abzug MJ. The enteroviruses: Problems in need of treatments. *The Journal of Infection*, 68(Suppl. 1), S108–S114 (2014).
170. Jensen LM, Walker EJ, Jans DA, Ghildyal R. Proteases of human rhinovirus: Role in infection. *Methods in Molecular Biology*, 1221, 129–141 (2015).
171. Mello C, Aguayo E, Rodriguez M et al. Multiple classes of antiviral agents exhibit *in vitro* activity against human rhinovirus type C. *Antimicrobial Agents and Chemotherapy*, 58(3), 1546–1555 (2014).
172. Zhang X, Song Z, Qin B et al. Rupintrivir is a promising candidate for treating severe cases of enterovirus-71 infection: Evaluation of antiviral efficacy in a murine infection model. *Antiviral Research*, 97(3), 264–269 (2013).
173. Lin HL, Harwood RJ, Fink JB, Goodfellow LT, Ari A. *In vitro* comparison of aerosol delivery using different face masks and flow rates with a high-flow humidity system. *Respiratory Care*, 60(9), 1215–1219 (2015).
174. Kleinstreuer C, Feng Y, Childress E. Drug-targeting methodologies with applications: A review. *World Journal of Clinical Cases*, 2(12), 742–756 (2014).
175. Cheng YS. Mechanisms of pharmaceutical aerosol deposition in the respiratory tract. *AAPS PharmSciTech*, 15(3), 630–640 (2014).
176. Myers TR. Year in review 2014: Aerosol delivery devices. *Respiratory Care*, 60(8), 1190–1196 (2015).

177. Merkel OM, Rubinstein I, Kissel T. siRNA Delivery to the lung: What's new? *Advanced Drug Delivery Reviews*, 0, 112–128 (2014).
178. Ari A, Atalay OT, Harwood R, Sheard MM, Aljamhan EA, Fink JB. Influence of nebulizer type, position, and bias flow on aerosol drug delivery in simulated pediatric and adult lung models during mechanical ventilation. *Respiratory Care*, 55(7), 845–851 (2010).
179. Myers TR. The science guiding selection of an aerosol delivery device. *Respiratory Care*, 58(11), 1963–1973 (2013).
180. Londahl J, Moller W, Pagels JH, Kreyling WG, Swietlicki E, Schmid O. Measurement techniques for respiratory tract deposition of airborne nanoparticles: A critical review. *Journal of Aerosol Medicine and Pulmonary Drug Delivery*, 27(4), 229–254 (2014).
181. Sanchis J, Corrigan C, Levy ML, Viejo JL, Group A. Inhaler devices—From theory to practice. *Respiratory Medicine*, 107(4), 495–502 (2013).
182. Dunbar C, Mitchell J. Analysis of cascade impactor mass distributions. *Journal of Aerosol Medicine: The Official Journal of the International Society for Aerosols in Medicine*, 18(4), 439–451 (2005).
183. Misra A, Jinturkar K, Patel D, Lalani J, Chougule M. Recent advances in liposomal dry powder formulations: Preparation and evaluation. *Expert Opinion on Drug Delivery*, 6(1), 71–89 (2009).
184. Tellier R. Review of aerosol transmission of influenza A virus. *Emerging Infectious Diseases*, 12(11), 1657–1662 (2006).
185. Denyer J, Dyche T. The Adaptive Aerosol Delivery (AAD) technology: Past, present, and future. *Journal of Aerosol Medicine and Pulmonary Drug Delivery*, 23(Suppl. 1), S1–S10 (2010).
186. Zheng M, Librizzi D, Kılıç A et al. Enhancing *in vivo* circulation and siRNA delivery with biodegradable polyethylenimine-graft-polycaprolactone-block-poly(ethylene glycol) copolymers. *Biomaterials*, 33(27), 6551–6558 (2012).
187. Martin AR, Finlay WH. Nebulizers for drug delivery to the lungs. *Expert Opinion on Drug Delivery*, 12(6), 889–900 (2015).
188. Djupesland PG, Skretting A. Nasal deposition and clearance in man: Comparison of a bidirectional powder device and a traditional liquid spray pump. *Journal of Aerosol Medicine and Pulmonary Drug Delivery*, 25(5), 280–289 (2012).
189. Chen C, Przedpelski A, Tepp WH, Pellett S, Johnson EA, Barbieri JT. Heat-labile enterotoxin IIa, a platform to deliver heterologous proteins into neurons. *mBio*, 6(4), e00734 (2015).
190. Jefferson T, Di Pietrantonj C, Rivetti A, Bawazeer GA, Al-Ansary LA, Ferroni E. Vaccines for preventing influenza in healthy adults. *The Cochrane Database of Systematic Reviews*, 3, CD001269 (2014).
191. Diaz-Ortega JL, Bennett JV, Castaneda D, Martinez D, Fernandez de Castro J. Aerosolized MMR vaccine: Evaluating potential transmission of components to vaccine administrators and contacts of vaccinees. *Biologicals*, 40(4), 278–281 (2012).
192. Chokephaibulkit K, Perng GC. Challenges for the formulation of a universal vaccine against dengue. *Experimental Biology and Medicine*, 238(5), 566–578 (2013).
193. Su YC, Townsend D, Herrero LJ et al. Dual proinflammatory and antiviral properties of pulmonary eosinophils in respiratory syncytial virus vaccine-enhanced disease. *Journal of Virology*, 89(3), 1564–1578 (2015).
194. Kapikian AZ, Mitchell RH, Chanock RM, Shvedoff RA, Stewart CE. An epidemiologic study of altered clinical reactivity to respiratory syncytial (RS) virus infection in children previously vaccinated with an inactivated RS virus vaccine. *American Journal of Epidemiology*, 89(4), 405–421 (1969).
195. Rey GU, Miao C, Caidi H et al. Decrease in formalin-inactivated respiratory syncytial virus (FI-RSV) enhanced disease with RSV G glycoprotein peptide immunization in BALB/c mice. *PLOS ONE*, 8(12), e83075 (2013).

196. Radu GU, Caidi H, Miao C, Tripp RA, Anderson LJ, Haynes LM. Prophylactic treatment with a G glycoprotein monoclonal antibody reduces pulmonary inflammation in respiratory syncytial virus (RSV)-challenged naive and formalin-inactivated RSV-immunized BALB/c mice. *Journal of Virology*, 84(18), 9632–9636 (2010).

197. Haynes LM, Jones LP, Barskey A, Anderson LJ, Tripp RA. Enhanced disease and pulmonary eosinophilia associated with formalin-inactivated respiratory syncytial virus vaccination are linked to G glycoprotein CX3C-CX3CR1 interaction and expression of substance P. *Journal of Virology*, 77(18), 9831–9844 (2003).

198. Wei J, Chen H, An J. Recent progress in dengue vaccine development. *Virologica Sinica*, 29(6), 353–363 (2014).

199. Yauch LE, Shresta S. Dengue virus vaccine development. *Advances in Virus Research*, 88, 315–372 (2014).

200. Shriver Z, Trevejo JM, Sasisekharan R. Antibody-based strategies to prevent and treat influenza. *Frontiers in Immunology*, 6, 315 (2015).

201. Barban V, Munoz-Jordan JL, Santiago GA et al. Broad neutralization of wild-type dengue virus isolates following immunization in monkeys with a tetravalent dengue vaccine based on chimeric yellow fever 17D/dengue viruses. *Virology*, 429(2), 91–98 (2012).

202. Guy B, Guirakhoo F, Barban V, Higgs S, Monath TP, Lang J. Preclinical and clinical development of YFV 17D-based chimeric vaccines against dengue, West Nile and Japanese encephalitis viruses. *Vaccine*, 28(3), 632–649 (2010).

203. Mantis NJ, Morici LA, Roy CJ. Mucosal vaccines for biodefense. *Current Topics in Microbiology and Immunology*, 354, 181–195 (2012).

204. Willson DF. Aerosolized surfactants, anti-inflammatory drugs, and analgesics. *Respiratory Care*, 60(6), 774–790; discussion 790–793 (2015).

205. Agu RU, Ugwoke MI, Armand M, Kinget R, Verbeke N. The lung as a route for systemic delivery of therapeutic proteins and peptides. *Respiratory Research*, 2(4), 198–209 (2001).

206. Hagenaars N, Mastrobattista E, Glansbeek H et al. Head-to-head comparison of four nonadjuvanted inactivated cell culture-derived influenza vaccines: Effect of composition, spatial organization and immunization route on the immunogenicity in a murine challenge model. *Vaccine*, 26(51), 6555–6563 (2008).

207. Thiam F, Charpilienne A, Poncet D, Kohli E, Basset C. B subunits of cholera toxin and thermolabile enterotoxin of Escherichia coli have similar adjuvant effect as whole molecules on rotavirus 2/6-VLP specific antibody responses and induce a Th17-like response after intrarectal immunization. *Microbial Pathogenesis*, 89, 27–34 (2015).

208. Claus S, Weiler C, Schiewe J, Friess W. How can we bring high drug doses to the lung? *European Journal of Pharmaceutics and Biopharmaceutics*, 86(1), 1–6 (2014).

209. Labiris NR, Dolovich MB. Pulmonary drug delivery. Part I: Physiological factors affecting therapeutic effectiveness of aerosolized medications. *British Journal of Clinical Pharmacology*, 56(6), 588–599 (2003).

210. Griffin DE. Current progress in pulmonary delivery of measles vaccine. *Expert Review of Vaccines*, 13(6), 751–759 (2014).

211. Lin W-H, Griffin DE, Rota PA et al. Successful respiratory immunization with dry powder live-attenuated measles virus vaccine in rhesus macaques. *Proceedings of the National Academy of Sciences of the United States of America*, 108(7), 2987–2992 (2011).

7 Pulmonary Delivery of Antibiotics for Respiratory Infections

Qi (Tony) Zhou, Li Qu, and Hak-Kim Chan

CONTENTS

INTRODUCTION

Respiratory infections are one of the major health problems. Lower respiratory infections were the fourth leading cause of death worldwide and the top leading cause of death in the low-income countries in 2012 (WHO 2014). In 2012, approximately 3.1 million lives were taken by lower respiratory infections. Besides the high mortality and morbidity rates, respiratory infections are also responsible for increasing financial burden to the healthcare system (Birnbaum et al. 2002). The discovery of antibiotics has saved billions of lives from infections, including those occurring in the airways. However, since the 1990s, there has been a marked decline in the discovery of new antibiotics, and unfortunately, this is accompanied by a significant increase in resistance to current antibiotics. We are facing a growing threat from the emergence of bacteria that are resistant to almost all available antibiotics (Boucher et al. 2013). Antimicrobial resistance has been identified by the World Health Organization as one of the three greatest threats to human health (Infectious Diseases Society of America 2010).

The most common practice for the treatment of respiratory infections is oral or parenteral administration of antibiotics to the patients. However, these traditional therapies may not be efficient to generate effective drug concentration in the airways. Consequently, high doses of antibiotics are required to provide local drug concentrations above the minimum inhibitory concentration (MIC) to kill the bacteria. Such high doses could result in serious systemic toxicity. For example, parenteral administration of colistin (a polypeptide antibiotic) resulted in severe nephrotoxicity in up to 50% of cystic fibrosis (CF) patients in the clinical studies (Garonzik et al. 2011b, Sandri et al. 2013). Alternatively, inhalation therapy has recently gained increasing interests to deliver antimicrobials directly to the infection sites. Both preclinical and clinical studies have demonstrated that through inhalation, drug concentrations in the airways can be significantly higher with a remarkable reduction in systemic exposure compared to parenteral administrations (Velkov et al. 2015). Such high exposure of drug at the sites of infection is well transferred into maximized antimicrobial efficacy and decreased systemic exposure (Velkov et al. 2015).

Nowadays, inhalation as the route to deliver some antibiotics has been recognized as a safe and efficacious way against respiratory infections (Zhou et al. 2014c). There are a few inhaled antibiotic products approved by the regulatory agencies. Inhaled tobramycin nebulization and dry powder were approved in the United States, inhaled aztreonam solution was also approved in the United States, while inhaled colistimethate sodium (CMS) nebulization and dry powder were approved in some European countries. There are also some other inhaled antibiotics in the late stage of development (Tables 7.1 and 7.2). Most of the approved and developed inhaled

TABLE 7.1
Development Status of the Nebulized Antibiotic Products

Drug	Brand Name	Manufacturer	Approval Status	Dose (mg)
Amikacin	ARIKACE®	Insmed	Clinical trial Phase 1b/2a	280, 560
		Bayer	Clinical trial Phase 3	400
Amikacin + Fosfomycin		Cardeas	Clinical trial Phase 2	300 + 120
Aztreonam	Cayston®	Gilead	Approved	75
Ciprofloxacin	Lipoquin®	Aradigm	Clinical trial Phase 2	150
	Pulmaquin®	Aradigm	Clinical trial Phase 3	210
Colistimethate sodium	Promixin®	Profile	Approved	80
Levofloxacin	Aeroquin™	Aptalis	Clinical trial Phase 3	240
Tobramycin	Bethkis®	Cornerstone	Approved	300
	Bramitob®	Chiesi	Approved	300
	Fluidosome™	Axentis	Clinical trial Phase 2	150/300
	TOBI®	Novartis	Approved	300
Tobramycin + Fosfomycin	FTI	Gilead	Clinical trial Phase 2	20 + 80/40 + 160

Note: Data are collected from the website of either the corresponding company or ClinicalTrials.gov.

TABLE 7.2

Development Status of Dry Powder Inhaler Antibiotic Products

Drug	Brand Name	Manufacturer	Approval Status	Dose (mg)
Ciprofloxacin		Bayer	Clinical trial Phase 2	32.5
Colistimethate sodium	Colobreathe®	Forest	Approved	125
Tobramycin	TOBI® Podhaler®	Novartis	Approved	112
Vancomycin	AeroVanc™	Savara	Clinical trial Phase 2	32/64

Note: Data are collected from the website of either the corresponding company or ClinicalTrials.gov.

antibiotic products aim for infections in CF patients. CF is a genetic disease, and one of its clinical manifestations is thick mucus in the airways along with compromised mucociliary clearance. Infections are prone to occur in the lungs of CF patients, and the bacteria are difficult or even impossible to be eradicated. Antimicrobial resistance is easy to develop in these recurring infections, and thus, periodic or long-term antibiotic treatments are necessary to prolong the lifetime and quality of life of CF patients. Long-term use of parenteral antibiotics can cause severe systemic toxicities, but inhalation therapy can solve this problem to a large extent by reducing the systemic exposure. Noteworthily, the research of inhaled antibiotics for CF patients mainly focuses on clinical studies; there is a lack of fundamental understanding on the drug distribution, transport, action, and local cytotoxicity in the airways at the molecular level. Future works in these areas are needed to understand the drug delivery process and to optimize inhalation therapy of antimicrobials. This is particularly important as inhaled therapy for respiratory infection has expanded beyond CF into non-CF bronchiectasis (Sugianto and Chan, 2015).

There are three main forms of inhalation products: nebulizer, pressurized metered dose inhaler (pMDI), and dry powder inhaler (DPI). pMDI was popular in the past to deliver low-dose medications for asthma or chronic obstructive pulmonary diseases. However, pMDI is not able to deliver high-dose drugs such as antibiotics. In contrast, nebulizer and DPI have been successfully used to administer antibiotics to the lungs. In general, traditional nebulizers such as jet nebulizers are bulking and have low delivery efficacy. Newer nebulization devices such as mesh vibrating or ultrasonic devices can be much smaller and have higher delivery efficiency; on the other hand, the cost can be a concern particularly for the low-income countries (Zhou et al. 2014c). DPI is promising to deliver high-dose antimicrobials into the respiratory tract, while there is a concern on the local adverse effects induced by inhaling high-dose powders. The pros and cons of each type of devices are discussed in this chapter.

NEBULIZATION

Inhaling wet aerosols of antibiotic solution produced by a nebulizer has become a common clinical treatment for respiratory infections in the patients with CF. In principle, antibiotics are dissolved or suspended in an isotonic solvent. An external mechanical or electric energy is applied to break up the liquid and form aerosols.

Jet nebulizers are the most common type of device utilizing compressed air or oxygen to aerosolize drug solutions at high velocities. The conventional jet nebulizers are bulky and generally have low drug delivery efficiency. The proportion of the drug delivered to lower airways can be as low as <20% of the loaded dose using a jet nebulizer (Reychler et al. 2004).

However, with the technological advances in nebulizer design, delivery efficiency and device portability have been considerably improved. Vibrating mesh nebulizers, which have minimal residual volume and rapid output, utilize a vibrating membrane with holes sized 1000–7000 μm to extrude the liquid through these holes to generate the drug aerosol. Digital software control of vibrating mesh nebulization, such as in the I-neb Adaptive Aerosol Delivery nebulizer system, can further improve the drug deposition by optimizing the drug release during the inhalation cycle. Nebulization of radiolabeled diethylenetriaminepentaacetic acid in normal saline solution by the I-neb achieved an FPFemitted (<4.6 μm) of 56.8% in an *in vitro* study (Nikander et al. 2010).

Traditional nebulization of antibiotics requires a relatively long administration time. As the antibiotic doses are usually more than 100 mg, the administration time can be over 20 min depending on the dose and concentration. Commercial nebulization products such as TOBI® (tobramycin) or Cayston® (aztreonam) contain highly concentrated drug solutions (>50 mg/mL) to reduce the volume and administration time (Coates et al. 2011).

For nebulized antibiotic products, so far, only tobramycin and aztreonam were approved in the United States. Colistin methanesulfonate (also known as colistimethate sodium) was approved only in some European countries. Other antibiotics are under development in the clinical trial Phase II or Phase III including amikacin, ciprofloxacin, and levofloxacin (Table 7.1). Most inhaled antibiotic products focus on the treatment of chronic respiratory infections such as in patients with CF. Clinical *in vivo* data have shown that inhaled antibiotics can decrease the colonization of the difficult-to-treat Gram-negative bacteria such as *Pseudomonas aeruginosa* and delay the onset of infections (Hoiby 2011). Consequently, improved lung function and quality of life can be achieved along with reduced numbers of morbidity and hospital admission. Nebulized antibiotics can also be used for non-CF bronchiectasis although no product has yet been approved for such indication. One possible adverse effect for non-CF bronchiectasis treatment is irritation, which may cause bronchospasm, cough, and wheeze. Pretreatment with bronchodilator or encapsulated drugs in liposomes may reduce the chance of such adverse effects (Cipolla and Chan 2013).

Pharmacokinetic studies have shown that local drug concentrations in the respiratory tract by inhaled therapy are much higher than those by parenteral administrations. Colistin is a typical example that is suitable for inhalation therapy. It is the last-line antibiotic for multidrug-resistant Gram-negative "superbugs" but can cause severe nephrotoxicity and neurotoxicity when administrated parenterally at high doses (Garonzik et al. 2011a). Ratjen et al. has reported in a clinical study of CF patients that the inhaled therapy obtained higher colistin concentrations (C_{max} 40 mg/L) in sputum and colistin concentrations were maintained above MICs for 12 h; negligible serum C_{max} 0.15 mg/L (Ratjen et al. 2006) was measured compared to intravenous administration (serum C_{max} 3–5 mg/L, $T_{1/2}$ 7.5 h) (Markou et al. 2008). High drug concentrations at the local infection sites are critical to reduce the total drug dose, to minimize the systemic adverse effects, and to reduce the risk of drug resistance.

The benefits of inhaled antibiotics are more obvious for the CF patients in whom biofilm formation is a common phenomenon. In the biofilms, bacteria are protected by a dense polysaccharide matrix, which prevents or decreases the penetration of antibiotics. As a result, the minimum biofilm inhibitory concentrations are generally several folds higher than the MICs of the planktonic bacteria. Direct delivery of antibiotics to the respiratory infection sites generates a much higher local drug concentration to offer enhanced antibiofilm activity. The superior antibiofilm effects of inhaled therapy can be further enhanced by advanced formulation strategies such as liposomes or polymeric nanoparticles (Yang et al. 2012).

DPI

DPIs allow the administration of high-dose antibiotics. Most DPI devices are in portable sizes and convenient to carry (Zhou et al. 2014c). Drugs and excipients are present in a powder form, which is generally more stable than solutions or suspensions. Administration of DPI can be achieved within 1–2 min. These advantages provide superior patient compliance as exemplified by CMS and tobramycin DPIs (Geller et al. 2007). Passive DPI devices require the inspiration airflow generated by the patients to aerosolize the powder and thus are not suitable to deliver powder aerosols to infants and incubated patients. Recently, a novel powder aerosol system has been developed to administer high doses (up to 320 mg) of mannitol powder from a passive DPI to the distal end of tracheal tubes in critically ill patients (Tang et al. 2011, Chan et al. 2012) (Figure 7.1).

DPI DEVICES

Only one antibiotic DPI of tobramycin (TOBI® Podhaler®) has been approved in the United States. DPI of CMS (Colobreathe®) was only approved in Europe. Two more (ciprofloxacin and vancomycin) are in the advanced development stage (Table 7.2). Both approved antibiotic DPIs of TOBI Podhaler and Colobreathe are using single-dose reloadable capsule-based devices with drug powders packaged and stored separately. Multidose inhalers are not suitable for high-dose antibiotics because accommodating a large amount of powder inside the inhaler would make the device too bulky to handle. In Colobreathe, each capsule contains 125 mg of colistimethate sodium powder. A single inhalation may not complete the dose; multiple inhalations are often needed. In TOBI Podhaler, 28 mg of drug is prefilled in a capsule and four capsules are administrated sequentially (112 mg per dose). One concern on the usage of this product is that it requires repeating procedures for four capsules, which is an onerous process for patients with a higher risk of misuse. Another device, Orbital® inhaler, could also deliver 200 mg of powder by multiple inhalations. High emitted

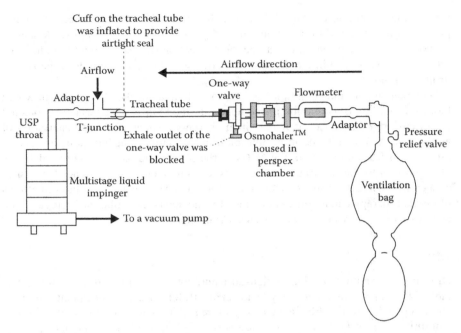

FIGURE 7.1 Experimental setup to determine the dose and particle size distribution of mannitol aerosol coming out from the tracheal tube via a novel powder aerosol delivery system designed for the incubated patients. (Reprinted from Tang, P. et al., *J. Aerosol Med. Pulmon. Drug Deliv.*, 24(1), 1, 2011. With permission from Mary Ann Liebert, Inc.)

doses (>90%) were obtained within <10 inhalations for the spray-dried ciprofloxacin or mannitol powders (Young et al. 2014). In addition, single-use disposable devices have been developed for antibiotics. Twincer® is a disposable device used to deliver colistin for CF patients and has potential also for antituberculosis formulations. It has only three simple parts and can be easily assembled. A multiple air classifier technology is built in the Twincer for powder dispersion (de Boer et al. 2006).

POWDER PRODUCTION AND PARTICLE ENGINEERING

Milling is a common technique to produce fine drug powder for inhalation, but the milled powder is generally cohesive since the new surfaces generated during milling usually have high surface free energy. Manufacturing of such cohesive drug powders is highly challenging due to their poor flowability, fluidization, and dispersion performance (Zhou et al. 2010b). In industrial practice, milled drug particles are blended with coarse carriers (notably lactose) to improve their manufacturability (Zhou and Morton 2012). For low-dose products such as most of the bronchodilators and steroids, carriers are also used as a filler to promote the manufacturing. However, for high-dose DPIs, high aerosol efficiency is preferred to minimize drug dose. It has been reported the FPF of a jet-milled colistin powder with lactose carrier was around 40% when aerosolized using a Cyclohaler®

(de Boer et al. 2002). When using a more efficient device such as the Twincer, the aerosol performance of CMS formulation containing jet-milled drug powder was improved with an FPF of 59%–67% of the loaded dose (10–50 mg) (de Boer et al. 2012, Grasmeijer et al. 2012). Nevertheless, in these two studies, mass losses (drug deposited on inhaler and USP induction port) were as high as 26.3%–29.1% even when coarse lactose powder (2 mg) was added as carrier (de Boer et al. 2012, Grasmeijer et al. 2012).

Particle engineering has been extensively explored to reduce powder cohesion and improve aerosolization (Lin et al. 2015). One of the effective strategies to reduce cohesion of milled drug powders is to coat high-surface-energy surfaces with low-surface-energy materials (Qu and Morton 2015). Such materials are also called force control agents and typically are pharmaceutical lubricants such as magnesium stearate (Zhou et al. 2010c). Magnesium stearate is highly hydrophobic and has low surface energy. Importantly, magnesium stearate is generally considered safe for inhalation and its use has been approved in commercial products such as Pulmicort®, CFC-free metered dose inhaler, and Foradil® Certihaler®. Attributable to the laminar structure and hydrophobicity of magnesium stearate, a low-surface-energy coating layer of coating materials with a relatively large particle size can form on the fine drug particles by means of high-shear dry coating (Zhou et al. 2013b). Traditional low-shear blending cannot offer sufficient shear and energy to deagglomerate the cohesive powder and to delaminate the magnesium stearate on the cohesive particle surface (Zhou et al. 2010a). Via high-shear dry coating, strong agglomerates of cohesive drug powder can be broken and surface of individual particles can be exposed and coated (Zhou et al. 2010a). Zhou et al. demonstrated after coating jet-milled drug particles with only 1% w/w of magnesium stearate, FPF was increased significantly for salbutamol sulfate (51.4%–68.6%), salmeterol xinafoate (59.9%–73.1%), and triamcinolone acetonide (26.4%–48.3%). Such enhancement in aerosol performance was contributable to the reduced surface energy and powder cohesion (Zhou et al. 2011). Advanced surface chemistry characterization measurements of x-ray photoelectron spectroscopy (XPS) and time-of-flight secondary ion mass spectrometry (ToF-SIMS) indicated the importance of coating parameters on coating quality and formulation performance (Zhou et al. 2013b). Another technique, co-jet-milling, also showed its potential to coat inhalable drug particles with magnesium stearate (Stank and Steckel 2013).

Spray-drying is attractive to produce fine drug powders for inhalation purpose by both academic and industrial scientists (Lin et al. 2015). In the pharmaceutical industry, spray-drying has become popular in manufacturing DPI products, as evidenced by the production of inhaled insulin (Exubera®), mannitol (Aridol®), and tobramycin (TOBI Podhaler). Since spray-drying is a continuous manufacturing process, the production efficiency can be improved and cost of the products can be reduced. Another advantage of spray-drying technique is its ability to manipulate the particle properties to achieve high aerosol performance. The operating conditions and formulations can be adjusted to produce spherical (Chew et al. 2005), porous (Geller et al. 2011), wrinkled (Chew et al. 2005, Zhou et al. 2014a), and dimpled (Master 1991, Vehring et al. 2007) particles, which have reduced contact areas and minimized interparticulate attractive forces. For example, Zhou et al. has spray-dried a colistin powder without adding any external excipient. The spray-dried colistin particles have rough surfaces and relatively high aerosol performance (FPFtotal > 82%) (Zhou et al. 2013a). Co-spray-drying of colistin and rifampicin without any excipients has also produced wrinkled particles with enhanced antimicrobial activity, high aerosol efficiency (FPFtotal > 90%), and moisture protection (Zhou et al. 2014b). In this study, XPS and ToF-SIMS have confirmed a coating layer of hydrophobic rifampicin on the colistin particle surface, which may also contribute to the high FPF of the formulation. An inhalable powder formulation of combination antituberculosis drugs containing rifapentine, moxifloxacin, and pyrazinamide was also prepared via spray-drying (Lee et al. 2013). In this study, addition of 10% (w/w) leucine was demonstrated to avoid recrystallization of pyrazinamide after storage (Lee et al. 2013) (Figure 7.2).

Addition of functional excipients in the spray-drying feed solution or suspension allows flexible engineering of particles. The excipients can either serve as a filler for low-dose drugs or act as an aerosolization enhancer. For example, spray-dried mannitol has been developed as a commercial DPI for asthma diagnosis (Aridol); on the other hand, the spherical and hollow microparticles of spray-dried mannitol can also act as a carrier for low-dose therapeutics such as peptide (Liang et al. 2014), siRNA (Liang et al. 2015), or combination of two small-molecule drugs (Kumon et al. 2010). Co-spray-drying of antibiotics with mannitol was shown to reduce the moisture absorption of the composite powder (Adi et al. 2010). Leucine is a well-known aerosolization enhancer. A relatively small amount of leucine (typically 5%–20% w/w) may result in a significant improvement in emitted dose and FPF (Rabbani and Seville 2005). Such reductions in cohesion and improvement in flowability and dispersion are the consequences of enrichment of low-surface-energy leucine on the spray-dried particle surface, supported by IGC, XPS, and ToF-SIMS data (Mangal et al. 2015). It is interesting to note in a recent study, the spray-dried pure colistin powder had a much higher emitted dose and FPF than the jet-milled powder; surprisingly, addition of leucine (20% w/w) did not further improve the aerosol performance (Jong et al. 2015). The mechanism of such abnormal phenomenon is unknown but was proposed due to the self-assembling behavior of amphiphilic colistin molecules. IGC data showed spray-dried colistin particles have surface free energy levels similar to that of leucine-coated particles, but a much higher surface free energy than the jet-milled colistin (Jong et al. 2015).

Porous particles have been used for inhalation because they have relatively large physical sizes, which promote the flowability; also they exhibit small aerodynamic sizes due to low density, which are favorable for aerosolization (Edwards et al. 1997). Innovation in production of porous inhalable particles has been soon transferred to the products. In the first marketed antibiotic DPI product, TOBI Podhaler, tobramycin porous particles are generated by spray-drying emulsion via PulmoSphere™ technology (Geller et al. 2011). By using this innovative porous-particle production technique, consistent aerosol performance can be achieved for the high-dose

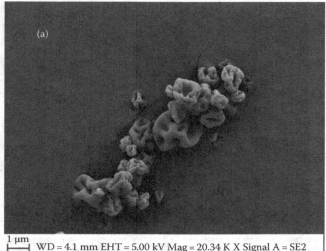

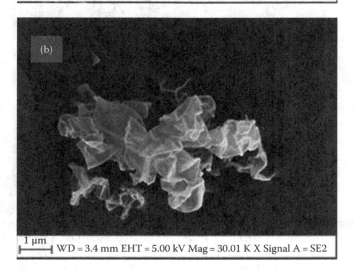

FIGURE 7.2 Scanning electron microscopy images of spray-dried powder formulations of (a) pure colistin. (From Zhou, Q., Morton, D., Yu, H.H., Jacob, J., Wang, J.P., Li, J., and Chan, H.K.: Colistin powders with high aerosolisation efficiency for respiratory infection: Preparation and *in vitro* evaluation. *J. Pharm. Sci.* 2013a. 102(10). 3736–3747. Copyright Wiley-VCH Verlag GmbH & Co. KGaA. Reproduced with permission.) (b) Combination of colistin and rifampicin. (With kind permission from Springer Science+Business Media: *AAPS J.*, Synergistic antibiotic combination powders of colistin and rifampicin provide high aerosolization efficiency and moisture protection, 16(1), 2014, 37–47, Zhou, Q.T., Gengenbach, T, Denman, J.A., Yu Heidi, H., Li, J., and Chan, H.K.)   (*Continued*)

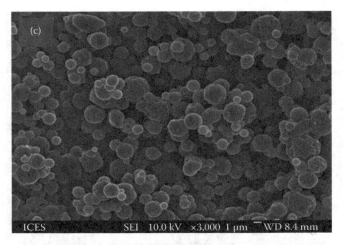

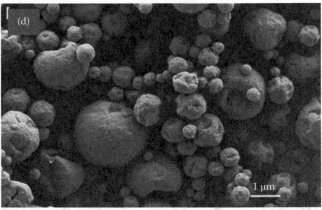

FIGURE 7.2 (*Continued*)   Scanning electron microscopy images of spray-dried powder formulations of (c) Combination of ciprofloxacin hydrochloride, gatifloxacin hydrochloride, and lysozyme. (Reprinted from *Eur. J. Pharm. Biopharm.*, 83(2), Lee, S.H., Teo, J., Heng, D., Ng, W.K., Chan, H.-K., and Tan, R.B.H., Synergistic combination dry powders for inhaled antimicrobial therapy: Formulation, characterization and *in vitro* evaluation, 275–284. Copyright 2013, with permission from Elsevier.) (d) Combination of moxifloxacin, rifa-pentine, pyrazinamide, and leucine. (Reprint from *Eur. J. Pharm. Biopharm.*, 83(2), Chan, J.G.Y., Chan, H.-K., Prestidge, C.A., Denman, J.A., Young, P.M., and Traini, D., A novel dry powder inhalable formulation incorporating three first-line anti-tubercular antibiotics, 285–292. Copyright 2013, with permission from Elsevier.)

antibiotic powders at different airflow rates (40–85 L/min), humidity (10%–65%), and temperatures (10°C–40°C) (Haynes et al. 2010), which is attributed to their superior flowability and aerosolization properties. This is a milestone for the phar-maceutical inhalation industry that novel benchtop technology can be successfully transferred to efficacious bedside products.

ADVERSE EFFECTS AND PATIENT COMPLIANCE

The main goal of using inhaled antibiotics is to maximize drug concentration in the respiratory tract and to minimize systemic exposure, therefore reducing systemic adverse effects. However, local side effects of inhaling high-dose antibiotics such as cough and throat irritation have been frequently reported in the clinical studies (Velkov et al. 2015). There is a long-term debate in the pharmaceutical inhalation industry as to what aerosol, that is, dry powder or liquid form, would cause more severe local side effects (Weers 2015). The clinical data obtained in the currently available literature are insufficient to draw a clear conclusion because a double-blind clinical trial is not feasible between two different forms. The results from different clinical studies vary largely due to the study design, evaluation method, and subject population (Table 7.3). On the other hand, the influence of delivery form on local side effects may also be drug dependent; thus, the data of one antibiotic may not be simply transferred to other antibiotics. Nevertheless, the chemical entity of the antibiotics appears to exhibit more significant impact on the local side effects than the form of delivery.

Oropharyngeal irritation and cough are the two most common adverse events upon inhalation of antibiotics. The frequency of these two side effects in the clinical trials has been reported to be associated with the chemical nature of the drug, mass of the dose, and location of drug deposition. For example, severe cough and throat irritation was reported for inhalation of colistin sulfate (Le Brun et al. 2002), while using its prodrug, CMS, has alleviated the severity of respiratory side effects (Westerman et al. 2007). Formulating inhaled antibiotics into liposomes is another plausible strategy to reduce airway irritation. The materials used for producing liposomes are mostly endogenous lipids and in general are safe and less irritative. In a randomized, double-blind, placebo-controlled clinical trial in non-CF bronchiectasis patients, Pulmaquin™ (containing liposomal and free ciprofloxacin) was even better tolerated than the liposome placebo (Serisier et al. 2013).

Another practical way to reduce the possibility of oropharyngeal irritation is to decrease the oropharyngeal deposition of the drug through optimal formulation design or to improve the performance of inhalers. To achieve a more accurate *in vitro* evaluation of oropharyngeal deposition of aerosols, a more realistic Alberta throat has been invented for use together with impactors or impingers (Mitchell et al. 2012).

ADVANCED FORMULATIONS FOR PULMONARY DELIVERY OF ANTIMICROBIALS

To achieve desirable therapeutic efficacy, advanced formulations including liposome, nanoparticle, and controlled-release systems have been explored for inhalation therapies in the past decade. The employment of such advanced formulations has potential to improve drug delivery efficiency, enhance *in vivo* efficacy, reduce adverse effects, and increase patient compliance. Some commercial inhalation products manufactured by the advanced formulation techniques are in the late development stage and not far away from regulatory approval. The usefulness of advanced formulation strategies in developing new inhalation therapies is discussed in this section.

TABLE 7.3
Cough Incidence during Use of Inhaled Antibiotics from the Clinical Trials

Drug	Formulation	Dose	Subject	Sample Size (Treatment Group)	Percentage of Cough	References
Tobramycin	DPI by PulmoSphere	300 mg/12 h	CF	46	26.1% vs. 24.4% in the placebo group	Konstan et al. (2011)
	Solution	300 mg/12 h	Bronchiectasis	37	41% vs. 24% for placebo	Barker et al. (2000)
	Solution	300 mg/12 h	CF	193	43.5	Schuster et al. (2013)
	Solution	300 mg/12 h	CF	53	9.4	Hodson et al. (2002)
Aztreonam	Solution	75 mg/12 h	CF	80	35% vs. 29.8% in the placebo group	Retsch-Bogart et al. (2009)
	Solution	75 mg/12 h and 75 mg/8 h	CF	69 for twice daily and 66 for three times daily	27.5% for twice daily and 36.4% for three times daily vs. 34.2% in the placebo group	McCoy et al. (2008)
Colistimethate sodium	DPI	125 mg/12 h	CF	186	75.4	Schuster et al. (2013)
	Nebulization	80 mg/12 h	CF	62	17.7	Hodson et al. (2002)
Ciprofloxacin	DPI by PulmoSphere	32.5 mg/single dose	Healthy adults	6	0	Stass et al. (2013a)
	DPI by PulmoSphere	32.5 mg daily, 65 mg daily and 32.5 mg/12 h	CF	6 for each dose	33% (2/6) for 32.5 mg daily and none for other two doses	Stass et al. (2013b)

Source: Reprinted from *Adv. Drug Deliv. Rev.*, 85, Velkov, T., Rahim, N.A., Zhou, Q.T., Chan, H.-K., and Li, J., Inhaled anti-infective chemotherapy for respiratory tract infections: Successes, challenges and the road ahead, 65–82. Copyright 2015, with permission from Elsevier.

LIPOSOMAL FORMULATION

The use of liposomal formulation for drug delivery in the pharmaceutical sector has been examined for a long time, with the first product of such kind, Doxil® (doxorubicin HCl liposome injection), being approved by the FDA in 1995. Twenty years later, there are two inhaled liposomal antibiotic products in the late stage of development: liposomal amikacin and ciprofloxacin. The major benefit of inhaled liposomal antibiotics is their superior tolerability profile. Clinical trials for both aforementioned antibiotics have shown the improved safety and tolerability of the liposomal products. For example, patients with nontuberculous mycobacterial lung diseases did not tolerate nonliposomal amikacin and 35% of 20 patients ceased the trial due to severe side effects such as hemoptysis, nephrotoxicity, ototoxicity, persistent dysphonia, and vertigo (Olivier et al. 2014). A Phase II, placebo-controlled, randomized study showed that inhalation of liposomal amikacin once daily was well tolerated by the non-CF bronchiectasis patients (2009).

Other advantages of liposomal antibiotic formulations are potentially enhanced antimicrobial activities and prolonged action time in the airways. Liposomes were reported to have better penetration into biofilm, hence enhanced bacterial killing (Meers et al. 2008). Furthermore, controlled release of antibiotics in the airways may be achieved by the liposomal formulation, which can be transferred to reduced dosing frequency and PK/PD benefits (Ong et al. 2014).

NANOPARTICLES

There are increasing interests to deliver drug nanoparticles to the lungs to achieve superior *in vivo* efficacy and minimized lung clearance. The rationales to design nanoparticle formulation for inhaled antibiotics include prolonged airway retention by reducing mucociliary clearance, increased solubility and dissolution rate of poorly water-soluble drugs, and superior penetration into biofilm and bacteria cells. Cefuroxime axetil nanoparticles were generated by sonoprecipitation (Dhumal et al. 2008) and high-gravity antisolvent precipitation (Heng et al. 2008) with enhanced dissolution. Polymeric antibiotic nanoparticles made of poly (lactic-co-glycolic) acid and chitosan (Abdelghany et al. 2012, Grumezescu et al. 2013) and solid lipid nanoparticles (Ghaffari et al. 2010, Varshosaz et al. 2012) have shown improved antimicrobial efficiency.

Due to the extremely small mass, there is a concern that nanosized particles may be exhaled. This problem can be solved by either holding the breath postinhalation or forming matrix microparticles. Yamasaki et al. produced a mannitol matrix microparticle containing cyclosporine nanoparticles with enhanced dissolution (Yamasaki et al. 2011). The strategy of forming inhalable matrix microparticles can also be applied to antibiotic nanoparticles.

INHALED BACTERIOPHAGE

Bacteriophage is a natural virus that infects and damages bacterial cells. The nature and mechanism of antimicrobial action by the bacteriophage are totally different to the traditional antibiotics. A benefit of bacteriophage therapy is that the virus will replicate *in vivo*. A small delivered dose of live bacteriophage can replicate to the effective dose. Facing the rapid declining number of new antibiotics and alarmingly increasing drug resistance, bacteriophage therapy can be a vital alternative to combating airway "superbugs" because bacteriophages can also evolve like bacteria.

Like many other biologics, stability of bacteriophage formulations during production, transport, and storage is a major challenge. Regarding storage, powder form is usually preferred to the liquid counterparts. There are several attempts aiming to formulate novel inhalable powders of bacteriophages as an alternative effective antimicrobial inhalation therapy (Matinkhoo et al. 2011). Apparently traditional production method by milling is not a viable option for biologics such as bacteriophage. Golshahi et al. produced a powder form of bacteriophages KS4-M and ΦKZ by lyophilization with lactose/lactoferrin (60:40, w/w) (Golshahi et al. 2011). The lyophilized powder underwent milling to produce the inhalable particle size; unfortunately, the aerosol performance of such milled powder was relatively low with an FPF of 32%–34% over the loaded dose via the Aerolizer® at 60 L/min. Further studies by the same group have utilized low-temperature spray-drying to improve aerosolization (FPF 70% via the Aerolizer at 90 L/min) and titer loss (<0.5 log) (Matinkhoo et al. 2011) for bacteriophage KS4-M, KS14, and cocktails of phages ΦKZ/D3 and ΦKZ/D3/KS4-M.

CONCLUSIONS

Respiratory infections remain a global critical health challenge. Pulmonary delivery of antimicrobials via inhalation therapy has been well accepted as an alternative or adjunctive treatment for respiratory infections. Recent advances in the design of inhaler and inhaled formulation have enabled convenient nebulization and DPI products with maximized therapeutic efficacy, minimized systemic adverse effects, and improved patient acceptability. The development of intelligent inhaled antimicrobial products will continue to play a vital role against life-threatening respiratory infections.

REFERENCES

Abdelghany, S. M., D. J. Quinn, R. J. Ingram, B. F. Gilmore, R. F. Donnelly, C. C. Taggart, and C. J. Scott. 2012. Gentamicin-loaded nanoparticles show improved antimicrobial effects towards *Pseudomonas aeruginosa* infection. *International Journal of Nanomedicine* 7:4053–4063.

Adi, H., P. M. Young, H.-K. Chan, H. Agus, and D. Traini. 2010. Co-spray-dried mannitol–ciprofloxacin dry powder inhaler formulation for cystic fibrosis and chronic obstructive pulmonary disease. *European Journal of Pharmaceutical Sciences* 40(3):239–247.

Barker, A. F., L. Couch, S. B. Fiel, M. H. Gotfried, J. Ilowite, K. C. Meyer, A. O'Donnell et al. 2000. Tobramycin solution for inhalation reduces sputum *Pseudomonas aeruginosa* density in bronchiectasis. *American Journal of Respiratory and Critical Care Medicine* 162:481–485.

Birnbaum, H. G., M. Morley, P. E. Greenberg, and G. L. Colice. 2002. Economic burden of respiratory infections in an employed population. *Chest* 122(2):603–611.

Boucher, H. W., G. H. Talbot, D. K. Benjamin, Jr., J. Bradley, R. J. Guidos, R. N. Jones, B. E. Murray, R. A. Bonomo, D. Gilbert, and Infectious Diseases Society of America. 2013. 10 × '20 progress-development of new drugs active against gram-negative bacilli: An update from the IDSA. *Clinical Infectious Diseases* 56(12):1685–1694.

Chan, H.-K., D. Rajbhandari, P. Tang, J. D. Brannan, and P. Phipps. 2012. Safety of administering dry powder mannitol to stimulate sputum clearance in intubated intensive care patients with sputum retention: A pilot study. *American Journal of Respiratory and Critical Care Medicine* 185:A6809.

Chan, J. G. Y., H.-K. Chan, C. A. Prestidge, J. A. Denman, P. M. Young, and D. Traini. 2013. A novel dry powder inhalable formulation incorporating three first-line antitubercular antibiotics. *European Journal of Pharmaceutics and Biopharmaceutics* 83(2):285–292.

Chew, N. Y. K, P. Tang, H.-K. Chan, and J. A. Raper. 2005. How much particle surface corrugation is sufficient to improve aerosol performance of powders? *Pharmaceutical Research* 22(1):148–152.

Cipolla, D. and H.-K. Chan. 2013. Inhaled antibiotics to treat lung infection. *Pharmaceutical Patent Analyst* 2(5):647–663.

Coates, A. L., O. Denk, K. Leung, N. Ribeiro, J. Chan, M. Green, S. Martin, M. Charron, M. Edwardes, and M. Keller. 2011. Higher tobramycin concentration and vibrating mesh technology can shorten antibiotic treatment time in cystic fibrosis. *Pediatric Pulmonology* 46(4):401–408.

de Boer, A. H., P. Hagedoorn, E. M. Westerman, P. P. H. Le Brun, H. G. M. Heijerman, and H. W. Frijlink. 2006. Design and *in vitro* performance testing of multiple air classifier technology in a new disposable inhaler concept (Twincer®) for high powder doses. *European Journal of Pharmaceutical Sciences* 28(3):171–178.

de Boer, A. H., P. Hagedoorn, R. Woolhouse, and E. Wynn. 2012. Computational fluid dynamics (CFD) assisted performance evaluation of the Twincer (TM) disposable high-dose dry powder inhaler. *Journal of Pharmacy and Pharmacology* 64(9):1316–1325.

de Boer, A. H., P. P. H. Le Brun, H. G. van der Woude, P. Hagedoorn, H. G. M. Heijerman, and H. W. Frijlink. 2002. Dry powder inhalation of antibiotics in cystic fibrosis therapy, part 1: Development of a powder formulation with colistin sulfate for a special test inhaler with an air classifier as de-agglomeration principle. *European Journal of Pharmaceutics and Biopharmaceutics* 54(1):17–24.

Dhumal, R. S., S. V. Biradar, S. Yamamura, A. R. Paradkar, and P. York. 2008. Preparation of amorphous cefuroxime axetil nanoparticles by sonoprecipitation for enhancement of bioavailability. *European Journal of Pharmaceutics and Biopharmaceutics* 70(1):109–115.

Edwards, D. A, J. Hanes, G. Caponetti, J. Hrkach, A. Ben-Jebria, M. L. Eskew, J. Mintzes, D. Deaver, N. Lotan, and R. Langer. 1997. Large porous particles for pulmonary drug delivery. *Science* 276(5320):1868–1872.

Garonzik, S. M., J. Li, V. Thamlikitkul, D. L. Paterson, S. Shoham, J. Jacob, F. P. Silveira, A. Forrest, and R. L. Nation. 2011a. Population pharmacokinetics of colistin methanesulfonate and formed colistin in critically ill patients from a multicenter study provide dosing suggestions for various categories of patients. *Antimicrobial Agents and Chemotherapy* 55(7):3284–3294.

Garonzik, S. M., J. Li, V. Thamlikitkul, D. L. Paterson, S. Shoham, J. Jacob, F. P. Silveira, A. Forrest, and R. L. Nation. 2011b. Population PK of CMS and formed colistin in critically ill patients from a multicenter study provide dosing suggestions for various categories of patients. *Antimicrobial Agents and Chemotherapy* 55(7):3284–3294.

Geller, D. E., J. Weers, and S. Heuerding. 2011. Development of an inhaled dry-powder formulation of tobramycin using PulmoSphere (TM) technology. *Journal of Aerosol Medicine and Pulmonary Drug Delivery* 24(4):175–182.

Geller, D. E., M. W. Konstan, S. B. Noonberg, and C. Conrad. 2007. Novel tobramycin inhalation powder in cystic fibrosis subjects: Pharmacokinetics and safety. *Pediatric Pulmonology* 42(4):307–313.

Ghaffari, S., J. Varshosaz, A. Saadat, and F. Atyabi. 2010. Stability and antimicrobial effect of amikacin-loaded solid lipid nanoparticles. *International Journal of Nanomedicine* 6:35–43.

Golshahi, L., K. H. Lynch, J. J. Dennis, and W. H. Finlay. 2011. *In vitro* lung delivery of bacteriophages KS4-M and ΦKZ using dry powder inhalers for treatment of Burkholderia cepacia complex and *Pseudomonas aeruginosa* infections in cystic fibrosis. *Journal of Applied Microbiology* 110(1):106–117.

Grasmeijer, F., P. Hagedoorn, H. W. Frijlink, and A. H. de Boer. 2012. Characterisation of high dose aerosols from dry powder inhalers. *International Journal of Pharmaceutics* 437(1–2):242–249.

Grumezescu, A. M., E. Andronescu, A. M. Holban, A. Ficai, D. Ficai, G. Voicu, V. Grumezescu, P. C. Balaure, and C. M. Chifiriuc. 2013. Water dispersible cross-linked magnetic chitosan beads for increasing the antimicrobial efficiency of aminoglycoside antibiotics. *International Journal of Pharmaceutics* 454(1):233–240.

Haynes, A., J. Nakamura, C. Heng, S. Heuerding, G. Thompson, and R. Malcolmson. 2010. Aerosol performance of tobramycin inhalation powder. *Respiratory Drug Delivery* April:25–29.

Heng, D., D. J. Cutler, H. K. Chan, J. Yun, and J. A. Raper. 2008. What is a suitable dissolution method for drug nanoparticles? *Pharmaceutical Research* 25(7):1696–1701.

Hodson, M. E., C. G. Gallagher, and J. R. Govan. 2002. A randomised clinical trial of nebulised tobramycin or colistin in cystic fibrosis. *European Respiratory Journal* 20(3):658–664.

Hoiby, N. 2011. Recent advances in the treatment of *Pseudomonas aeruginosa* infections in cystic fibrosis. *BMC Medicine* 9:32.

Infectious Diseases Society of America. 2010. The 10 × '20 Initiative: Pursuing a global commitment to develop 10 new antibacterial drugs by 2020. *Clinical Infectious Diseases* 50(8):1081–1083.

Insmed. 2009. A placebo controlled, randomized, parallel cohort, safety and tolerability study of two dose levels of liposomal amikacin for inhalation (Arikace™) in patients with bronchiectasis complicated by chronic infection due to *Pseudomonas aeruginosa*. https://www.google.com/url?sa=t&rct=j&q=&esrc=s&source=web&cd=2&cad=rja&uact=8&ved=0ahUKEwiLva3725DKAhVKJCYKHcXjCTYQFggIMAE&url=http%3A%2F%2Fwww.insmed.com%2Fpdf%2FPub9%25209_13_09.pdf&usg=AFQjCNHUyMeCaL5_rOfNyyGx0ykYo6L9Mg&sig2=1VpVvrGWOXYj4Z2F3VolUQ. Protocol Number: TR02-107. Accessed September 22, 2014.

Jong, T., J. Li, D. A. V. Morton, Q. T. Zhou, and I. Larson. 2015. Investigation of the changes in aerosolization behavior between the jet-milled and spray-dried colistin powders through surface energy characterization. *Journal of Pharmaceutical Sciences* 105(3):1156–1163.

Konstan, M. W., D. E. Geller, P. Minic, F. Brockhaus, J. Zhang, and G. Angyalosi. 2011. Tobramycin inhalation powder for *P. aeruginosa* infection in cystic fibrosis: The EVOLVE trial. *Pediatric Pulmonology* 46(3):230–238.

Kumon, M., P. C. L. Kwok, H. Adi, D. Heng, and H.-K. Chan. 2010. Can low-dose combination products for inhalation be formulated in single crystalline particles? *European Journal of Pharmaceutical Sciences* 40(1):16–24.

Le Brun, P. P. H., A. H. De Boer, G. P. M. Mannes, D. M. I. De Fraître, R. W. Brimicombe, D. J. Touw, A. A. Vinks, H. W. Frijlink, and H. G. M. Heijerman. 2002. Dry powder inhalation of antibiotics in cystic fibrosis therapy: Part 2: Inhalation of a novel colistin dry powder formulation: A feasibility study in healthy volunteers and patients. *European Journal of Pharmaceutics and Biopharmaceutics* 54(1):25–32.

Lee, S. H., J. Teo, D. Heng, W. K. Ng, H.-K. Chan, and R. B. H. Tan. 2013. Synergistic combination dry powders for inhaled antimicrobial therapy: Formulation, characterization and *in vitro* evaluation. *European Journal of Pharmaceutics and Biopharmaceutics* 83(2):275–284.

Liang, W., P. C. Kwok, M. Y. Chow, P. Tang, A. J. Mason, H. K. Chan, and J. K. Lam. 2014. Formulation of pH responsive peptides as inhalable dry powders for pulmonary delivery of nucleic acids. *European Journal of Pharmaceutics and Biopharmaceutics* 86(1):64–73.

Liang, W., M. Y. T. Chow, P. N. Lau, Q. T. Zhou, P. C. L. Kwok, G. P. H. Leung, A. J. Mason, H.-K. Chan, L. L. M. Poon, and J. K. W. Lam. 2015. Inhalable dry powder formulations of siRNA and pH-responsive peptides with antiviral activity against H1N1 influenza virus. *Molecular Pharmaceutics* 12(3):910–921.

Lin, Y.-W., J. Wong, L. Qu, H.-K. Chan, and Q. T. Zhou. 2015. Powder production and particle engineering for dry powder inhaler formulations. *Current Pharmaceutical Design* 21(27):3902–3916.

Mangal, S., F. Meiser, G. Tan, T. Gengenbach, J. Denman, M. R. Rowles, I. Larson, and D. A. V. Morton. 2015. Relationship between surface concentration of l-leucine and bulk powder properties in spray dried formulations. *European Journal of Pharmaceutics and Biopharmaceutics* 94:160–169.

Markou, N., S. L. Markantonis, E. Dirnitrakis, D. Panidis, E. Boutzouka, S. Karatzas, P. Rafailidis, H. Apostolakos, and G. Baltopoulos. 2008. Colistin serum concentrations after intravenous administration in critically ill patients with serious multidrug-resistant, gram-negative bacilli infections: A prospective, open-label, uncontrolled study. *Clinical Therapeutics* 30(1):143–151.

Master, K. 1991. *Spray Drying Handbook*. New York: John Wiley & Sons Inc.

Matinkhoo, S., K. H. Lynch, J. J. Dennis, W. H. Finlay, and R. Vehring. 2011. Spray-dried respirable powders containing bacteriophages for the treatment of pulmonary infections. *Journal of Pharmaceutical Sciences* 100(12):5197–5205.

McCoy, K. S., A. L. Quittner, C. M. Oermann, R. L. Gibson, G. Z. Retsch-Bogart, and A. B. Montgomery. 2008. Inhaled aztreonam lysine for chronic airway *Pseudomonas aeruginosa* in cystic fibrosis. *American Journal of Respiratory and Critical Care Medicine* 178(9):921–928.

Meers, P., M. Neville, V. Malinin, A. W. Scotto, G. Sardaryan, R. Kurumunda, C. Mackinson, G. James, S. Fisher, and W. R. Perkins. 2008. Biofilm penetration, triggered release and *in vivo* activity of inhaled liposomal amikacin in chronic *Pseudomonas aeruginosa* lung infections. *Journal of Antimicrobial Chemotherapy* 61(4):859–868.

Mitchell, J., M. Copley, Y. Sizer, T. Russell, and D. Solomon. 2012. Adapting the Abbreviated Impactor Measurement (AIM) concept to make appropriate inhaler aerosol measurements to compare with clinical data: A scoping study with the "Alberta" idealized throat (AIT) inlet. *Journal of Aerosol Medicine and Pulmonary Drug Delivery* 25(4):188–197.

Nikander, K., I. Prince, S. Coughlin, S. Warren, and G. Taylor. 2010. Mode of breathing-tidal or slow and deep-through the I-neb Adaptive Aerosol Delivery (AAD) system affects lung deposition of (99m)Tc-DTPA. *Journal of Aerosol Medicine and Pulmonary Drug Delivery* 23(Suppl. 1):S37–S43.

Olivier, K. N., P. A. Shaw, T. S. Glaser, D. Bhattacharyya, M. Fleshner, C. C. Brewer, C. K. Zalewski, L. R. Folio et al. 2014. Inhaled amikacin for treatment of refractory pulmonary nontuberculous mycobacterial disease. *Annals of the American Thoracic Society* 11(1):30–35.

Ong, H. X., F. Benaouda, D. Traini, D. Cipolla, I. Gonda, M. Bebawy, B. Forbes, and P. M. Young. 2014. *In vitro* and ex vivo methods predict the enhanced lung residence time of liposomal ciprofloxacin formulations for nebulisation. *European Journal of Pharmaceutics and Biopharmaceutics* 86(1):83–89.

Qu, L. and D. A. V. Morton. 2015. Particle engineering via mechanical dry coating in the design of pharmaceutical solid dosage forms. *Current Pharmaceutical Design* 21(40):5802–5814.

Rabbani, N. R. and P. C. Seville. 2005. The influence of formulation components on the aerosolisation properties of spray-dried powders. *Journal of Controlled Release* 110(1):130–140.

Ratjen, F., E. Rietschel, D. Kasel, R. Schwiertz, K. Starke, H. Beier, S. van Koningsbruggen, and H. Grasemann. 2006. Pharmacokinetics of inhaled colistin in patients with cystic fibrosis. *Journal of Antimicrobial Chemotherapy* 57(2):306–311.

Retsch-Bogart, G. Z., A. L. Quittner, R. L. Gibson, C. M. Oermann, K. S. McCoy, A. B. Montgomery, and P. J. Cooper. 2009. Efficacy and safety of inhaled aztreonam lysine for airway pseudomonas in cystic fibrosis. *Chest* 135(5):1223–1232.

Reychler, G., A. Keyeux, C. Cremers, C. Veriter, D. O. Rodenstein, and G. Liistro. 2004. Comparison of lung deposition in two types of nebulization: Intrapulmonary percussive ventilation vs jet nebulization. *Chest* 125(2):502–508.

Sandri, A. M., C. B. Landersdorfer, J. Jacob, M. M. Boniatti, M. G. Dalarosa, D. R. Falci, T. F. Behle et al. 2013. Population PK of intravenous polymyxin B in critically ill patients: Implications for selection of dosage regimens. *Clinical Infectious Diseases* 57(4):524–531.

Schuster, A., C. Haliburn, G. Doring, M. H. Goldman, and Group Freedom Study. 2013. Safety, efficacy and convenience of colistimethate sodium dry powder for inhalation (Colobreathe DPI) in patients with cystic fibrosis: A randomised study. *Thorax* 68(4):344–350.

Serisier, D. J., D. Bilton, A. De Soyza, P. J. Thompson, J. Kolbe, H. W. Greville, D. Cipolla, P. Bruinenberg, I. Gonda, and Orbit-Investigators. 2013. Inhaled, dual release liposomal ciprofloxacin in non-cystic fibrosis bronchiectasis (ORBIT-2): A randomised, double-blind, placebo-controlled trial. *Thorax* 68(9):812–817.

Stank, K. and H. Steckel. 2013. Physico-chemical characterisation of surface modified particles for inhalation. *International Journal of Pharmaceutics* 448(1):9–18.

Stass, H., J. Nagelschmitz, S. Willmann, H. Delesen, A. Gupta, and S. Baumann. 2013a. Inhalation of a dry powder ciprofloxacin formulation in healthy subjects: A phase I study. *Clinical Drug Investigation* 33(6):419–427.

Stass, H., B. Weimann, J. Nagelschmitz, C. Rolinck-Werninghaus, and D. Staab. 2013b. Tolerability and pharmacokinetic properties of ciprofloxacin dry powder for inhalation in patients with cystic fibrosis: A phase I, randomized, dose-escalation study. *Clinical Therapeutics* 35(10):1571–1581.

Sugianto, T.D., H. K. Chan. 2016. Inhaled antibiotics in the treatment of non-cystic fibrosis bronchiectasis: *Clinical and drug delivery perspectives*. Expert Opinion on Drug Delivery 13:7–22.

Tang, P., H. K. Chan, D. Rajbhandari, and P. Phipps. 2011. Method to introduce mannitol powder to intubated patients to improve sputum clearance. *Journal of Aerosol Medicine and Pulmonary Drug Delivery* 24(1):1–9.

Varshosaz, J., S. Ghaffari, M. R. Khoshayand, F. Atyabi, A. J. Dehkordi, and F. Kobarfard. 2012. Optimization of freeze-drying condition of amikacin solid lipid nanoparticles using D-optimal experimental design. *Pharmaceutical Development and Technology* 17(2):187–194.

Vehring, R., W. R. Foss, and D. Lechuga-Ballesteros. 2007. Particle formation in spray drying. *Journal of Aerosol Science* 38:728–746.

Velkov, T., N. A. Rahim, Q. T. Zhou, H.-K. Chan, and J. Li. 2015. Inhaled anti-infective chemotherapy for respiratory tract infections: Successes, challenges and the road ahead. *Advanced Drug Delivery Reviews* 85:65–82.

Weers, J. 2015. Inhaled antimicrobial therapy—Barriers to effective treatment. *Advanced Drug Delivery Reviews* 85:24–43.

Westerman, E. M., A. H. De Boer, P. P. H. Le Brun, D. J. Touw, A. C. Roldaan, H. W. Frijlink, and H. G. M. Heijerman. 2007. Dry powder inhalation of colistin in cystic fibrosis patients: A single dose pilot study. *Journal of Cystic Fibrosis* 6(4):284–292.

WHO. May 2014. The 10 leading causes of death in the world, 2000 and 2012. who.int/media-centre/factsheets/fs310/en/. Accessed 23 August, 2016.

Yamasaki, K., P. C. L. Kwok, K. Fukushige, R. K. Prud'homme, and H.-K. Chan. 2011. Enhanced dissolution of inhalable cyclosporine nano-matrix particles with mannitol as matrix former. *International Journal of Pharmaceutics* 420(1):34–42.

Yang, L., Y. Liu, H. Wu, Z. J. Song, N. Hoiby, S. Molin, and M. Givskov. 2012. Combating biofilms. *FEMS Immunology and Medical Microbiology* 65(2):146–157.

Young, P. M., J. Crapper, G. Philips, K. Sharma, H. K. Chan, and D. Traini. 2014. Overcoming dose limitations using the orbital multi-breath dry powder inhaler. *Journal of Aerosol Medicine and Pulmonary Drug Delivery* 27(2):138–147.

Zhou, Q. and D. Morton. 2012. Drug-lactose binding aspects in adhesive mixtures: Controlling performance in dry powder inhaler formulations by altering lactose carrier surfaces. *Advanced Drug Delivery Reviews* 64(3):275–284.

Zhou, Q., B. Armstrong, I. Larson, P. J. Stewart, and D. A. V. Morton. 2010a. Effect of host particle size on the modification of powder flow behaviours for lactose monohydrate following dry coating. *Dairy Science and Technology* 90(2–3):237–251.

Zhou, Q., T. Gengenbach, J. A. Denman, H. H. Yu, J. Li, and H. K. Chan. 2014a. Synergistic antibiotic combination powders of colistin and rifampicin provide high aerosolization efficiency and moisture protection. *The AAPS Journal* 16(1):37–47.

Zhou, Q., D. Morton, H. H. Yu, J. Jacob, J. P. Wang, J. Li, and H. K. Chan. 2013a. Colistin powders with high aerosolisation efficiency for respiratory infection: Preparation and *in vitro* evaluation. *Journal of Pharmaceutical Sciences* 102(10):3736–3747.

Zhou, Q. T., B. Armstrong, I. Larson, P. J. Stewart, and D. A. V. Morton. 2010b. Understanding the influence of powder flowability, fluidization and de-agglomeration character-istics on the aerosolization of pharmaceutical model powders. *European Journal of Pharmaceutical Sciences* 40(5):412–421.

Zhou, Q. T., J. A. Denman, T. Gengenbach, S. Das, L. Qu, H. Zhang, I. Larson, P. J. Stewart, and D. A. V. Morton. 2011. Characterization of the surface properties of a model pharmaceutical fine powder modified with a pharmaceutical lubricant to improve flow via a mechanical dry coating approach. *Journal of Pharmaceutical Sciences* 100(8):3421–3430.

Zhou, Q. T., T. Gengenbach, J. A. Denman, H. Yu Heidi, J. Li, and H. K. Chan. 2014b. Synergistic antibiotic combination powders of colistin and rifampicin provide high aerosolization efficiency and moisture protection. *The AAPS Journal* 16(1):37–47.

Zhou, Q. T., L. Qu, T. Gengenbach, I. Larson, P. J. Stewart, and D. A. V. Morton. 2013b. Effect of surface coating with magnesium stearate via mechanical dry powder coating approach on the aerosol performance of micronized drug powders from dry powder inhalers. *AAPS PharmSciTech* 14(1):38–44.

Zhou, Q. T., P. Tang, S. S. Y. Leung, J. G. Y. Chan, and H.-K. Chan. 2014c. Emerging inhala-tion aerosol devices and strategies: Where are we headed? *Advanced Drug Delivery Reviews* 75:3–17.

Zhou, Q. T., L. Qu, I. Larson, P. J. Stewart, and D. Morton. 2010c. Improving aerosolization of drug powders by reducing powder intrinsic cohesion via a mechanical dry coating approach. *International Journal of Pharmaceutics* 394(1–2):50–59.

8 Inhaled Liposomes

David Cipolla

CONTENTS

INTRODUCTION

Liposomes are supramolecular aggregates possessing one or more closed lipid bilayers and thus can vary in a number of attributes, including bilayer thickness, number of lamellae, and overall size and shape (usually spherical) depending upon their composition and how the formulation has been processed [1]. These lipid vesicles are typically composed of phospholipids and sterols in which both hydrophobic fatty acid tails of each phospholipid molecule are oriented toward the center of the bilayer, while the hydrophilic head group, for example, the phosphatidylcholine (PC) moiety, is oriented toward the internal or external aqueous phases [1,2]. The formation and stabilization of these bilayers is driven both by entropic factors related to the sequestration of the hydrophobic fatty acid tails from the aqueous medium as well as enthalpic elements due to hydrogen bonding between the hydrophilic head groups and van der Waals interactions between the aligned acyl groups of the fatty acid chains. Even for a specific liposomal formulation manufactured under controlled conditions, a range of liposome sizes and shapes will be present. The selection of the manufacturing processes, the controls over the various processing steps, and the ingredients that constitute the liposome as well as the solvents and buffers used during manufacturing will determine the extent of this heterogeneity and the reproducibility from batch to batch.

The pharmaceutical interest in liposomes arises because these lipid vesicles can be utilized to package drug molecules with superior pharmacologic properties relative to the unencapsulated drug alone. Two key attributes of liposomes are their size and morphology; liposomes can be produced spanning two orders of magnitude in size with unilamellar liposomes typically around 100 nm or smaller, while multilamellar liposomes can be as large as a few microns in size [1]. Another important parameter for liposomes is the ratio of drug to lipid; larger liposomes have the potential to encapsulate a greater amount of drug relative to lipid, but this advantage can be undermined if the larger liposomes are not stable or do not release drug at the appropriate rate to achieve safe and efficacious levels in the target organ. Thus, many liposomal products on the market or in development utilize unilamellar liposomes even though the potential drug payload on a per weight basis (and per liposome) is smaller [1].

The formulation development and the manufacturing process for liposomes are more complex and costly than for standard pharmaceutical products and so would not be utilized unless liposomal formulations provided an inherent advantage over that for the free drug alone. In spite of these challenges, liposomes are now well accepted as drug delivery vehicles with the potential to change the *in vivo* distribution of the encapsulated drug relative to that of the unencapsulated drug [1,3–5]. However, it is important to recognize that the drug can only assert its effect once it is released from the liposome, so the rate of release of the drug is a critical parameter that determines whether the liposome composition will be pharmaceutically efficacious.

More than ten pharmaceutical products utilizing liposomes have been approved in the United States for intravenous (IV) or subcutaneous administration [1]. The first one, liposomal amphotericin B (AmBisome®, Gilead Sciences) [6–8], was approved for the treatment of fungal infections in 1990 (in Europe), 29 years after Dr. Alec Bangham and colleagues first discovered liposomes [9]. AmBisome was followed in 1995 by liposomal doxorubicin HCl (DOXIL®, Centocor), which is now labeled for the treatment of ovarian cancer, Kaposi's sarcoma, and myeloma [10–12]. A liposomal formulation of vincristine (Marqibo®, Talon Therapeutics) was approved in 2012 to treat a leukemia indication, Philadelphia chromosome–negative acute lymphoblastic leukemia, given via IV administration [1,13–16]. For these products, the liposomes provide an altered pharmacokinetic (PK) profile that leads to improved safety and efficacy and a reduction in side effects. For AmBisome, the liposomes also serve as a solubilizing matrix with the amphiphilic amphotericin B intercalated within the membrane bilayer. While hydrophobic drugs can be "solubilized" within the lipid bilayer, hydrophilic drugs can be compartmentalized within the interior of the liposome, either by passive encapsulation or by active transport [17], and in some cases form precipitates that can lead to a depot effect upon release [18].

The physicochemical properties of liposomes, and in particular their drug release profile, can be engineered into the formulation via a variety of strategies, including the following:

- Modification of the liposomal composition: An increase in the acyl chain length of PC can reduce the drug release rate of a liposomal formulation as was observed for liposomal vincristine [19].

- Addition of sterol: The presence of moderate amounts of cholesterol (e.g., 30%) reduces membrane permeability [20], leading to a slower drug release rate for many liposomal formulations, including adriamycin [21] and doxorubicin [22]. Cholesterol also increases membrane rigidity and thus the liposomes are more likely to retain their physical integrity in response to stress encountered during nebulization [23,24].
- Surface modification with polyethyleneglycol (PEG): The presence of covalently attached PEG groups can lead to longer circulation half-lives and slower release as was observed for doxorubicin from hydrogenated soy phosphatidylcholine (HSPC)/cholesterol liposomes containing PEG (DOXIL) versus egg PC/cholesterol liposomes without PEG (Myocet®) [12].
- Liposomal size and lamellarity: Unilamellar liposomes typically release their contents at a faster rate than multilamellar vesicles because each bilayer represents a barrier to transport or diffusion.
- Drug to lipid ratio: Higher drug to lipid ratios reduced the release rate of liposomal vincristine that was associated with an increase in efficacy [25].
- State of the drug inside the vesicle: Liposomes can be designed with drug in either a soluble or a precipitated form resulting in different release rates. For example, liposomes containing precipitated doxorubicin had slower release than those with doxorubicin in solution [18]. Similarly, liposomes containing ciprofloxacin in nanocrystalline form also had slower release than those with ciprofloxacin in solution [26,27].
- Choice of drug loading method: A larger transmembrane pH gradient reduced the release rate of liposomal doxorubicin [28].
- Other factors can influence the release rate, including osmolarity, pH, and choice of buffer and excipients encapsulated within the liposome.

For liposomes given systemically, other features have been exploited, including the addition of antibodies on the surface to target-specific receptors or PEG groups (producing "stealth" liposomes) to prevent uptake by the mononuclear phagocyte system. Stealth liposomes have a longer circulating half-life and enhanced localization in tumors and other pathological tissues with increased vascular permeability [1]. A good example of a product adopting this strategy is pegylated liposomal doxorubicin [10–12].

PULMONARY RATIONALE AND HISTORY

The primary rationale to develop an inhaled liposomal product has not changed in the past 25 years since the development of inhaled liposomal formulations were first considered [4,5,29]. Similar to most inhaled products, the goal is to combat lung disease by delivering high concentrations of the therapeutic agent directly to the treatment site [3,24,30–32]. In contrast to oral or IV administration, which requires much higher doses to achieve the same drug concentration in the lung, the inhalation route of delivery results in lower systemic exposure [30,33]. The benefits described earlier for the IV-administered liposomal products may also apply to liposomal formulations delivered as aerosols to the respiratory tract—modified PK and reduced side effects.

The modified release profile of small molecule drugs from liposomes may allow for less frequent dosing compared to that of the unencapsulated form that would be rapidly absorbed from the lungs and need to be replaced more often (by more frequent administration events). In addition, for compounds that are bitter, cause cough, or have vesicant properties (e.g., cancer compounds), inhaled liposomal formulations may reduce local irritation in the airways and thus increase their tolerability, allowing for higher doses to be delivered, thus increasing the likelihood of achieving efficacy [32]. Furthermore, to treat intracellular pathogens, including nontuberculous mycobacteria (NTM), or bioterrorism threats like tularemia and pneumonic plague, appropriately designed liposomal formulations may be more effective due to their propensity to accumulate in alveolar macrophages [34].

Researchers targeting lung disease have used liposomes to encapsulate a wide variety of agents including small molecule drugs, peptides, proteins, and nucleic acids [24]. Initial efforts included attempts to improve asthma therapy by formulating steroids [35–37], bronchodilators [38,39], and cromolyn [40] in liposomes with the goal to extend their duration of effect. Additionally, oncology drugs (e.g., 9-nitrocamptothecin [41,42], IL-2 [43], and cisplatin [44]) were encapsulated in liposomes to treat lung cancer more effectively by allowing higher doses to be administered with reduced side effects. Some of these inhaled liposomal products were evaluated in human subjects or patients, but none remained in clinical development, for a variety of reasons. For asthma treatment, long-acting beta agonists (e.g., salmeterol [Serevent Diskus®, Advair®] and formoterol [Foradil Aerolizer®]) and long-acting muscarinic antagonists (e.g., tiotropium, Spiriva®) were developed with a greater duration of effect, thus reducing the business proposition for formulation strategies using liposomes in this therapeutic area.

During the 1990s, after safety concerns arose with the use of viral vectors for the delivery of gene therapy products, interest in the use of liposomes and lipid complexes for gene therapy applications exploded. However, the interest was relatively short-lived due to the difficulties in showing correlations between *in vitro* transfection and *in vivo* effect, as well as toxicities associated with some of these charged lipid complexes [32].

The development activity of inhaled liposomal products waned for a period of time in the early 2000s, but interest in using these formulations to address unmet needs in the field of lung infection and lung transplantation gradually emerged. AmBisome, a liposomal amphotericin B, is used off-label by nebulizer to *treat* patients with fungal infections in the lung and was found to be better tolerated than formulations of "free" amphotericin B [32]. As a prophylactic therapy, AmBisome is also inhaled to *prevent* fungal infections in lung transplant patients [45–47].

Cyclosporine, an immunosuppressive, has been delivered by nebulizer to prevent rejection in lung transplant patients. Due to cyclosporine's poor aqueous solubility, the nebulizer formulation contained propylene glycol, which was irritating and may have contributed to its failure in the clinic [48]. Liposomal formulations of cyclosporine have been developed and found to be well tolerated by inhalation [49,50]; however, the clinical failure of the propylene glycol formulation—possibly due to poor compliance in response to its poor tolerability, rather than a true lack of efficacy—may have blunted enthusiasm for continued development of a liposomal cyclosporine product [32].

There are now two liposomal products in the late stages of clinical evaluation to treat lung infection and these will be described more thoroughly later in this chapter: liposomal amikacin [51–55] and liposomal ciprofloxacin [30,56–59].

CHALLENGES IN DEVELOPING PHARMACEUTICAL LIPOSOME FORMULATIONS

ANALYTICAL CHALLENGES

In the early stages of clinical development, research scientists typically determine the requirements for the drug product (e.g., therapeutic window, frequency of administration, patient population constraints) and the various formulation and delivery options that may best meet those diverse product requirement specifications. If a liposome formulation is utilized, it should be designed so that the *in vivo* rate of drug release results in drug levels falling within the therapeutic window until the next administration event: high enough to provide therapeutic benefit but not so high that pernicious side effects result. An *in vitro* release (IVR) assay can be utilized to evaluate various liposome compositions and rank order their relative release rates; however, it is unlikely that the results of the IVR assay alone can be used to select a single composition to move into clinical development. Instead, the IVR assay is typically used to exclude liposome formulations that are unacceptable (e.g., possess a high initial burst or do not release at all) and narrow down the list of compositions to be evaluated in a preclinical setting. If the relative release rates in the *in vivo* preclinical setting mirror that in the IVR assay, then the IVR assay may be utilized more fully to fine-tune formulation compositions and understand the effects of manufacturing changes (e.g., an increase in the scale of operations or a change in a process step) or CMC changes (e.g., alternative excipient suppliers) on the release profile [60]. Preclinical PK data can be used to further exclude undesirable formulations, but depending upon the choice of animal model and the route of delivery, PK data in animals may not be fully predictive of the disposition in humans. Because of this uncertainty, the lead formulation(s) will need to be tested in human clinical studies to provide assurance that the *in vivo* PK meets the design requirements.

The FDA has specific recommendations for additional content to be provided in the regulatory submission of a liposomal product due to its unique technical aspects [60]. These include characterization of the following physicochemical properties: the liposome structure, liposome integrity, liposome morphology and lamellarity, the encapsulated drug, the viscosity, the surface charge or zeta potential, the drug leakage rate, the vesicle size distribution, the lipid composition, and the IVR of drug using an appropriate physiological medium [60]. Assurance also needs to be provided that the physicochemical properties do not change over the shelf life of the liposomal product [60].

Focusing first on the IVR methodology, the test method should measure the amount of the released (free) drug over a time scale to cover the complete release of the drug [61–63]. In practice, this may be challenging for a liposomal product because it can often be difficult to differentiate the free drug from that remaining encapsulated in the liposomes by routine analytical methods. There are three general methodologies that have been developed to measure the IVR of a drug from liposomal products [63]. For drugs that fluoresce, the change in fluorescence can be translated into a drug release rate—this is termed an *in situ* method as the amount of fluorescence is directly measured without further sample manipulation. The advantage of the *in situ* IVR method is its simplicity (rapid data output), but unfortunately, most drugs do not have properties that are amenable to measurement *in situ*. Thus, a number of specific dissolution or IVR test methodologies have been developed for liposomal products [61–63]. A second class of methods utilizes membrane dialysis to physically separate the released drug from the encapsulated drug [61,63]. Dialysis methods are appropriate when the rate of drug release from the liposomes is slow compared to the time to diffuse across the membrane—otherwise, the measured release rate may not reflect the true release rate from the liposomes [63]. The third class of IVR methods is the "sample and separate" method: samples are periodically removed from the IVR vessel and the free drug is separated from the encapsulated drug (often by chromatography, centrifugation, or filtration), thus allowing for quantitation by HPLC or another analytical assay [63].

The liposome formulation should also be robust to the delivery method and procedure; for example, a formulation that requires dilution for IV administration should be evaluated to ensure that it retains its physical properties at the lower (diluted) concentration and in contact with the materials in the IV bag and line. For an inhaled liposomal product, the liposomal formulation will be inhaled into the lung. The *in vivo* release in the lung fluid may be very different from that for an IV product that is injected into the bloodstream. The relative dilution into the bodily fluids and the composition of the biological milieu are different; for example, the dilution in the lung fluid (ca. 50 mL) is one hundredth that of dilution into the bloodstream (ca. 5 L). The site of deposition in the lung, for example, peripheral versus bronchial airways, and the presence of lung disease will also affect the fluid volume and composition [61]. Ideally the IVR assay should be developed using an appropriate simulated physiological medium or human plasma to mimic the *in vivo* situation [60]. However, there is no recognized standard simulated lung fluid [61–63]. Many of the simulated lung fluids in the published literature do not contain components that are naturally present in the lung, which may interact with liposomes, for example, proteins, surfactant, or lipids, and result in modulation of the rate of drug release [61–63]. For many of these simulated lung fluids, the IVR data may have little relevance to the *in vivo* release kinetics [61].

One IVR assay was developed specifically for an inhaled liposomal product utilizing bovine serum as the release vehicle [63]. Bovine serum was chosen because it is biological in composition, it is inexpensive to obtain in large quantities from established suppliers, and the components in serum may be relevant to the release mechanisms in the lung [63]. Most serum proteins including albumin, trypsin, and ovalbumin do not induce release from liposomes [64]. The components in serum that do have a destabilizing effect on liposomes, causing drug release, are lipoproteins and apolipoproteins [64,65]. All serum lipoproteins and apolipoproteins induce drug release from liposomes and these components are present in lung fluid at about half the concentration in serum and thus are relevant as release agents for inhaled liposomal products [63,64]. In this IVR assay, after the liposomes are diluted into bovine serum and incubated for varying times at 37°C, the released drug is separated from

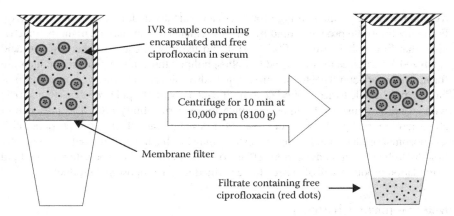

FIGURE 8.1 Schematic of the centrifugal filtration device to separate free drug (dots) from liposomally encapsulated drug (circles containing dots). (Reprinted from Cipolla, D. et al., *J. Pharm. Sci.*, 103(1), 314, 2014. With permission.)

the encapsulated drug using centrifugal filtration [63] (Figure 8.1). This IVR assay has been used to discriminate between liposome formulations with different release rates [26,27,30,66]. However, the drawback to utilizing bovine serum or any other biological source as a release medium is at least twofold: there is the possibility of a supply disruption and the potency may change batch to batch, for example, if the amount of lipoproteins and apolipoproteins (which are not typically measured or reported) were to change in the bovine serum.

During pharmaceutical development, the critical quality attributes (CQAs) of a liposomal product, like all pharmaceutical products, must be identified to establish product quality [67]. The CQAs of the drug product represent the physical, chemical, biological, or microbiological properties or characteristics that should be monitored and verified to remain within an appropriate range to provide assurance of product purity, strength, and performance at the time of release and on stability. In addition to the standard CQAs that are typical for most pharmaceutical products, a liposomal product may require additional CQAs to ensure maintenance of liposome integrity, vesicle size, and drug release rate, among other functional attributes [60].

Analytical assays need to be established to verify that the drug product's CQAs remain within the acceptable range over the shelf life required to cover manufacturing, distribution, and use of the product by the patient—most marketing organizations typically require a shelf life of at least 18 months and preferably 2 years or more to ensure that the supply chain can be effectively managed. A number of analytical methods and procedures have been developed that are specific to liposomal products and many are described in these references [68–71].

In addition to verifying that the active pharmaceutical ingredient retains its purity within acceptable levels, for liposome products, the functional excipients (e.g., lipids) must also be monitored to ensure that degradation products are not formed that compromise the safety or performance of the drug product [72]. While lipid oxidation is a possible degradation route [70], the use of high-purity excipients and the elimination of oxidants from the manufacturing processes can typically address this concern [32,70]. For many liposome products, lipid hydrolysis remains the primary degradation mechanism that limits shelf life [69,70,73,74]. Lipid hydrolysis can be either base or acid catalyzed to form free fatty acid and lysophospholipid; thus, most liposome products are formulated near neutral pH to minimize lipid hydrolysis [75]. However, liposome formulations may be able to accommodate a significant amount of lipid hydrolysis (e.g., 10%) without compromise to the liposome integrity or permeability [70]. The presence of cholesterol in the lipid bilayer counteracts the destabilizing effect of lysophospholipids so liposomal products containing cholesterol may be able to accommodate even greater lipid hydrolysis without deleterious effects on functionality [73]. The safety of the lipid degradation products will also need to be verified for each liposomal product.

MANUFACTURING CHALLENGES

Inhaled liposomal products are not as straightforward to develop as some other inhaled dosage forms, like nebulizer solutions, and may have more complex and expensive manufacturing processes, so would only be exploited when the simpler formulation alternatives are either unsafe, less effective, or not viable [24,32]. Prior to entering the clinic with the liposomal formulation, the manufacturing conditions and choice of lipids should be identified that produce liposomes of the appropriate size, that are safe for inhalation, and that contain the appropriate amount of drug so it is released at the proper time and at a rate that is both safe and therapeutic. Furthermore, the manufacturing processes should be well characterized so that each batch of the liposomal product is comparable and possesses an adequate shelf life.

While it is true that pharmaceutical preparations of liposomes require a sophisticated manufacturing process, and not all CMOs have the expertise or the equipment in house, these processes are now becoming increasingly well accepted given that liposome products have been on the market for more than 20 years. There are many ways to prepare liposomes [76–78]: they form spontaneously when lipid mixtures are hydrated in excess water yielding a heterogeneous size distribution. The micron-sized multilamellar liposomes that are generated can subsequently be processed to reduce their size distribution by a variety of means including sonication, homogenization, microfluidization, or extrusion through filters or via a combination of these processes. Many drug products can be terminally sterilized after manufacture to assure sterility, but that is not generally the case for liposomes [79–81]. Instead, two options are available to provide assurance of sterility. For larger liposomes that cannot be sterile filtered, every step of the manufacturing process must be conducted in an aseptic environment, which requires specialized manufacturing facilities and may be labor intensive. In contrast, unilamellar liposomes can often be sterile filtered and only the subsequent vial or ampule filling step of the process needs to be conducted under aseptic conditions, which reduces the manufacturing burden.

The purity of the lipid and sterol excipients is critical to the ability to manufacture liposomes that possess acceptable long-term stability. Fortunately, there are now multiple suppliers of high-quality lipid and sterol excipients. More than 75 registered Drug Master Files (DMFs) for pharmaceutical grade lipids exist in the United States [32] and an abbreviated list of some of the more commonly used excipients is shown in Table 8.1.

TABLE 8.1
Selected Pharmaceutical Grade Lipids with the U.S. Drug Master Files

Product Name/#	Supplier	U.S. DMF #	Type[a]	Date
Cholesterol				
770,000 (ovine wool)	Avanti	9,285	II	8/12/1991
Cholesterol HP	Dishman	14,346	II	8/3/1999
770,100 (plant)	Avanti	23,761	II	4/28/2010
DMPG: dimyristoyl phosphatidylglycerol				
770,445	Avanti	7,369	IV	3/7/1988
Lipoid PG 14:0/14:0	Lipoid	8,463	IV	3/5/1990
Coatsome MG-4040LS	Nippon Oil & Fats Co.	9,578	IV	2/21/1992
Coatsome MG-4040LS	Nippon Oil & Fats Co.	17,807	II	11/2/2004
DPPC: dipalmitoyl phosphatidylcholine				
770,355	Avanti	7,187	II	7/18/1987
Coatsome MC-6060	Nippon Oil & Fats Co.	8,403	IV	1/27/1990
Coatsome MC-6060	Nippon Oil & Fats Co.	9,263	II	7/30/1991
LP-04-057	Genzyme	12,555	II	6/23/1997
Lipoid PC 16:0/16:0	Lipoid	13,000	IV	5/19/1998
Lipoid PC 16:0/16:0	Lipoid	13,001	II	5/19/1998
Coatsome MC-6060EX	Nippon Oil & Fats Co.	20,876	II	9/24/2007
DPPG: dipalmitoyl phosphatidylglycerol				
770,455	Avanti	9,727	II	6/9/1992
LP-04-016	Genzyme	14,837	II	4/17/2000
Coatsome MG-6060LS	Nippon Oil & Fats Co.	22,318	II	12/17/2008
EPC: egg phosphatidylcholine				
Lipoid E PC	Lipoid	8,657	II	7/16/1990
770,051	Avanti	12,760	II	11/25/1997
Coatsome NC-50	Nippon Oil & Fats Co.	17,404	IV	5/17/2004
Coatsome PC-98SR	Nippon Oil & Fats Co.	22,208	IV	11/19/2008
ESM: egg sphingomyelin				
Lipoid E SM	Lipoid	14,414	IV	9/24/1999
Coatsome NM-10	Nippon Oil & Fats Co.	17,234	II	3/8/2004
HSPC: hydrogenated soy phosphatidylcholine				
Lipoid S PC-3	Lipoid	8,907	IV	12/27/1990
Coatsome NC-21E	Nippon Oil & Fats Co.	20,764	II	8/8/2007

Source: Cipolla, D. et al., Liposomes, niosomes and proniosomes—A critical update of their (commercial) development as inhaled products, in *Respiratory Drug Delivery Europe 2011*, Davis Healthcare Int'l Publishing, River Grove, IL, 2011. With permission.

[a] Type II DMF refers to drug substance, drug substance intermediate, and the material used in their preparation or drug product; Type IV DMF refers to excipient, colorant, flavor, essence, or material used in their preparation.

CONSIDERATIONS FOR INHALED PRODUCTS

In addition to the challenges mentioned earlier, to develop an inhaled product, the formulation must also be tailored to a specific delivery device modality, for example, dry powder inhaler (DPI), metered dose inhaler, or nebulizer [24,33]. Nebulized formulations may be the most straightforward choice with the broadest range of formulation options and least complex manufacturing processes. However, liposomal solutions for nebulization will likely require refrigerated storage to ensure long-term physical and chemical stability. One alternative is to develop a lyophilized formulation [82–85] that can be reconstituted just prior to nebulizer administration by the patient. However, identifying a liposomal formulation that maintains its physical integrity during exposure to the drying processes and subsequent reconstitution may be challenging. If efforts are successful, as was the case for the injectable products, such as AmBisome and Visudyne [32], a lyophilized product may have less restrictive storage conditions. A third option is to create a respirable, powder formulation for use in a DPI. However, this strategy may increase development risk and manufacturing complexity. Drying technologies that have been evaluated include spray-drying, spray-freeze-drying, supercritical fluid extraction, and freeze-drying followed by micronization [82]. As with the case for lyophilized products, the DPI formulations of liposomes must be stabilized with excipients so that the liposome bilayers are not disrupted during drying [82]. In addition, the dried powder must be dispersible into respirable-sized particles during inhalation to ensure reproducible lung delivery.

For any of these product formats, the formulation should be robust to the aerosolization process. Disruption of the liposome vesicles could lead to premature release of drug and/or inconsistent performance *in vivo* [24]. Historically, most liposome formulations developed for inhalation have been nebulizer solutions. The energetics of the nebulization process, involving exposure to shear and air–liquid interface, can cause changes in vesicle size distribution and/or loss of encapsulated drug (Figure 8.2). Whether using a jet, ultrasonic, or mesh nebulizer, large multilamellar vesicles typically are less stable to the nebulization process with large losses of encapsulated drug (Figure 8.3) and changes in vesicle size distribution. The minority of liposomal formulations that are stable to nebulization with retention of both vesicle size and drug encapsulation have all been unilamellar liposomes of ~100 nm in size (Figure 8.3).

BIOCOMPATIBILITY AND FATE OF LIPOSOMES IN THE LUNG

Surfactant and lipids, including both cholesterol and phospholipids, are endogenous to the lung. Of the phospholipids, PC is the major component in the lung and for this reason many inhaled liposomal formulations utilize a form of PC in their composition. Thus, it is expected that liposomes that are composed of sterols and natural phospholipids should be biocompatible. There is a long history of safe and efficacious administration of inhaled or instilled formulations of surfactants, lipids, and liposomes. Synthetic dipalmitoyl PC (DPPC) was delivered by aerosol to infants with respiratory distress syndrome (RDS) as early as 1964. This was followed by studies that demonstrated an improvement in symptoms for babies and infants with RDS after inhalation of DPPC and dipalmitoyl phosphatidylglycerol (DPPG) [24].

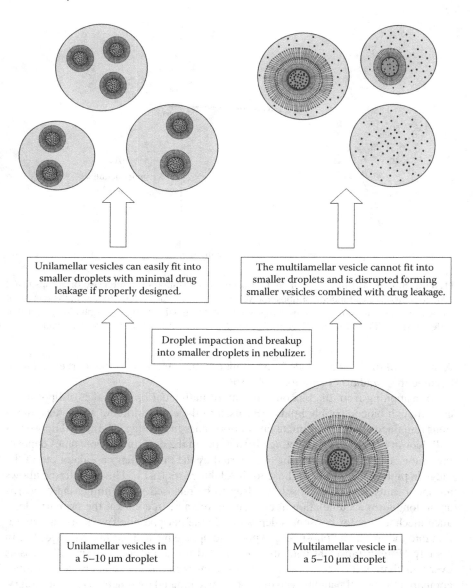

FIGURE 8.2 Schematic of nebulization of liposomes. During nebulization, many of the primary droplets impact within the nebulizer and form smaller droplets or are exposed to shear during droplet formation. This process may be deleterious to the large multilamellar vesicles but unilamellar liposomes have a greater likelihood of being uncompromised. The drug molecules are represented by the dots. (From Cipolla, D. et al., *Ther. Deliv.*, 4(8), 1047, 2013. With permission.)

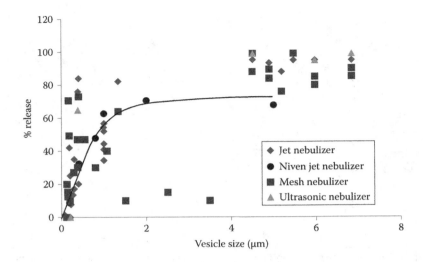

FIGURE 8.3 Effect of jet, mesh, and ultrasonic nebulization on the release of encapsulated drug (or marker) as a function of liposome vesicle size. The black circles represent the release of carboxyfluorescein from liposomes comprised of soyPC and dipalmitoyl phosphatidylglycerol of different sizes. (From Cipolla, D. et al., *Pharm. Res.*, 11(4), 491, 1994. With permission.)

A number of instilled or inhaled surfactant products are now on the market and have become the standard of care for RDS [86].

Transitioning from the biocompatibility of individual lipids to that of liposomes, even though biocompatible lipids were used in the composition of liposomes, questions remained about the ultimate fate of liposomes in the lung [5]. Inhaled liposomes will deposit both in the conducting airways and in the deep lung. Liposomes depositing in the central airways will be transported by the mucociliary escalator out of the lungs in time spans similar to those for insoluble particles [5]. This time frame allows an opportunity for the encapsulated drug to be released while mitigating concerns about long-term accumulation in the central airways. In contrast, the primary clearance mechanisms for liposomes depositing in the peripheral airways are incorporation into the surfactant phospholipid pool and uptake by alveolar macrophages [5]. In a study of lung transplant patients who inhaled liposomal amphotericin B aerosols over a median of 24 weeks, there were no changes in the lipid content in their lungs compared to control patients who did not receive inhaled treatment [47]. In summary, inhaled liposomes do not appear to accumulate in the lungs and their lipids are most likely processed and recycled similar to that for endogenous surfactant.

The safety of inhaled empty liposomes (without drug) has been assessed in a number of studies in animals and humans and no changes in lung function have been reported [5,24]. Other subjective measures of safety and tolerability have also been monitored and found to be acceptable [5,24]. For inhaled products to proceed into human clinical trials, inhalation toxicity studies in animals must be completed at doses severalfold higher than those in humans. While no inhalation toxicity studies have been published for the inhaled liposomal products in late-stage development due to their proprietary nature, presumably they have been reviewed by the regulators and the liposomal products have been deemed adequately safe to continue their evaluation in human clinical trials.

TREATMENT OF LUNG INFECTIONS WITH INHALED LIPOSOMAL ANTIBIOTICS

The rationale for an inhaled antibiotic formulation to treat lung infections is straightforward: lower doses can be delivered by inhalation than via the oral or IV routes while still achieving lung concentrations that exceed the minimum inhibitory concentration (MIC) of the bacteria of interest [30]. Additionally, the potential for side effects may be reduced for an inhaled product due to lower systemic drug levels [30]. The higher lung and lower systemic drug levels for inhaled ciprofloxacin formulations compared to oral or IV formulations of ciprofloxacin confirms this premise (Figure 8.4). Inhaled antibiotics have been approved by the FDA to treat patients with cystic fibrosis (CF); those include tobramycin, with its twice-daily treatment regimen, and aztreonam, with a thrice-daily treatment regimen [34,87]. Inhaled twice-daily colistin and its prodrug are also approved in the European Union for this same patient population [34,87].

Since the approval of inhaled tobramycin more than 15 years ago, the clinical benefit of inhaled antibiotic treatments in CF patients has long been established [34]. Recognized benefits include a delay in the onset of chronic colonization with

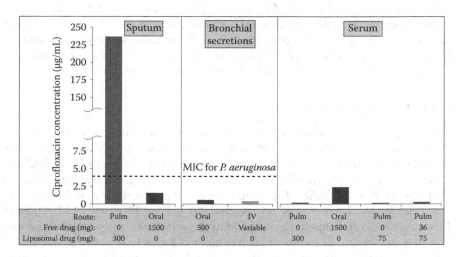

FIGURE 8.4 The concentration of ciprofloxacin in lung sputum (Cmax), bronchial secretions (mean concentration), and serum (Cmax) following inhaled (Pulm), oral, or IV administration. The oral dose leads to a maximum drug concentration in the sputum that falls below the *Pseudomonas aeruginosa* minimum inhibitory concentration (MIC). In contrast, the maximum drug concentration in the sputum by inhalation exceeds the MIC by more than 50-fold and the mean concentration over the 24 h dosing period exceeds the MIC by 20-fold. (From Cipolla, D. et al., *Pharmaceutics*, 8(1), 6, 2016. With permission.)

Pseudomonas aeruginosa (PA), an improvement in the quality of life, and a reduction in the rate of decline of lung function, exacerbations, and hospital admissions [34]. The lifespan of CF patients has increased by more than 10 years during these past two decades due in part to inhaled antibiotic therapy becoming a standard of treatment [34]. However, there are a number of other patient populations with PA lung infections for whom inhaled antibiotics have not yet been approved, including COPD and non-CF bronchiectasis (NCFB) [30,87]. Trials with the inhaled antibiotics approved in CF have so far been unsuccessful in those patient populations likely due to tolerability issues, including cough, hoarseness, dysgeusia, and voice alteration and increases in the number of respiratory adverse events [30,88]. There are also other patient populations with severe lung infections that have no approved treatment options, including those infected with NTM [30]. NTM can be difficult to treat due to its ability to flourish in airway fluid, in biofilms, and within alveolar macrophages [30]. Thus, the development of improved inhaled antibiotic therapies with promise in these patient populations is warranted.

A *liposomal* antibiotic formulation may be better tolerated than the conventional liquid or dry powder formulations because they are unlikely to cause significant perturbations in pH or osmolarity, which can lead to cough or bronchoconstriction [88,89]. Additionally, a liposomal formulation with an appropriately designed sustained release profile has the potential to reduce the frequency of administration to once daily [30,34]. Products that are administered once daily generally have superior compliance to those requiring multiple administration events daily, which may translate into improved efficacy [34,90]. A recent trial with inhaled colistin in NCFB patients colonized with PA failed to meet the primary endpoint of delay in the time to first exacerbation; however, the primary endpoint was met in a post hoc analysis of patients that were at least 80% compliant [91]. This suggests that an inhaled antibiotic regimen that is convenient and well tolerated, leading to improved adherence, may demonstrate efficacy in NCFB patients colonized with PA, among other indications.

LIPOSOMAL CIPROFLOXACIN

There are two preparations of liposomal ciprofloxacin that have been evaluated in human subjects: Lipoquin®, which is comprised of ~90 nm unilamellar liposomes containing 50 mg/mL ciprofloxacin HCl [24,26,30,32,34,58], and Pulmaquin, which is a 1:1 mixture of Lipoquin and 20 mg/mL free ciprofloxacin HCl [24,26,30,32,34,56,58]. Lipoquin's vesicle size distribution and encapsulation state are unchanged after refrigerated storage for 24 months [30,92]. Both Lipoquin and Pulmaquin are also stable to the nebulization process without loss of structural integrity or encapsulated drug or changes to the vesicle size distribution or their IVR profiles [30,93]. Additional studies in cell cultures and preclinical models demonstrated sustained release of ciprofloxacin and antibacterial activity [30,59,94,95].

Both liposomal ciprofloxacin formulations have been evaluated in the clinical setting using the PARI LC Sprint nebulizer. Lipoquin aerosols have been inhaled by healthy subjects and patients with CF and NCFB and were well tolerated, with no clinically relevant changes in routine laboratory and spirometry tests and an improved tolerability profile compared to inhalation of free antibiotics [30,32,56,58]. The drug release profile, with an *in vivo* half-life of ~10 h (as measured by systemic clearance), supports a once-daily inhaled format. Inhalation of 300 mg Lipoquin, once daily, for 14 days in CF patients, resulted in an increase in lung function of 6.9% ($p = 0.04$), over the baseline with no serious adverse events, as well as a 1.43 log reduction in PA colony-forming units (CFUs) ($p < 0.01$) [30,58]. In a 28-day Phase 2 trial in non-CF BE, Lipoquin doses of 150 and 300 mg were also well tolerated with reductions in PA colonization of 4.0 and 3.5 log CFUs, respectively, versus baseline ($p < 0.001$ for both) [30,58].

Once-daily inhalation of Pulmaquin (210 mg), or placebo, in NCFB patients was well tolerated over three cycles of a 28-day on/28-day off therapy [30,56]. There were fewer pulmonary adverse events in the Pulmaquin group compared to placebo [30,56]. In the primary endpoint of antimicrobial efficacy, Pulmaquin demonstrated a reduction of 4.2 log CFU at 28 days, versus an increase of 0.1 log CFU for placebo ($p = 0.002$) (Figure 8.5). In addition, the median time to first pulmonary exacerbation increased from 58 days for placebo to 134 days for Pulmaquin ($p = 0.046$), meeting the secondary efficacy endpoint (Figure 8.6) [30,56]. Pulmaquin is currently being evaluated in two Phase 3 efficacy trials in NCFB with data expected in the second half of 2016.

While not yet tested in human subjects with NTM, liposomal ciprofloxacin has also demonstrated efficacy against *Mycobacterium avium* and *Mycobacteria*

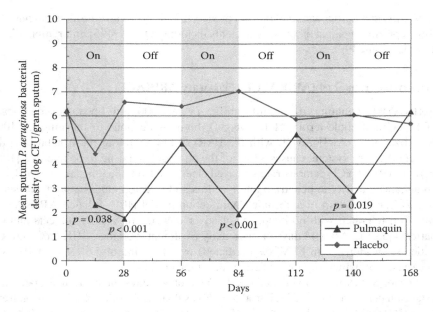

FIGURE 8.5 Change in mean sputum *P. aeruginosa* bacterial density (as $\log_{10}$ colony-forming unit/gram of sputum) across the 24 weeks of the study comparing Pulmaquin and placebo groups. (From Serisier, D.J. et al., *Thorax*, 68(9), 812, 2013. With permission.)

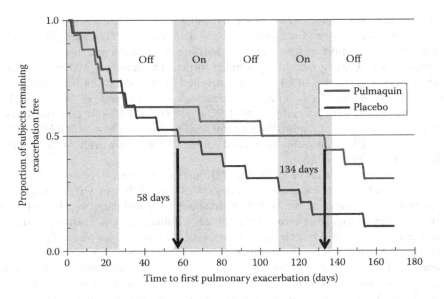

FIGURE 8.6 Kaplan–Meier curves comparing Pulmaquin and placebo groups for time to first pulmonary exacerbation. (From Serisier, D.J. et al., *Thorax*, 68(9), 812, 2013. With permission.)

abscessus in macrophages and biofilm models [57]. Liposomal ciprofloxacin has also shown promise against bioterrorism agents including Q-fever [96], tularemia [97,98], and the plague [99].

Liposomal Amikacin (ARIKAYCE® Formerly ARIKACE)

ARIKAYCE contains 70 mg/mL amikacin in ~300 nm liposomes composed of DPPC and cholesterol (2:1 by weight), both endogenous to the lung [32,100]. Nebulization of ARIKAYCE with the PARI eFlow vibrating mesh nebulizer, the current delivery system, causes ~30% of the encapsulated drug to be released [100]. In rats, ARIKAYCE demonstrated delayed clearance from the lung, as designed, and an enhanced ability to penetrate into biofilms and infected mucus, and it was superior to free amikacin in a chronic PA infection model [101]. Inhaled ARIKAYCE was well tolerated with no incidence of adverse events in healthy subjects and CF patients [53,55]. After 14 days of once-daily treatment (500 mg ARIKAYCE) in CF patients, an increase in FEV_1 (% predicted) over baseline of 5.6% ($p = 0.03$) was observed [53], which supported further development in CF.

The longest exposure to inhaled ARIKAYCE of 504 days comes from an open-label extension period in a Phase 2 CF trial ($n = 49$) evaluating 6 cycles of a 28-day on treatment (560 mg) followed by a 56-day off treatment [52]. There was a mean 0.6 log CFU reduction over baseline ($p = 0.003$) at the end of each of the six 28-day dosing periods [52]. There was also a statistically significant improvement in lung function compared to baselines of 7.9% ($p < 0.0001$) and 5.9% ($p = 0.0001$) at the end of each 28-day

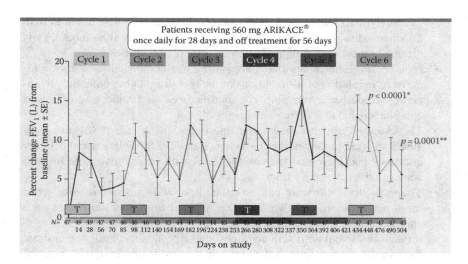

FIGURE 8.7 Change in lung function (FEV_1, % predicted) from baseline through cycle 6 for 49 cystic fibrosis patients in an open-label extension. Each cycle consists of once-daily administration of 560 mg ARIKACE for 28 days followed by a 56-day off treatment. (From Okusanya, O.O. et al., *Antimicrob. Agents Chemother.*, 53(9), 3847, 2009. With permission.)

treatment cycle and 56-day off-treatment cycle, respectively (Figure 8.7). ARIKAYCE met the primary endpoint of noninferiority to TOBI (tobramycin inhalation solution) in a phase 3 trial of ARIKAYCE in CF [51]. These data supported regulatory filings with the EMA [102]; however, approval in the EU is not anticipated in 2016.

In NCFB, inhaled once-daily ARIKACE (280 or 560 mg) was shown to be safe and well tolerated versus placebo after 28 days [24]. However, there has been no further recent activity in this patient population.

As discussed earlier, there are no approved inhaled treatments for NTM infections in the lung. The ability of liposomes to accumulate in alveolar macrophages, the site of NTM infections, provides strong rationale for an inhaled liposomal anti-infective to combat this disease. To that end, a Phase 2 trial evaluating once-daily inhaled ARIKACE for 84 days in NTM was recently completed [103]. While the primary efficacy endpoint of a change in mycobacterial density was not met, a secondary endpoint of culture conversion was achieved with 11 out of 44 patients treated with ARIKAYCE demonstrating negative cultures by day 84 of the study compared to 3 out of 45 patients treated with placebo ($p = 0.01$) [103]. A Phase 3 trial in treatment refractory patients with NTM lung infections is ongoing [102].

SUMMARY

- With more than 10 liposomal products on the market and a greater than 20-year history for one (AmBisome), liposomes have a good track record of safety.
- High-quality lipids with registered DMFs are available from multiple suppliers. Manufacturing of liposomes has become routine and predictable.

The analytical characterization of liposomal products is more complex than for standard solution formulations; however, the analytical methodology is routine in most well-equipped pharmaceutical laboratories.

- *Inhaled* liposome-encapsulated drugs offer reduced systemic toxicity compared to inhalation of formulations of the free drug. Other potential advantages include better tolerability, a modified release profile, and improved compliance due to less frequent dosing.
- The extensive interest in *inhaled* liposomes in the late 1980s and early 1990s answered many of the fundamental *in vitro* formulation and delivery questions and increased the comfort level with *in vivo* exposure to liposomes in the respiratory tract.
- The most straightforward path to create liposomal aerosols is using jet or mesh nebulization, and two late-stage inhaled liposomal antibiotics have chosen these delivery modalities.
- *Inhaled* liposomal amikacin and liposomal ciprofloxacin both demonstrate increased residence time in the lung and delayed systemic uptake, as compared to unencapsulated antibiotic formulations, and may be approved to treat lung infections in the near future.

REFERENCES

1. Allen, T.M. and P.R. Cullis. Liposomal drug delivery systems: From concept to clinical applications. *Adv Drug Deliv Rev*, 2013. **65**(1): 36–48.
2. Allen, T.M. and P.R. Cullis. Drug delivery systems: Entering the mainstream. *Science*, 2004. **303**(5665): 1818–1822.
3. Loira-Pastoriza, C., J. Todoroff, and R. Vanbever. Delivery strategies for sustained drug release in the lungs. *Adv Drug Deliv Rev*, 2014. **75**: 81–91.
4. Schreier, H. Liposome aerosols. *J Liposome Res*, 1992. **2**(2): 145–184.
5. Schreier, H., R.J. Gonzalez-Rothi, and A.A. Stecenko. Pulmonary delivery of liposomes. *J Control Release*, 1993. **24**(1): 209–223.
6. Dupont, B. Overview of the lipid formulations of amphotericin B. *J Antimicrob Chemother*, 2002. **49**(Suppl. 1): 31–36.
7. Adler-Moore, J. and R.T. Proffitt. AmBisome: Liposomal formulation, structure, mechanism of action and pre-clinical experience. *J Antimicrob Chemother*, 2002. **49**(Suppl. 1): 21–30.
8. Stone, N.R. et al. Liposomal amphotericin B (AmBisome): A review of the pharmacokinetics, pharmacodynamics, clinical experience and future directions. *Drugs*, 2016. **76**(4): 485–500
9. Bangham, A.D., M.M. Standish, and J.C. Watkins. Diffusion of univalent ions across the lamellae of swollen phospholipids. *J Mol Biol*, 1965. **13**: 238–252.
10. Fugit, K.D. et al. Mechanistic model and analysis of doxorubicin release from liposomal formulations. *J Control Release*, 2015. **217**: 82–91.
11. Tardi, P.G., N.L. Boman, and P.R. Cullis. Liposomal doxorubicin. *J Drug Target*, 1996. **4**(3): 129–140.
12. Abraham, S.A. et al. The liposomal formulation of doxorubicin. *Methods Enzymol*, 2005. **391**: 71–97.
13. Rodriguez, M.A. et al. Vincristine sulfate liposomes injection (Marqibo) in heavily pretreated patients with refractory aggressive non-Hodgkin lymphoma: Report of the pivotal phase 2 study. *Cancer*, 2009. **115**(15): 3475–3482.

14. Hagemeister, F. et al. Long term results of a phase 2 study of vincristine sulfate liposome injection (Marqibo((R))) substituted for non-liposomal vincristine in cyclophosphamide, doxorubicin, vincristine, prednisone with or without rituximab for patients with untreated aggressive non-Hodgkin lymphomas. *Br J Haematol*, 2013. **162**(5): 631–638.

15. Silverman, J.A. and S.R. Deitcher. Marqibo(R) (vincristine sulfate liposome injection) improves the pharmacokinetics and pharmacodynamics of vincristine. *Cancer Chemother Pharmacol*, 2013. **71**(3): 555–564.

16. Kaplan, L.D. et al. Phase II study of vincristine sulfate liposome injection (Marqibo) and rituximab for patients with relapsed and refractory diffuse large B-Cell lymphoma or mantle cell lymphoma in need of palliative therapy. *Clin Lymphoma Myeloma Leuk*, 2014. **14**(1): 37–42.

17. Mayer, L.D. et al. Techniques for encapsulating bioactive agents into liposomes. *Chem Phys Lipids*, 1986. **40**(2–4): 333–345.

18. Lasic, D.D. et al. Transmembrane gradient driven phase transitions within vesicles: Lessons for drug delivery. *Biochim Biophys Acta*, 1995. **1239**(2): 145–156.

19. Boman, N.L., L.D. Mayer, and P.R. Cullis. Optimization of the retention properties of vincristine in liposomal systems. *Biochim Biophys Acta*, 1993. **1152**(2): 253–258.

20. de Gier, J., J.G. Mandersloot, and L.L. van Deenen. Lipid composition and permeability of liposomes. *Biochim Biophys Acta*, 1968. **150**(4): 666–675.

21. Mayer, L.D. et al. Uptake of antineoplastic agents into large unilamellar vesicles in response to a membrane potential. *Biochim Biophys Acta*, 1985. **816**(2): 294–302.

22. Mohammadi ZA et al. Liposomal doxorubicin delivery systems: Effects of formulation and processing parameters on drug loading and release behavior. *Curr Drug Deliv*, 2015. **13**: 1–1. The doi is: 10.2174/1567201813666151228104643.

23. Niven, R.W. and H. Schreier. Nebulization of liposomes. I. Effects of lipid composition. *Pharm Res*, 1990. **7**(11): 1127–1133.

24. Cipolla, D., I. Gonda, and H.K. Chan. Liposomal formulations for inhalation. *Ther Deliv*, 2013. **4**(8): 1047–1072.

25. Johnston, M.J.W. et al. Therapeutically optimized rates of drug release can be achieved by varying the drug-to-lipid ratio in liposomal vincristine formulations. *Biochim Biophys Acta Biomembr*, 2006. **1758**(1): 55–64.

26. Cipolla, D., J. Froehlich, and I. Gonda. Emerging opportunities for inhaled antimicrobial therapy. *J Antimicro*, 2015. **1**(1): 104.

27. Cipolla, D. et al. Formation of drug nanocrystals under nanoconfinement afforded by liposomes. *RSC Adv*, 2016. **6**(8): 6223–6233.

28. Mayer, L.D. et al. Comparison of free and liposome encapsulated doxorubicin tumor drug uptake and antitumor efficacy in the SC115 murine mammary tumor. *Cancer Lett*, 1990. **53**(2–3): 183–190.

29. Kellaway, I.W. and S.J. Farr. Liposomes as drug delivery systems to the lung. *Adv Drug Deliv Rev*, 1990. **5**(1): 149–161.

30. Cipolla, D., J. Blanchard, and I. Gonda. Development of liposomal ciprofloxacin to treat lung infections. *Pharmaceutics*, 2016. **8**(1): 6.

31. Cipolla, D. et al. Lipid-based carriers for pulmonary products: Preclinical development and case studies in humans. *Adv Drug Deliv Rev*, 2014. **75**: 53–80.

32. Cipolla, D., T. Redelmeier, S. Eastman, P. Bruinenberg, and I. Gonda. Liposomes, niosomes and proniosomes—A critical update of their (commercial) development as inhaled products. In *Respiratory Drug Delivery Europe 2011*, P.R. Byron, R.N. Dalby, J. Peart, J.D. Suman, S.J. Farr, P.M. Young, eds. River Grove, IL: Davis Healthcare Int'l Publishing, 2011, pp 41–54.

33. Cipolla, D.C. and I. Gonda. Formulation technology to repurpose drugs for inhalation delivery. *Drug Discov Today*, 2011. **8**(3–4): 123–130.

34. Cipolla, D. and H.-K. Chan. Inhaled antibiotics to treat lung infection. *Pharm Patent Analyst*, 2013. **2**(5): 647–663.
35. Waldrep, J.C. et al. Pulmonary delivery of beclomethasone liposome aerosol in volunteers: Tolerance and safety. *Chest*, 1997. **111**(2): 316–323.
36. Saari, S.M. et al. Regional lung deposition and clearance of 99mTc-labeled beclomethasone-DLPC liposomes in mild and severe asthma. *Chest*, 1998. **113**(6): 1573–1579.
37. Saari, M. et al. Pulmonary distribution and clearance of two beclomethasone liposome formulations in healthy volunteers. *Int J Pharm*, 1999. **181**(1): 1–9.
38. Abra, R.M., P.J. Mihalko, and H. Schreier. The effect of lipid composition upon the encapsulation and *in vitro* leakage of metaproterenol sulfate from 0.2μm diameter, extruded, multilamellar liposomes. *J Control Release*, 1990. **14**(1): 71–78.
39. Fielding, R.M. and R.M. Abra. Factors affecting the release rate of terbutaline from liposome formulations after intratracheal instillation in the guinea pig. *Pharm Res*, 1992. **9**(2): 220–223.
40. Taylor, K.M. et al. The influence of liposomal encapsulation on sodium cromoglycate pharmacokinetics in man. *Pharm Res*, 1989. **6**(7): 633–636.
41. Verschraegen, C.F. et al. Feasibility, phase I, and pharmacological study of aerosolized liposomal 9-nitro-20(S)-camptothecin in patients with advanced malignancies in the lungs. *Ann N Y Acad Sci*, 2000. **922**: 352–354.
42. Verschraegen, C.F. et al. Clinical evaluation of the delivery and safety of aerosolized liposomal 9-nitro-20(s)-camptothecin in patients with advanced pulmonary malignancies. *Clin Cancer Res*, 2004. **10**(7): 2319–2326.
43. Skubitz, K.M. and P.M. Anderson. Inhalational interleukin-2 liposomes for pulmonary metastases: A phase I clinical trial. *Anticancer Drugs*, 2000. **11**(7): 555–563.
44. Wittgen, B.P. et al. Assessing a system to capture stray aerosol during inhalation of nebulized liposomal cisplatin. *J Aerosol Med*, 2006. **19**(3): 385–391.
45. Monforte, V. et al. Feasibility, tolerability, and outcomes of nebulized liposomal amphotericin B for Aspergillus infection prevention in lung transplantation. *J Heart Lung Transplant*, 2010. **29**(5): 523–530.
46. Monforte, V. et al. Nebulized liposomal amphotericin B prophylaxis for Aspergillus infection in lung transplantation: Pharmacokinetics and safety. *J Heart Lung Transplant*, 2009. **28**(2): 170–175.
47. Monforte, V. et al. Prophylaxis with nebulized liposomal amphotericin B for Aspergillus infection in lung transplant patients does not cause changes in the lipid content of pulmonary surfactant. *J Heart Lung Transplant*, 2013. **32**(3): 313–319.
48. Niven, R.W., W. Verret, H. Raff, T.E. Corcoran, and S.G. Dilly. The challenges of developing an inhaled cyclosporine product for lung transplant patients. In *Respiratory Drug Delivery 2012*, P.R. Byron, R.N. Dalby, J. Peart, J.D. Suman, S.J. Farr, P.M. Young, eds. River Grove, IL: Davis Healthcare Int'l Publishing, pp. 51–60, 2012.
49. Gilbert, B.E. et al. Tolerance of volunteers to cyclosporine A-dilauroylphosphatidylcholine liposome aerosol. *Am J Respir Crit Care Med*, 1997. **156**(6): 1789–1793.
50. Behr, J. et al. Lung deposition of a liposomal cyclosporine A inhalation solution in patients after lung transplantation. *J Aerosol Med Pulm Drug Deliv*, 2009. **22**(2): 121–130.
51. Bilton, D. et al. Phase 3 efficacy and safety data from randomized, multicenter study of liposomal amikacin for inhalation. In *NACF Conference*, Salt Lake City, UT, 2013.
52. Clancy, J.P. et al. Phase II studies of nebulised Arikace in CF patients with *Pseudomonas aeruginosa* infection. *Thorax*, 2013. **68**(9): 818–825.
53. Okusanya, O.O. et al. Pharmacokinetic and pharmacodynamic evaluation of liposomal amikacin for inhalation in cystic fibrosis patients with chronic pseudomonal infection. *Antimicrob Agents Chemother*, 2009. **53**(9): 3847–3854.

54. Okusanya, O.O. et al. Evaluation of the pharmacokinetics and pharmacodynamics of liposomal amikacin for inhalation in cystic fibrosis patients with chronic pseudomonal infections using data from two phase 2 clinical studies. *Antimicrob Agents Chemother*, 2014. **58**(9): 5005–5015.

55. Weers, J. et al. A gamma scintigraphy study to investigate lung deposition and clearance of inhaled amikacin-loaded liposomes in healthy male volunteers. *J Aerosol Med Pulm Drug Deliv*, 2009. **22**(2): 131–138.

56. Serisier, D.J. et al. Inhaled, dual release liposomal ciprofloxacin in non-cystic fibrosis bronchiectasis (ORBIT-2): A randomised, double-blind, placebo-controlled trial. *Thorax*, 2013. **68**(9): 812–817.

57. Blanchard, J., L. Danelishvili, I. Gonda, and L. Bermudez. Liposomal ciprofloxacin preparation is active against mycobacterium avium subsp hominissuis and mycobacterium abscessus in macrophages and in biofilm. In *ATS Conference*, San Diego 2014.

58. Bruinenberg, P., J. Blanchard, D.C. Cipolla, F. Dayton, S. Mudumba, and I. Gonda. Inhaled liposomal ciprofloxacin: Once a day management of respiratory infections. In *Respiratory Drug Delivery 2010*, P.R. Byron, R.N. Dalby, J. Peart, J.D. Suman, S.J. Farr, P.M. Young, eds. River Grove, IL: Davis Healthcare Int'l Publishing, 2010. 73–81.

59. Yim, D., J. Blanchard, S. Mudumba, S. Eastman, K. Manda, T. Redelmeier, and S. Farr. The development of inhaled liposome-encapsulated ciprofloxacin to treat cystic fibrosis. In *Respiratory Drug Delivery X*, P.R. Byron, R.N. Dalby, J. Peart, J.D. Suman, S.J. Farr, P.M. Young, eds. River Grove, IL: Davis Healthcare International Publishing, 2005. 425–428.

60. US FDA CDER. Draft guidance: Liposome drug products. Silver Spring, Maryland, 2015.

61. Riley, T. et al. Challenges with developing *in vitro* dissolution tests for orally inhaled products (OIPs). *AAPS PharmSciTech*, 2012. **13**(3): 978–989.

62. Marques, M.R.C., R. Loebenberg, and M. Almukainzi. Simulated biological fluids wih possible application in dissolution testing. *Dissolut Technol*, 2011. **18**(3): 14–28.

63. Cipolla, D. et al. Development and characterization of an *in vitro* release assay for liposomal ciprofloxacin for inhalation. *J Pharm Sci*, 2014. **103**(1): 314–327.

64. Weinstein, J.N. et al. Phase transition release, a new approach to the interaction of proteins with lipid vesicles: Application to lipoproteins. *Biochim Biophys Acta*, 1981. **647**(2): 270–284.

65. Allen, T.M. A study of phospholipid interactions between high-density lipoproteins and small unilamellar vesicles. *Biochim Biophys Acta*, 1981. **640**(2): 385–397.

66. Cipolla, D. et al. Modifying the release properties of liposomes toward personalized medicine. *J Pharm Sci*, 2014. **103**(6): 1851–1862.

67. Center for Drug Evaluation and Research (U.S.), Center for Biologics Evaluation and Research (U.S.), International Conference on Harmonisation. *Pharmaceutical Development Q8(R2)*. Rockville, MD: U.S. Department of Health and Human Services, Food and Drug Administration, Center for Drug Evaluation and Research, 2009.

68. Edwards, K.A. and A.J. Baeumner. Analysis of liposomes. *Talanta*, 2006. **68**(5): 1432–1441.

69. Crommelin, D.J. and E.M. van Bommel. Stability of liposomes on storage: Freeze dried, frozen or as an aqueous dispersion. *Pharm Res*, 1984. **1**(4): 159–163.

70. Grit, M. and D.J. Crommelin. Chemical stability of liposomes: Implications for their physical stability. *Chem Phys Lipids*, 1993. **64**(1–3): 3–18.

71. Crommelin, D.J.A. and G. Storm. Liposomes: From the bench to the bed. *J Liposome Res*, 2003. **13**(1): 33–36.

72. Meers, P.R. and P.L. Ahl. Stress testing to determine liposome degradation mechanisms. In *Pharmaceutical Stress Testing*. CRC Press, Boca Raton, Florida. pp. 426–446, 2011.

73. Grit, M. and D.J. Crommelin. The effect of aging on the physical stability of liposome dispersions. *Chem Phys Lipids*, 1992. **62**(2): 113–122.
74. Zuidam, N.J. et al. Physical (in) stability of liposomes upon chemical hydrolysis: The role of lysophospholipids and fatty acids. *Biochim Biophys Acta*, 1995. **1240**(1): 101–110.
75. Zuidam, N.J. and D.J. Crommelin. Chemical hydrolysis of phospholipids. *J Pharm Sci*, 1995. **84**(9): 1113–1119.
76. Gregoriadis, G., ed. *Liposome Technology*, 3rd edn. Vol. 1: Liposome preparation and related techniques. New York: Informa Healthcare USA, Inc., 2007.
77. Mozafari, M.R. Liposomes: An overview of manufacturing techniques. *Cell Mol Biol Lett*, 2005. **10**(4): 711–719.
78. Gregoriadis, G., ed. *Liposome Technology*, 3rd edn. Vol. 2: Entrapment of drugs and other materials into liposomes. New York: Informa Healthcare USA, Inc., 2007.
79. Zuidam, N.J., S.S. Lee, and D.J. Crommelin. Gamma-irradiation of non-frozen, frozen, and freeze-dried liposomes. *Pharm Res*, 1995. **12**(11): 1761–1768.
80. Zuidam, N.J., S.S. Lee, and D.J. Crommelin. Sterilization of liposomes by heat treatment. *Pharm Res*, 1993. **10**(11): 1591–1596.
81. Zuidam, N.J. et al. Gamma-irradiation of liposomes composed of saturated phospholipids: Effect of bilayer composition, size, concentration and absorbed dose on chemical degradation and physical destabilization of liposomes. *Biochim Biophys Acta*, 1996. **1280**(1): 135–148.
82. Ingvarsson, P.T. et al. Stabilization of liposomes during drying. *Expert Opin Drug Deliv*, 2011. **8**(3): 375–388.
83. Misra, A. et al. Recent advances in liposomal dry powder formulations: Preparation and evaluation. *Expert Opin Drug Deliv*, 2009. **6**(1): 71–89.
84. Mansour, H.M., Y.S. Rhee, and X. Wu. Nanomedicine in pulmonary delivery. *Int J Nanomed*, 2009. **4**: 299–319.
85. Willis, L., D. Hayes, Jr., and H.M. Mansour. Therapeutic liposomal dry powder inhalation aerosols for targeted lung delivery. *Lung*, 2012. **190**(3): 251–262.
86. Polin, R.A. and W.A. Carlo. Surfactant replacement therapy for preterm and term neonates with respiratory distress. *Pediatrics*, 2014. **133**(1): 156–163.
87. Zhou, Q.T. et al. Inhaled formulations and pulmonary drug delivery systems for respiratory infections. *Adv Drug Deliv Rev*, 2015. **85**: 83–99.
88. Weers, J. Inhaled antimicrobial therapy—Barriers to effective treatment. *Adv Drug Deliv Rev*, 2015. **85**: 24–43.
89. Cipolla, D., J. Froehlich, and I. Gonda. Comment on: Inhaled antimicrobial therapy—Barriers to effective treatment, by J. Weers, inhaled antimicrobial therapy—Barriers to effective treatment, *Adv Drug Deliv Rev*, 2015. **85**: e6–e7.
90. Kardas, P. Comparison of patient compliance with once-daily and twice-daily antibiotic regimens in respiratory tract infections: Results of a randomized trial. *J Antimicrob Chemother*, 2007. **59**(3): 531–536.
91. Haworth, C.S. et al. Inhaled colistin in patients with bronchiectasis and chronic *Pseudomonas aeruginosa* infection. *Am J Respir Crit Care Med*, 2014. **189**(8): 975–982.
92. Cipolla, D.C., F. Dayton, S. Fulzele, E. Gabatan, S. Mudumba, D. Yim, H. Wu, and R. Zwolinski. Inhaled liposomal ciprofloxacin: *In vitro* properties and aerosol performance. In *Respiratory Drug Delivery 2010*, P.R. Byron, R.N. Dalby, J. Peart, J.D. Suman, S.J. Farr, P.M. Young, eds. River Grove, IL: Davis Healthcare Int'l Publishing, 2010. 409–414.
93. Cipolla, D., H. Wu, J. Chan, H.-K. Chan, and I. Gonda. Liposomal ciprofloxacin for inhalation retains integrity following nebulization. In *Respiratory Drug Delivery Europe 2013*, P.R. Byron, R.N. Dalby, J. Peart, J.D. Suman, S.J. Farr, P.M. Young, eds. River Grove, IL: Davis Healthcare Int'l Publishing, 2013. 237–242.

94. Ong, H.X. et al. Liposomal nanoparticles control the uptake of ciprofloxacin across respiratory epithelia. *Pharm Res*, 2012. **29**(12): 3335–3346.
95. Ong, H.X. et al. *In vitro* and ex vivo methods predict the enhanced lung residence time of liposomal ciprofloxacin formulations for nebulisation. *Eur J Pharm Biopharm*, 2014. **86**(1): 83–89.
96. Norville, I.H. et al. Efficacy of liposome-encapsulated ciprofloxacin in a murine model of Q fever. *Antimicrob Agents Chemother*, 2014. **58**(9): 5510–5518.
97. Hamblin, K.A. et al. The potential of liposome-encapsulated ciprofloxacin as a tularemia therapy. *Front Cell Infect Microbiol*, 2014. **4**: 79.
98. Hamblin, K.A. et al. Liposome encapsulation of ciprofloxacin improves protection against highly virulent *Francisella tularensis* strain Schu S4. *Antimicrob Agents Chemother*, 2014. **58**(6): 3053–3059.
99. Hamblin, K.A., J.D. Blanchard, C. Davis, S.V. Harding, A.J.H. Simpson. Efficacy of inhaled liposome-encapsulated ciprofloxacin against *Yersinia pestis*. *J Aerosol Med Pulm Drug Deliv*, 2013. **26**(2): A-16.
100. Li, Z. et al. Characterization of nebulized liposomal amikacin (Arikace) as a function of droplet size. *J Aerosol Med Pulm Drug Deliv*, 2008. **21**(3): 245–254.
101. Meers, P. et al. Biofilm penetration, triggered release and *in vivo* activity of inhaled liposomal amikacin in chronic *Pseudomonas aeruginosa* lung infections. *J Antimicrob Chemother*, 2008. **61**(4): 859–868.
102. Release, I.c.p. Insmed provides regulatory update for ARIKAYCE. August 4, 2014. Available from: http://investor.insmed.com/releasedetail.cfm?ReleaseID=863838.
103. Release, I.c.p. Insmed announces results from phase 2 clinical trial for treatment resistant nontuberculous mycobacterial lung infections. March 26, 2014. Available from: http://investor.insmed.com/releasedetail.cfm?ReleaseID=835499.
104. Cipolla, D., I. Gonda, and S.J. Shire. Characterization of aerosols of human recombinant deoxyribonuclease I (rhDNase) generated by jet nebulizers. *Pharm Res*, 1994. **11**(4): 491–498.

9 Inhaled Traditional Chinese Medicine for Respiratory Diseases

Yun Zhao, Jing Zhou, Yong-Hong Liao, and Ying Zheng

CONTENTS

Respiratory diseases, including asthma, chronic obstructive pulmonary disease (COPD), bronchitis, bronchiolitis, and respiratory tract infections, are one of the most common health problems in the world. Data from the World Health Organization [1] showed that lower respiratory tract infections (LRTI) and COPD are ranked third and fourth, respectively, in the top ten global death causes. In China, respiratory diseases are responsible for ~14% of hospitalizations and 13%–16% of deaths (excluding lung cancer). Uniquely, apart from conventional chemical drugs used for the standard treatment, *traditional Chinese medicine* (*TCM*) has also been playing an important role in the primary care and first-line treatment of patients with respiratory diseases in China [2]. Although the sales of TCMs accounted only for less than 20% of the total Chinese pharmaceutical market, the market share of TCMs for the treatment of respiratory diseases was as high as 45% in 2011. In particular, among the drug sales in hospitals, 10.88% of TCM were used for respiratory diseases, markedly higher than 2.71% of chemical drugs [3].

Clinically, TCM are generally administered by oral or intravenous routes. Compared to oral administration, TCM injections exhibit a rapid onset of effect and favorable efficacy. As a consequence, TCM injections are often preferred to the oral counterparts for hospitalized patients with respiratory diseases. Indeed, among the top five selling TCM products by annual sales in hospitals for respiratory diseases, four of them, namely, *Xiyanping, Tanreqing, Xuebijing,* and *Yanhuning,* are injectables, accounting for about 35% of the market share of respiratory diseases. However, with the increasingly wide application of TCM injections in clinical practice, the associated adverse drug reactions (ADRs) are becoming a worrisome issue and even the target of public criticism in the recent years [4]. The use of TCM injections has caused ~50% of ADR and 83%–87% of severe ADR associated with TCM, despite the fact that the former only accounts for a minor fraction of total TCM consumption in terms of the number of prescriptions. The occurrence of fatal ADR associated with TCM injections has resulted in not only the suspension of certain products, such as *Yuxingcao,* but also the damaged credibility of TCM injections as a whole. Although great efforts have been dedicated to reevaluate the clinical safety, the occurrence of ADR associated with TCM injections is yet largely unpredictable. Therefore, it is highly desirable to pursue alternative delivering means to injections of TCM so as to maintain the advantages of rapid onset and favorable efficacy and yet to minimize ADR associated with injections.

INHALATION DELIVERY OF TCM

Inhalation delivery represents the oldest modes of drug delivery and the therapeutic value of inhaled TCM, mainly practiced in the form of smoke and steam vapor together with medicated pillows and aromatic sachets, was well recognized in ancient China [5]. The earliest documented TCM inhalation therapy for respiratory disease might be the smoke inhalation of *Flos Farfarae (Tussilago farfara)* for the relief of chronic cough as recorded in the book *A Handbook of Prescriptions for Emergencies* (Zhou Hou Bei Ji Fang) by Ge Hong (284–346). Nowadays, inhaled TCMs are mainly delivered by metered-dose inhalers (MDIs) and nebulizers. There were four TCM MDI products, which were approved for treating respiratory disease, including asthma and influenza, by the China Food and Drug Administration (CFDA). However, these chlorofluorocarbon (CFC)-based MDI products are subjected to phaseout due to the implementation of the Montreal Protocol. In general, the availability and accessibility to TCM MDI products are negligible in the current market.

The off-label uses of TCM injections for nebulization have been extensively practiced in China for the last two decades and there have been a large number of randomized controlled trials and nonrandomized controlled studies of nebulized TCM for respiratory diseases. After searching the clinical studies of nebulized TCM therapy in the literature including Chinese publications in China National Knowledge Infrastructure electronic database (1979–October 2015), a total of 892 reports (involving 55,000 patients) including 695 randomized controlled trials and 197 nonrandomized controlled studies were retrieved. Among the published reports, 59 of them were documented for treating nonrespiratory diseases, such as heart disease, coronary heart disease, stroke, esophagitis, and cerebrovascular disease, whereas the rest were for respiratory diseases with the most frequent indications being upper respiratory tract infection (URTI, including pharyngitis, pharyngolaryngitis, oral mucositis,

TABLE 9.1

Summary of Traditional Chinese Medicine Nebulization Therapy in Active Control Trials

Indications	Number of Cases	Effective Rate Nebulization (%)	Controls (%)	Number of Reports
URTI	30,434	92.6	74.0	384
Bronchitis/ bronchiolitis	9,334	93.8	76.8	190
Pneumonia	7,217	92.3	73.9	153
Asthma	2,626	91.2	77.6	54
COPD	2,379	93.1	77.9	52
Others	3,010	85.9	80.2	59
Total	55,000	—	—	892

Notes: URTI, upper respiratory tract infection, including pharyngitis, pharyngolaryngitis, oral mucositis, and rhinitis; COPD, chronic obstructive pulmonary disease; others, nonrespiratory diseases.

rhinitis, and vocal cord disease), bronchitis, bronchiolitis, pneumonia, asthma, and COPD. These documented clinical studies have investigated the efficacy and safety of nebulized TCM, generally using *active control trials*. Substantial evidence from these trials supports that nebulized TCM conferred to significant therapeutic benefits in terms of reducing exacerbations; improving symptoms by relieving fever, cough, and sore throat and reducing bacterial or viral load and airway inflammation; and decreasing the disease course. As summarized in Table 9.1, the overall therapeutic efficiency conferred by the nebulized TCM appeared to be fairly positive, generally superior to that by the corresponding standard therapy in the control groups. For all the indications of respiratory diseases, nebulized TCM resulted in the *effective rates* [38] of more than 90%, whereas those conferred by standard treatments in the corresponding control groups were below 80%. Among the clinical reports, some trials (exemplified in Table 9.2) have directly compared nebulized TCM with the corresponding intravenously infused counterparts, and it is found that the nebulized route was associated with less ADRs and comparable or significantly better outcomes in terms of effective rates and symptom improvement. Nebulized TCMs are generally regarded safe and only induce very low incidence of minor ADRs. In particular, no case of severe allergic reactions, which are typically associated with TCM injections, has been recorded in the clinical studies of nebulized TCMs.

There are 176 TCM formulas that are intended for oral or parenteral administration and have been clinically utilized for nebulization therapy. Among these formulas, CFDA-approved injectable products of five formulas, namely, *Shuanghuanglian (SHL), Yuxingcao, Qingkailing, Tanreqing*, and *Andrographolides*, have been extensively studied for nebulization and each nebulized formula has been documented in more than 50 reports as summarized in Table 9.3. More details on the clinical applications of nebulized TCM are as follows.

TABLE 9.2
Example Trials Where Nebulized Traditional Chinese Medicine Was Compared with Intravenous Infused Traditional Chinese Medicine

Formula	Indication (n, neb./I.V.)	Neb. Dose	I.V. Dose	Outcome Measures	Conclusion
SHL [20]	Pneumonia (45/45)	600 mg in 30 mL, bid, 5–7 days	60 mg/kg, qd, 5–7 days	Clinical symptoms	Equivalent outcomes, 4 ADR cases in I.V., and 0 in neb.
[19]	Pneumonia (42/28)	30 mg/kg in 20 mL, qd or bid, 7–10 days	60 mg/kg, qd, 7–10 days	Clinical symptoms	Equivalent outcomes, no ADR
YXC [34]	Lower RTI (21/21)	30 mL diluted to 40 mL, bid, 7–10 days	50 mL, bid, 7–10 days, qd, 3–5 days	Clinical symptoms	Equivalent outcomes, no ADR
[35]	Upper RTI (35/48)	5 mL diluted to 20 mL, bid, 5–7 days	10–40 mL/day, qd, 3–5 days	Clinical symptoms	Equivalent outcomes, no ADR
QKL [51]	URTI (92/91)	10 mL diluted to 30 mL, bid, 5–7 days	10 mL diluted to 135 mL, bid, 5–7 days	Clinical symptoms and effective rate	Equivalent outcomes, 2 ADR cases in I.V., and 0 in neb.
[50]	URTI (40/60)	10 mL diluted to 30 mL, bid, 5–7 days	10 mL diluted to 125 mL, bid, 5–7 days	Clinical symptoms and effective rate	Neb. more efficacious, no ADR
TRQ [61]	Bronchitis (60/60)	5 mL diluted to 25 mL, bid, 7 days	0.5 mL/kg in 100 mL, qd, 7 days	Clinical symptoms and length of hospital stay	Neb. more efficacious, 16 ADR cases in I.V., and 5 in neb.
[62]	Chronic bronchitis (35/29)	10 mL, diluted to 25 mL, bid, up to 15 days	30 mL diluted to 300 mL, qd, up to 15 days	Effective rate	Neb. more efficacious, no ADR
AGP [71]	Pneumonia (75/75)	0.2 g in 50 mL, bid, 21 days	0.4 g in 250 mL, bid, 21 days	Clinical symptoms	Equivalent outcomes, 24 ADR cases including 1 case anaphylactic shock in I.V. and 0 in neb.
[69]	URTI (250/250)	4–5 mg/kg diluted to 20 mL, bid, 3–5 days	5–8 mg/kg diluted to 100 mL, qd, 3–5 days	Effective rate	Neb. more efficacious, no ADR

Notes: *SHL*, *Shuanghuanglian*; YXC, *Yuxingcao*; QKL, *Qingkailing*; TRQ, *Tanreqing*; AGP, *Andrographolides*; CAV, cough variant asthma; neb, nebulization; I.V., intravenous infusion; ADR, adverse reactions; qd, once a day; bid, twice a day.

TABLE 9.3
Clinical Applications of Five Main Nebulized Traditional Chinese Medicine Formulas

Formula	Indications (Number of Trials)	Number of Cases	Effective Rate		ADR in Neb.
			Neb. (%)	Controls (%)	
SHL	Bronchitis or bronchiolitis (40), pneumonia (27), asthma (2), URTI (85), COPD (1), others (7)	9590	92.5	73.5	117 trials recorded 12 ADR cases, for example, cough, diarrhea, rash, and skin redness.
YXC	Bronchitis or bronchiolitis (17), pneumonia (22), asthma (2), URTI (59), COPD (4), others (9)	9952	92.6	76.7	64 trials recorded 2 ADR cases, for example, mild diarrhea.
QKL	Bronchitis or bronchiolitis (8), pneumonia (3), URTI (38), COPD (7), others (11)	5392	94.3	72.3	39 trials recorded 33 ADR cases, for example, rash, diarrhea, and nausea.
TRQ	Bronchitis or bronchiolitis (8), pneumonia (28), asthma (6), URTI (25), COPD (12), others (8)	4493	96.6	80.4	65 trials recorded 8 ADR cases, for example, mild diarrhea.
AGP	Bronchitis or bronchiolitis (24), pneumonia (18), URTI (50), COPD (1), others (2)	5444	94.1	79.9	88 trials recorded 52 ADR cases, for example, mild diarrhea, nausea, and skin discomfort.

Notes: SHL, Shuanghuanglian; YXC, Yuxingcao; QKL, Qingkailing; TRQ, Tanreqing; AGP, Andrographolides; Neb., nebulization; ADR, adverse drug reaction.

NEBULIZED *SHL*

SHL is extracted and refined from honeysuckle flower, *Radix Scutellariae*, and *Fructus Forsythiae* and it was initially approved in an injectable formulation in the early 1970s for the treatment of influenza and respiratory infections in China, and later, the peroral and inhalation products were also developed. *SHL* contains various chemical ingredients, including phenolic acids, flavonoids, phenylethanoid glycosides, iridoid glycosides, and lignans, with chlorogenic acid, baicalin, and forsythia glycosides being used as chemical makers for quality control in the *Chinese Pharmacopoeia* [6]. Numerous pharmacological studies have demonstrated that the preparation and the containing ingredients have the ability of anti-inflammation, improving immunity, and inhibiting the growth of various viruses and bacteria [7–10]. In addition, a great number of randomized controlled trials have also confirmed the effectiveness of *SHL* injections for the treatment of acute URTIs, common cold, pneumonia, and other respiratory diseases caused by bacteria/viruses [11–13].

However, with the extensive application of *SHL* injections clinically, high incidence of ADRs associated with the injections was observed and severe ADRs, such as anaphylactic shock and dyspnea, were reported twice by the National ADR Monitoring Center of China. And hence the sales and application of *SHL* injections from certain companies were suspended by the CFDA in 2009 [14,15]. Since then, the number of annual prescriptions collapsed from 600 million to less than 100 million ampoules. Currently, the reasons underlying the ADRs are not completely clear, but they appeared to correlate with the "impurities" and the incompatibility with coadministered drugs and/or diluents. *SHL* has a complex composition, and it may remain a minor amount of tannins, proteins, and resins, which could not be completely removed during the manufacturing process. These "impurities" could cause allergic reactions and other ADRs when intravenously delivered. In addition, as suggested in a retrospective study of 4382 medical records, only 1.0% of *SHL* injections were used independently, whereas 82.8% of applications were combined with antibiotics [16]. Mixing *SHL* injections with other drug solutions or diluting solvents, such as glucose or sodium chloride solution, often resulted in increases in the insoluble particles [17–19]. In a systematic review of public references on ADRs associated with *SHL* injections, Wang and colleagues [15] found that coadministration of other medicines with *SHL* injections increased the ADR incidence by 2.69 times as compared to the single use of the injection.

SHL is the most extensively studied TCM formula for inhalation delivery and its CFC-based MDI was approved by the CFDA for the treatment of influenza, sore throat, and cough, but it was subjected to phaseout and the hydrofluoroalkane (HFA)-based alternative is yet registered. As for the nebulization therapy, the clinical effectiveness has been addressed in 123 randomized controlled trials (involving 6817 patients) and 39 nonrandomized controlled studies (2773 patients). Similar to the injections, nebulized *SHL* in these trials was mainly used for the treatment of acute URTIs, pneumonia, and bronchitis/bronchiolitis caused by bacteria/viruses. In the majority of the trials, effective rates were used to assess therapeutic outcome. The clinical efficacy of nebulized *SHL* is discussed in the present review using data from 162 published studies, which included a total of 9590 infant, children, or adult patients.

These studies suggested that treatment with nebulized *SHL*, which exhibited overall average effective rates of over 90%, has been shown to be more effective than the corresponding control groups dealt with standard treatment, which conferred to overall average effective rates of less than 80% (Table 9.3). The ADRs of nebulized *SHL* were largely uninvestigated in many of these trials. Only 12 cases of ADRs were reported in 117 trials and the incidence of ADRs was less than 0.2%, which was 10-fold lower than 3.25% of incidence associated with intravenous *SHL* reported by Wang et al. [15]. The main ADRs associated with nebulized *SHL* included cough, diarrhea, rash, and skin redness, but no typical severe ADRs associated with *SHL* injections were observed.

Several randomized controlled trials (e.g., Table 9.2) have been performed to directly compare the clinical efficacy of nebulized and intravenously infused *SHL* and have shown that nebulized *SHL* was equally as effective as or superior to infused *SHL* in infants, children, and adults with respiratory diseases caused by bacterial or viral infections [20]. For example, in a trial, 70 infants or children aged 2 months–2 years and with asthmatic pneumonia caused by viral infection were randomized to receive 7–10 days' treatment with nebulized *SHL* at 30 mg/kg once or twice daily ($n = 42$) or intravenously infused *SHL* at 60 mg/kg once daily ($n = 28$). The results showed that the length of hospital stay (7.5 ± 1.5 days) and the time for relieving symptoms including coughing (4.6 ± 1.3 days), shortness of breath (5.3 ± 1.1 days), and rales (6.2 ± 1.2 days) with nebulized *SHL* were significantly shorter than those (9.3 ± 2.5, 6.9 ± 1.5, 8.4 ± 2.0, 7.2 ± 1.0 days, respectively) with infused *SHL* [20]. In another similar trial [21], 90 infants or children aged <3 years and with asthmatic pneumonia caused by viral infection were treated with nebulized *SHL* at 5 mg/kg twice daily ($n = 45$) or intravenously infused *SHL* at 60 mg/kg once daily ($n = 45$). Over the course of the trial, statistically significant improvements in the symptoms including fever, coughing, shortness of breath, and rales were noted with no significant difference in the time for relieving symptoms between the two treatment regimens. In addition, 4 cases of ADRs were observed in the patients treated with infused *SHL*, whereas no ADR case was reported in the nebulized group.

However, it is worth noting that the nebulization parameters and protocols adopted in the clinical studies varied noticeably in terms of therapeutic dose, the concentration and fill volume of nebulizer solution, types of nebulizers, and nebulizer duration and frequency (Table 9.4). In the retrieved reports, the therapeutic dose varied from 5 to 100 mg/kg with varied nebulizer duration (10–30 min) and frequency (once to three times daily), whereas the concentration and fill volume of nebulizer solutions ranged from 12–100 mg/mL to 5–60 mL, respectively. There were 22 types of both ultrasonic and jet nebulizers used in these studies, but the aerodynamic properties and the particle size distribution of nebulized droplets were not analyzed.

NEBULIZED *YUXINGCAO*

Yuxingcao injection (also called Houttuynia injection) is the aqueous solution of the steam distillate from *Herba Houttuyniae* and it was initially approved via intramuscular injection in 1978 and then via intravenous injection in 1994 for the treatment of respiratory diseases. The formulation contains volatile oils from *Houttuynia cordata* as the

TABLE 9.4

Technical Aspects of Nebulization Used in the Clinical Studies

	Shuanghuanglian	Yuxingcao	Qingkailing	Tanreqing	Androgapholides
Formulation	Injection solution or reconstituted lyophilized powders	Injection solution	Injection solution or reconstituted lyophilized powders	Injection solution	Injection solution or reconstituted lyophilized powders
Dose	5–100 mg/kg	0.2–1.6 mL/kg	4–24 mg/kg	0.2–1.0 mL/kg	4–20 mg/kg
Fill volume (mL)	4–60	5–130	2–130	2–150	2–40
Drug concentration	12–180 mg/mL	10%–100% of the injection solution	20%–100% of the injection solution	10%–100% of the injection solution	1–40 mg/mL
Types of nebulizers used	22	21	10	6	12
Nebulizing time (min)	10–30	10–30	10–30	10–20	15–40
Dose frequency (times/daily)	1–3	1–4	1–3	1–4	1–3
Particle size distribution, output rate and yield, and residue volume	Not specified				

active ingredients, 0.5% Tween 80 as the solubilizer, and NaCl as the osmotic pressure regulator. The volatile oils have a complex composition with at least 30 ingredients being identified, such as methyl-*n*-nonylketone, decanoylacetaldehyde, bornyl acetate, β-linalool, 1-nonanol, 4-terpineol, and α-terpineol [22–24]. Methyl-*n*-nonylketone is regarded as one of the main active components, and the least of 0.8 μg/mL is required for the quality control of *Yuxingcao* injection. As a *heat-clearing and detoxifying* agent, *Yuxingcao* is traditionally used for the treatment of pneumonia, respiratory and urinary tract infections, refractory hemoptysis, and malignant pleural effusion. Pharmacological studies have demonstrated that *Yuxingcao* exhibited antiviral, anti-bacterial, anti-inflammatory, and immunomodulatory effects [25–28]. During the outbreak of severe acute respiratory syndrome (SARS) in 2003, it was short-listed by Chinese scientists to tackle SARS problem and had played a unique role in improving the immune system of SARS patients and alleviating the side effects associated with standard treatment [29]. The clinical efficacy has also been extensively studied. For example, in a meta-analysis on the efficacy of *Yuxingcao* injection for respiratory tract infections and pneumonia, the authors concluded that the injection resulted in superior therapeutic effect in adult trials but comparable efficacy in child trials to the antibiotics control treatment [30].

The clinical application of *Yuxingcao* injections was found to induce multiple ADRs. In a systematic review of 372 clinical reports involving 34,969 patients, the incidence of ADRs caused by intravenous *Yuxingcao* injections was about 0.87%. Although the incidence was lower than that of *SHL* injections, 59% of the ADR cases of *Yuxingcao* injections fell into the categories of severe ADRs, including 11 cases of death [31]. Due to the occurrence of serious and fatal ADRs, CFDA temporarily suspended the use of injections in early 2006, when *Yuxingcao* was one of the top-selling TCM injections with the number of annual prescriptions being more than 600 million ampoules. Yet, many clinicians believed that the unique therapeutic benefits of *Yuxingcao* injections cannot be fully replaced by current available medicine. As a consequence, in September 2006, the intramuscular formulations were allowed to be reregistered after the reevaluation of the safety, whereas as for the intravenous use of *Yuxingcao* injections, scientists, the Chinese government, and TCM industry have so far been making great efforts to reformulate and to reevaluate the clinical safety. The exact mechanism responsible for the ADRs associated with *Yuxingcao* injection is unclear; possible causes have been attributed to allergens arising from oxidation, polymerization, and hydrolysis of drug ingredients during heating sterilization and/or storage, impurities from drug and excipients, the incompatibility with coadministered drugs and/or diluents, and irrational use in clinical applications [32]. Intravenous administration could result in the higher exposure of particulates induced by incompatibility, impurities, and allergens, leading to 6.7-fold higher incidence of ADRs than intramuscular injections [31].

As shown in Table 9.3, nebulized *Yuxingcao* therapy has also been extensively studied for the treatment of various indications of respiratory diseases, mainly induced by infections. The results from 113 clinical reports involving 9952 patients have shown that aerosolized *Yuxingcao* treatment resulted in average effective rates of over 90% and significantly improved therapeutic outcomes relative to the standard treatment in the control groups. Two meta-analyses [33,34] have been performed to assess the benefits and risks of nebulized *Yuxingcao* in pneumonia and URTIs. The clinical efficacy of nebulized *Yuxingcao* in pneumonia was discussed in the meta-analysis using data from 6 published studies, which included 217 infants and children and 34 adults in the nebulized groups. In the study, the therapeutic outcomes were evaluated in terms of the effective rates, the clinical symptoms and signs, and the length of hospital stay, and the results suggested that nebulization significantly improved the outcomes compared to the control treatment [33]. The data used in the meta-analysis in URTIs were from 11 randomized clinical trials involving 901 infants, children, and adults in the nebulized groups. The control groups were mainly treated with antibiotics. The study concluded that nebulized *Yuxingcao* brought about significant increase in the effective rates and improvement in clinical symptoms and signs relative to the control treatment, but no reliable conclusion on the efficacy and safety of nebulized *Yuxingcao* could be drawn due to the low quality of the randomized clinical trials [34]. Among the 113 clinical reports, 64 of them mentioned ADRs and 2 minor ADR cases were observed, whereas the rest of the reports did not specify whether ADRs had occurred or not.

Three clinical studies suggested that the nebulized route was at least as efficacious as the intravenous infusion for the treatment of LRTIs and URTIs when the two routes were directly compared (Table 9.2). In the treatment of LRTI, the adult patients were treated with nebulized *Yuxingcao* at a dose of 30 mL once daily ($n = 20$), 30 mL three times daily ($n = 21$), or intravenous infusion at 50 mL twice daily ($n = 21$). Although the nebulization once daily was less efficacious than infusion, nebulized *Yuxingcao* three times daily conferred to comparable efficacy to the intravenously infused counterparts [35]. In another study, the results showed that the infants and children with URTI receiving 3–5 mL nebulized *Yuxingcao* ($n = 35$) twice daily exhibited comparable effective rates but better efficacy of coughing relief than those treated with 10–40 mL infused drug once daily ($n = 48$) [36]. The efficacy of nebulized *Yuxingcao* ($n = 40$) was also compared with that of intramuscular injection ($n = 40$) for the treatment of infants and children with LRTI in a clinical trial. The nebulized group offered significant better therapeutic outcomes than the injection group in terms of the time to relieve fever, cough, shortness of breath, and rales and to fully recover [37].

The technical aspects of nebulization in the clinical trials were generally not well controlled. The principal factors influencing aerosol performance such as initial fill volume, drug concentration, and nebulizer type varied from trial to trial, and the particle size distribution and output of aerosol and residual volume were not specified (Table 9.4).

Nebulized Qingkailing

Qingkailing injection is prepared from the extracts of five herbs, including *Radix Isatidis*, *Flos Lonicerae*, *Fructus Gardeniae*, and mother of pearl and buffalo horn, and three purified natural products, including baicalin, cholic acid, and hyodeoxycholic acid. The chemical composition of *Qingkailing* injection includes various types of ingredients including flavonoids (mainly baicalin), bile acids (mainly cholic and hyodeoxycholic acids), iridoid glycosides (mainly from gardenia), organic acids (mainly from honeysuckle and gardenia), amino acids (mainly from *Radix Isatidis* and mother of pearl and buffalo horn), nucleosides (mainly from *Radix Isatidis*), inorganic elements (mainly from mother of pearl and buffalo horn), and pigments (mainly from gardenia) [39]. Extensive *in vitro* and *in vivo* studies have demonstrated that the preparation and the containing ingredients have a variety of desirable biological and pharmacological actions including anti-inflammation, immunomodulation, antiviruses, antibacteria, antipyretic effect, and hepato- and neuroprotection [40–44]. It is the most widely prescribed TCM injection and more than 30 million patients are taking the drug annually in clinical practice for the treatment of respiratory diseases together with viral encephalitis, hepatitis, stoke, and cerebral thrombosis. Extensive clinical trials have been carried out to evaluate the clinical efficacy of *Qingkailing* injection for the treatment of respiratory diseases, such respiratory infections and pneumonia, and other disorders [45–47]. For instance, in a meta-analysis on treating respiratory system infections, intravenous infusion of *Qingkailing* injection was shown to confer to superior clinical outcomes to the control treatment mainly with antiviral agents or antibiotics based on the data from 22 clinical trials [47].

However, the injection-related ADRs can be *bothersome* and may even jeopardize the clinical use and sales [4]. In a systematic review of qualified clinical reports involving 4233 patients, the incidence of ADRs caused by intravenous infusion of *Qingkailing* injections was about 3.38% [48]. Another study has systematically analyzed the 1486 cases of ADRs associated with *Qingkailing* documented in 277 reports and concluded that 32.9% of severity-classifying cases were severe ADRs and 13 cases were fatal. Anaphylactic shock represents the major clinical manifestation, accounting for 55.5% of severe ADRs. In addition, among the 1486 cases, only 15 cases were from oral- and intramuscular-dosed patients and the rest intravenously administered the drug, suggesting that the ADRs were mainly associated with intravenous infusion/injection [49]. The authors also suggested that the irrational use and the incompatibility with coadministered drugs and/or diluents played a major role in the occurrence of ADRs. In order to evaluate the real situation of safety profile of *Qingkailing* injection, a large-scale, multicenter postmarketing safety monitoring was performed following a standard protocol excluding potential irrational use and incompatibility, and the incidence of ADRs associated with the injection was found to be 0.086% [50].

The clinical efficacy of nebulized *Qingkailing* has been addressed in 67 published studies, which included a total of 5392 patients. Nebulized *Qingkailing* were mainly used for the treatment of acute URTIs, pneumonia, bronchitis/bronchiolitis caused by bacteria/viruses, and acute exacerbation of COPD. Acute exacerbation of COPD is generally triggered by an infection with bacteria or viruses; the efficacy of nebulized *Qingkailing* might be attributable to the ability of anti-inflammation, antiviruses, and antibacteria. Data from the previous clinical studies indicated that nebulized *Qingkailing* has been shown to be more effective than the standard treatment with the overall average effective rates being 94.3% in the former treatment and 72.3% in the latter (Table 9.3). In addition, 39 clinical trials have reported the ADRs and 33 cases of minor ADRs, for example, rash, diarrhea, and nausea, were observed (Table 9.3). But no typical severe ADRs associated with injections such as anaphylaxis were observed in the nebulization therapy.

Four randomized controlled trials have been performed with a view to determining whether nebulized therapy is as efficacious as intravenously infused *Qingkailing* (e.g., Table 9.2). In one study, a dose of 10 mL *Qingkailing* injection was nebulized twice daily to adult patients ($n = 40$) hospitalized with bronchitis/bronchiolitis induced by parainfluenza virus, whereas the control group ($n = 60$) were treated with infusion of 10 mL *Qingkailing* twice daily. Nebulized *Qingkailing* was found to be superior to the control group in terms of clinical cure on Day 4 ($P < 0.01$); the time for relieving symptoms including coughing, hoarseness, and rales ($P < 0.01$); and the length of hospital stay ($P < 0.05$) [51]. In another study [52], infant and child patients hospitalized with URTI by virus were treated with either nebulized ($n = 92$) or intravenously infused *Qingkailing* ($n = 91$). The results suggested that the nebulized route resulted in comparable outcomes than intravenous dosing in terms of effective rates and the time to relieve symptoms. Four cases of ADRs were observed in the infused group, but no ADR case in the nebulized treatment.

The technical aspects of nebulization across the clinical trials have large variations in terms of fill volume, drug concentration, nebulizer type, dose frequency, and nebulizing duration, and the particle size distribution and output of aerosol and residual volume were not specified (Table 9.4).

NEBULIZED *TANREQING*

Tanreqing injection was approved by CFDA in 2003 for the treatment of respiratory tract infections, early pneumonia, and COPD, and it is a standardized formulation extracted and refined from *Radix Scutellariae*, bear bile powder, goat horn, *Flos Lonicerae japonicae*, and *Fructus Forsythiae*. The preparation has a complex composition and contains various types of ingredients, such as flavonoids, cholic acids, amino acids, and organic acids. Baicalin, chlorogenic acid, caffeic acid, ursodeoxycholic acid, and chenodeoxycholic acid have been used as the chemical makers for the quality control of the injection [53]. The pharmacological actions described in the drug label include antibacterial, antiviral, and anti-inflammatory effects and the ability to improve immunity. Unlike the TCM products approved in the 1980s or before, the approval of *Tanreqing* injection was subjected to relatively strict randomized clinical trials. Several systematic reviews have been performed to evaluate the clinical efficacy of *Tanreqing* injection for the treatment of respiratory tract infections, pneumonia, and COPD and have concluded that the injection may provide more benefits for patients compared to the control of standard treatment when used alone or as an add-on agent [54–57].

Similar to other TCM injections, *Tanreqing* injection may induce various ADRs including allergic reaction and anaphylactic shock. In a postmarketing safety surveillance study, the incidence of ADRs in children aged <16 years treated with *Tanreqing* injection was found to be ~2.54% and ADRs were mainly allergic reactions [58]. Yang and colleagues have analyzed 376 ADR cases of *Tanreqing* injection in Chongqing and found that 11 cases (2.9%) were severe ADRs [59]. The mechanism underlying the ADRs is unclear, but the occurrence of ADRs was generally related to the irrational use, the presence of impurities, and the incompatibility with coadministered drugs and/or diluents.

The efficacy and safety of nebulized *Tanreqing* in the treatment of the respiratory diseases have been documented in 87 clinical reports involving 4493 infant, children, and adult patients. Nebulized *Tanreqing* were mainly used for the treatment of URTIs, pneumonia, bronchitis/bronchiolitis caused by bacteria/viruses, asthma, and acute exacerbation of COPD. The previous clinical studies have shown that the overall effective rate of nebulized *Tanreqing* was as high as 96.6%, markedly higher than that of the control groups (80.4%). For example, a meta-analysis [60] was performed to evaluate the efficacy of nebulized *Tanreqing* for the treatment of the infections of the respiratory system and asthma based on the data from 16 randomized clinical trials involving 673 patients. It was found that for the treatment of pulmonary infections, nebulized *Tanreqing* was superior to gentamicin or gentamicin in combination with chymotrypsin in terms of effective rates and improved symptoms, whereas it was equivalent to nebulized budesonide when used for asthmatic patients [60]. As for the treatment of acute exacerbation of COPD, a clinical trial showed that nebulized *Tanreqing* as add-on therapy resulted in significant reduction in the serum level of interleukin-6 and tumor necrosis factor-α, leading to improved effective rates and symptoms compared to the standard treatment [61]. Clinical studies also suggested that nebulization appeared to have fewer side effects than intravenously infused *Tanreqing*. Among the documented clinical reports, 65 studies mentioned ADRs, and 8 cases of minor ADRs, including mild diarrhea and mouth discomfort, were observed and likely associated with nebulization, but no case of anaphylactic reaction, a severe ADR typically associated with *Tanreqing* injection, was observed.

To date, there have been six published reports (e.g., Table 9.2) that have directly compared the efficacy and safety between nebulized and intravenously infused *Tanreqing* and showed that patients receiving the nebulized treatment had comparable or greater improvement relative to those receiving infused *Tanreqing*. Nong and coauthors examined the impacts of the delivery routes on clinical outcome of infants with bronchiolitis caused by respiratory syncytial virus. The infants (mean age of 8.3 months) were randomized to receive 7 days' treatment with nebulization twice daily ($n = 60$) or infusion once daily ($n = 60$). The results showed that the nebulization treatment resulted in a significant reduction in the time to relieve shortness of breath ($P < 0.01$) and rales ($P < 0.05$), the length of hospital stay ($P < 0.01$), and the incidence of ADRs ($P < 0.01$) [62]. In another study, patients with chronic bronchitis were randomized to receive either nebulized ($n = 35$) or intravenously infused ($n = 30$) *Tanreqing* injection in addition to a regular treatment or a regular treatment only ($n = 29$) [63] for 15 days. The results showed that the nebulized group achieved an effective rate of 94.3%, significantly higher ($P < 0.05$) than 85.3% of the infusion, and 75.9% of the regular treatment only, respectively.

As shown in Table 9.4, the technical control of nebulization in the clinical trials was also poorly performed and varied from trial to trial.

NEBULIZED ANDROGRAPHOLIDES

Purified andrographolides, isolated from *Andrographis paniculata* (*Chuanxinlian*), which is a *heat-clearing and detoxifying* herb used for the treatment of common cold, fever, and detoxification in Chinese medicine, are the main ingredients of several

TCM injections, including *Xiyanping* (sulfonated derivatives of total andrographolides), *Yanhuning* (dehydroandrographolide disuccinate monopotassium salt), *Chuanhuning* (dehydroandrographolide disuccinate potassium–sodium salt), and *Lianbizhi* (andrographolide sodium bisulfate). Extensive studies have revealed that andrographolides have broad range of pharmacological effects such as antibacterial, antidiarrheal, antiviral, antimalarial, hepatoprotective, anti-inflammatory, immunostimulatory, and anticancer activity [64–66]. Clinically, andrographolide-based injections have been the best-selling TCM formula for respiratory diseases since the suspension of *Yuxingcao* in China. A great number of clinical studies have suggested that they are of more benefits to patients with respiratory system infections than the control groups. Take *Xiyanping* injection as an example; many randomized trials have been performed to evaluate the clinical efficacy in the treatment of viral pneumonia and bronchiolitis using ribavirin injection as a control in children. These previous studies demonstrated that *Xiyanping* injection appeared to be an effective and safe treatment option and significantly more effective than ribavirin injection in terms of the time to relieve symptoms and signs including fever, cough, shortness of breath, and rales and the length of hospital stay [67,68].

However, similar to other TCM injections, the use of andrographolides injections also led to high incidence of ADR. CFDA has issued ADR warning on *Lianbizhi* in 2005, *Yanhuning* and *Chuanhuning* in 2009, and *Xiyanping* in 2011 in the 8th, 23rd, and 48th issues of *Adverse Drug Reaction Information Bulletin*, respectively. For example, 1476 cases of ADRs including 49 severe cases were reported for *Xiyanping* in 2011 [69] and a systematic review suggested that the incidence of *Xiyanping* injection via intravenous administration was about 2% [70]. The key factors related to the occurrence of ADRs were attributed to the irrational use and the incompatibility with coadministered drugs.

The efficacy and safety of nebulized andrographolides have been evaluated in 94 clinical trials, involving 5444 infant, children, and adult patients. Most studies had reported better efficacy for the treatment of bronchitis or bronchiolitis, pneumonia, and URTI with nebulized therapy than with the control groups in terms of effective rates and improved symptoms and function. As shown in Table 9.3, the overall average effective rates of 94.1% for nebulized andrographolides were significantly higher than those of 79.9% for the control. In addition, these clinical studies also revealed that nebulization resulted in fewer side effects. Among the 88 clinical trials that had reported the ADRs, only 52 cases of minor ADRs, which also commonly occurred in standard treatment, were recorded with no case of serious allergic reaction being observed (e.g., Table 9.3).

Sixteen randomized controlled trials have been performed in an attempt to determine whether nebulized therapy is as efficacious and safe as intravenously infused andrographolides for the treatment of pneumonia, bronchitis, influenza, and other respiratory tract infections (e.g., Table 9.2 and [73]). In one of these trials [71], 500 children aged 1–4 years with URTIs received nebulized *Yanhuning* 4–5 mg/kg twice daily ($n = 250$) or *Yanhuning* 5–8 mg/kg intravenous infusion once daily ($n = 250$) for 3–5 days. The nebulized route was associated with more treatment successes (238/250 vs. 210/250) and significantly better responses in terms of time to relieve clinical symptoms, for example, fever, cough, and sore throat. In a meta-analysis based on the data from six clinical trials, Geng et al. have evaluated the effectiveness and safety of nebulization and intravenous infusion of *Xiyanping* injection for treatment of pediatric respiratory diseases and concluded that patients receiving the nebulized treatment had greater efficacy than those receiving the drug by the intravenous route [72]. In addition, apart from the improved effectiveness, nebulized therapy conferred to better safety profile than the treatment with infused andrographolides. Among the 1055 patients receiving intravenous treatment enrolled in the 16 trials, 125 ADR cases including 3 cases of anaphylactic shock were documented, whereas only 9 minor ADR cases were reported in 1087 patients receiving the nebulization of andrographolides.

Nonetheless, it should be noted that the importance of technical aspects of nebulization was often underestimated in clinical practice. The principal factors influencing nebulizer performance such as particle size distribution, output rate and yield, and residue volume were not mentioned at all in any of the studies. Although other factors including therapeutic dose, solution concentration, fill volume, nebulizer, and nebulizer duration and frequency were stated, large variations were found from trial to trial.

OTHER NEBULIZED TCMS

Besides the five TCM formulas described earlier, asarone and *Fufangdanshen* (also called "Xiangdan") injections represent the other main nebulized TCMs. In particular, 87 clinical reports have studied the efficacy and safety of nebulized asarone injection for the treatment of bronchitis or bronchiolitis (in 45 trials involving 2312 patients), pneumonia (in 21 trials involving 1307 patients), asthma and COPD (in 15 trials involving 762 patients), and respiratory system infection (in 6 trials involving 401 patients). Most of the studies suggested that nebulized asarone exerted improved clinical efficacy compared with the control groups, whereas two studies have shown the former resulted in significantly inferior therapeutic outcomes to nebulized budesonide when used for patients with bronchitis or bronchiolitis. Although asarone injection is regarded as a TCM injection, it is a pure compound–based preparation. As a result, no detailed description is present in this review.

Fufangdanshen injection is prepared from *Dalbergia odorifera* and *Salvia miltiorrhiza* (rosewood) by combining *Salvia* aqueous extracts and saturated distilled solutions of rosewood, and the major chemical ingredients include water-soluble phenolic compounds, such as salvianolic acids, and water-insoluble essential oils [74]. It is a TCM injection approved for the treatment of coronary heart and cerebrovascular diseases in China. The injection is often off-label used for respiratory diseases. However, the intravenous application of the injection, particularly for off-label use, is associated with high incidence of ADRs including severe ADRs as warned in the 45th issue of *Adverse Drug Reaction Information Bulletin* [75]. Nebulized *Fufangdanshen* has also been off-label used for the treatment of respiratory diseases, such as bronchitis or bronchiolitis, pneumonia, asthma and COPD, and respiratory system infection, in 37 clinical trials involving 1687 patients, together with systemic disorders in 5 trials involving 243 patients. Most studies tended to confirm the superior therapeutic outcomes of nebulized route to those of the control groups with very few ADR cases being recorded.

INHALED TCM VIA MDI OR DPI

MDI devices have been used for TCM delivery since the 1960s, and *Huashanshen* MDI, which contains atropine-type alkaloids of *Radix Physochlainae* as active ingredients for the treatment of asthma, was recorded in the *Chinese Pharmacopoeia 1977*. Atropine-type alkaloids are known anticholinergic agents, eliciting antiasthmatic effect like ipratropium. Later, *Zhichuanling* (containing a combination of clenbuterol and atropine-type alkaloids of *Datura stramonium* [*Yangjinhua*]) and *Yinhuangpingchuan* (containing extracts of ephedra, *Semen Ginkgo*, *Radix Sophorae*, and *Radix Scutellariae*) MDI were also approved by CFDA for the treatment of asthma, whereas *SHL* CFC MDI was registered for anti-influenza. Apart from these approved MDI products, other TCM formulas, such as *Fufang Shuanghua* (containing ephedrine analogues), tetrandrine, and *Yuchuan* (isoproterenol and guaifenesin), have also been formulated as CFC MDI in the literature. However, it should be noted that no evidence may demonstrate the improved efficacy of TCM except *SHL* in a CFC inhaler compared with the original oral or injectable forms [76]. As for *SHL*, a clinical trial has revealed that the MDI exhibited comparable effective rates but significantly better results in alleviating coughing and/or lung rales relative to the oral solution or intravenous infusion when used for treating acute respiratory tract infections [77]. With phasing out CFC use in TCM MDI, no progress has yet been made in the development of HFA-based MDI alternatives so far.

In the last decade, DPI devices are proposed to deliver several TCM formulas, including *Senecio cannabifolius* (*Fanhuncao*), alkaloids of *Radix Physochlainae* (*Huashanshen*), alkaloids of *Stephania japonica* (*Qianjinteng*), oligosaccharides of *Rehmannia glutinosa* (*Dihuang*), and *SHL*, but only the latter formula has studied the *in vitro* aerosol performance of the DPI [78]. In the study, results have shown that *SHL* might be developed as a DPI product, albeit not HFA MDI due to partial solubility in HFA, and the carrier-based DPI might lead to improved aerosol performance, independent of variation in constituent composition, when spray-dried as corrugated particles [78].

RATIONALE FOR TCM INHALATION THERAPY

Substantial available evidence from clinical studies tends to support that TCM inhalation therapy could represent an intriguing alternative to intravenous injections with numerous potential advantages. The first obvious justification is the maximization of the delivered dose to the respiratory tract, the intended target site of drug delivery, leading to positive therapeutic outcomes. For the treatment of asthma and COPD, the applicability of inhalation delivery has been well established in the literature. Although there is relatively little evidence for nebulized chemical drugs with regard to the treatment of respiratory airway infections and pneumonia, the use of nebulized TCM for the latter indications of respiratory diseases has been substantiated in clinical studies. The second advantage conferred by nebulized TCM is attributed to the ability to reduce typical ADR associated with TCM injections. Although the occurrence of ADRs associated with TCM injections is unpredictable and the reasons are not entirely clear, the presence of particulates and the high concentration of TCM constituents (impurities) in the blood during infusion may have play an important role [4]. A reduction of the risk of ADR induced by the presence of particulates and high concentration of impurities should be expected because TCM ingredient diffusion or particle penetration from bronchial and alveolar compartments to the systemic circulation is restricted by the presence of bronchial endothelium and alveolar–capillary barrier.

Nevertheless, it should be noted that the trial design and reporting in many clinical reports of nebulized TCM were generally poor. First, the efficacy and safety of nebulized TCM were assessed as add-on therapy to basic treatment in many clinical studies. Indeed, in the treatment groups, interventions that involved purely nebulized TCM only consisted of 27.5% of studies, whereas the majority of studies (72.5%) applied nebulized TCM in combination with conventional treatment. The cointerventions in the treatment groups can lead to difficulties in equivocal interpretation of outcome arising from inhaled TCM. Second, nebulization parameters were not well controlled and/or poorly specified in the clinical reports, and the conditions have varied from trial to trial. Taking nebulized *SHL* as an example, the output and particle size distribution have never been tested; the therapeutic dose and the concentration of nebulized solution have varied between 5 and 100 mg/kg and between 12 and 120 mg/mL; 22 different brands of nebulizers have been used in the 162 reports. Third, the information on ADRs was generally poorly documented and no detailed information on how to measure them was reported. In fact, the pulmonary biocompatibility of TCM preparations and containing ingredients has yet been fully confirmed in preclinical toxicological studies. For example, in a study of the pulmonary toxicity of *SHL in vitro* in respiratory cells following exposure and *in vivo* in rats following intratracheal spray, the authors found that *SHL* may exhibit a dose-dependent pulmonary toxicity and concluded that the inhalation therapy of SHL may be safe only if the inhaled dose is properly controlled [79]. Fourth, no blinding measurement was taken in the clinical trials, and hence, the subjective influence on the interpretation of outcome cannot be ignored. As a result, it is yet difficult to draw definite conclusions concerning to the clinical effectiveness and safety of nebulized TCM.

In addition, nebulized TCMs manifest their therapeutic efficacy in different respiratory conditions through a number of recognized or unclear potential mechanisms [5,80]. The main nebulized TCMs are classified into heat-clearing and detoxifying agents according to the TCM theory and the mechanism of actions have been generally attributed to their antibacterial, antiviral, and anti-inflammatory actions and/or the ability to improve immunity [5]. However, except the purified andrographolides, the rest of the TCM formulas consist of complex mixtures of numerous phytocomplexes and the active ingredients and site of action are not well elucidated. It is well known that the mode and site of action is highly relevant to optimization of the delivered site of the inhaled drug. Moreover, the pulmonary pharmacokinetic profiles of the active ingredients in the inhaled TCM are largely unknown and only a few studies have addressed the pulmonary absorption/elimination of these natural products [81]. An understanding of the pharmacokinetics is critical to the optimization of dose and dose frequency. Nonetheless, the frequency of drug administration, an important determinant of clinical outcome, was arbitrarily determined due to the lack of pharmacokinetic information in the previous clinical trials of nebulized TCM. Therefore, to develop nebulized TCM products meeting the international acceptable quality standards and subsequently to be accepted as standard therapy, substantial effort needs to be made in understanding the mode and site of action, and randomized controlled trials with scientifically rigorous methodology are warranted to further decisively confirm the efficacy and safety.

SUMMARY

- TCM, particularly TCM injections, is widely applied in the standard treatment for hospitalized patients with respiratory diseases in China, but ADRs associated with TCM injections are worrisome.
- Nebulized TCMs, when used alone or as add-on therapy, have positive therapeutic benefits for patients with respiratory diseases.
- Nebulized TCMs lead to comparable or superior efficacy to the intravenously infused counterparts.
- Nebulized TCM treatments generally have fewer side effects than intravenously infused TCM and are free of severe ADR associated with TCM injections.
- The inhalation route may provide a viable, noninvasive, safe, and efficacious means as an alternative to TCM injections.

REFERENCES

1. World Health Organization. 2014. The top 10 causes of death. http://who.int/media-centre/factsheets/fs310/en/index.html. Accessed August 25, 2016.
2. Wang, X., Jia, W., Zhao, A. H., Wang, X. R. 2006. Anti-influenza agents from plants and traditional Chinese medicine. *Phytother. Res.* 20:335–341.
3. Cheng, J. Z., Zhu, H. P. 2013. *The Blue Book of Medicine and Pharmaceuticals: Annual Report on China's Pharmaceutical Market in 2012*. Social Sciences Academic Press, Beijing, China.
4. Wang, L., Yuan, Q., Marshall, G., Cui, X. H., Cheng, L., Li, Y. Y., Shang, H. C., Zhang, B. L., Li Y. P. 2010. Adverse drug reactions and adverse events of 33 varieties of traditional Chinese medicine injections on National Essential medicines List (2004 edition) of China: An overview on published literatures. *J. Evid. Based Med.* 3:95–104.
5. Miao, X. Q., Zhou, J., Li, J., Liao, Y. H., Zheng, Y. 2015. Chinese medicine in inhalation therapy: A review of clinical application and formulation development. *Curr. Pharm. Des.* 21:3917–3931.

6. Sun, H. Y., Liu, M. X., Lin, Z. T., Jiang, H. X., Niu, Y. Y., Wang, H., Chen, S. Z. 2015. Comprehensive identification of 125 multifarious constituents in Shuang-huang-lian powder injection by HPLC-DAD-ESI-IT-TOF-MS. *J. Pharm. Biomed. Anal.* 115:86–106.

7. Li, H. W., Wu, J. F., Zhang, Z. W., Ma, Y. Y., Liao, F. F., Zhang, Y., Wu, G. J. 2011. Forsythoside a inhibits the avian infectious bronchitis virus in cell culture. *Phytother. Res.* 25:338–342.

8. Song, Z. J., Johansen, H. K., Moser, C., Faber, V., Kharazmi, A., Rygaard, J., Høiby, N. 2000. Effects of Radix *Angelicae sinensis* and *Shuanghuanglian* on a rat model of chronic *Pseudomonas aeruginosa* pneumonia. *Chin. Med. Sci. J.* 15:83–88.

9. Gao, Y., Fang, L., Cai, R. L., Zong, C. J., Chen, X., Lu, J., Qi, Y. 2014. Shuang-Huang-Lian exerts anti-inflammatory and anti-oxidative activities in lipopolysaccharide-stimulated murine alveolar macrophages. *Phytomedicine* 21:461–469.

10. Chen, X., Howard, O. M., Yang, X., Wang, L., Oppenheim, J. J., Krakauer, T. 2002. Effects of *Shuanghuanglian* and *Qingkailing*, two multi-components of traditional Chinese medicinal preparations, on human leukocyte function. *Life Sci.* 70:2897–2913.

11. Zhang, H. W., Chen, Q., Zhou, W. W., Gao, S., Lin, H. G., Ye, S. F., Xu, Y. H., Cai, J. 2013. Chinese medicine injection *Shuanghuanglian* for treatment of acute upper respiratory tract infection: A systematic review of randomized controlled trials. *Evid. Based Complement. Alternat. Med.* 2013:987326.

12. Chen, W., Liu, B., Wang, L. Q., Ren, J., Liu, J. P. 2014. Chinese patent medicines for the treatment of the common cold: A systematic review of randomized clinical trials. *BMC Complement Altern. Med.* 14:273.

13. Zhang, H.Y., Ren, X. L., Li, Y. Z. 2010. Meta-analysis of efficacy of *Shuanghuanglian* for children pneumonia. *Chin. Pharm.* 21:4205–4208.

14. Shi, Q. P., Jiang, X. D., Ding, F., Liu, Y., Yu, M. L., Zhu, J. X., Zhang, S. Q. 2014. Consequences, measurement, and evaluation of the costs associated with adverse drug reactions among hospitalized patients in China. *BMC Health Serv. Res.* 14:73.

15. Wang, L., Cheng, L., Yuan, Q., Cui, X. H., Shang, H. C., Zhang, B. L., Li, Y. P. 2010. Adverse drug reactions of *Shuanghuanglian* injection: A systematic review of public literatures. *J. Evid. Based Med.* 3:18–26.

16. Wu, Y., Ren, J. T., Yan, M., Guo, X. X., Zhang, C. X., Cao, L. Y. 2004. Investigation of the clinical situation of *Shuanghuanglian* injection in six cities during 2001–2002. *Chin. J. Pharmacovigil.* 1:21–23.

17. Zhang, J. H., Shang, H. C., Zheng, W. K., Hu, J., Xu, H. J., Wang, H., Zhang, L., Ren, M., Zhang, B. L. 2010. Systematic review on the compatibility of *Shuanghuanglian* injection combined with western medical injections. *J. Evid. Based Med.* 3:27–36.

18. Yang, C. P. 2004. Observation on insoluble particles due to compatibility of *Shuanghuanglian* or *Qingkailing* injection with glucose or sodium injection. *J. Henan Univ. Chin. Med.* 19:18.

19. Zhai, L., Liu, Z. M., Guo, R. H., Han, G., Liu, G. J. 2007. The variations in quantity of insoluble particles of *Shuanghuanglian* injection after mixed with four antibiotics. *Lishizhen Med. Mater. Med. Res.* 18:1951–1952.

20. Liu, Z. C., Tang, Y. L. 1996. Effect of delivery routes on the clinical efficacy of *Shuanghuanglian*. *J. Appl. Clin. Pediatr.* 11:49.

21. Li, H. M., Zhang, X. M. 2007. *Shuanghuanglian* inhalation in treating asthmatic pneumonia of 45 cases. *Chin. J. Integr. Tradit. West. Med. Intensive Crit. Care* 14:302.

22. Zhang, J. J., Wu, Y. 2012. HS-GC-MS analysis of the volatile ingredients in *Yuxingcao* injection. *J. Chin. Med. Mater.* 31:1858–1860.

23. Lu, H. M., Liang, Y. Z., Qian, P. 2005. Profile-effect on quality control of *Houttuynia cordata* injection. *Yao Xue Xue Bao* 40:1147–1150.

24. Lu, H. M., Liang, Y. Z., Chen, S. 2006. Identification and quality assessment of *Houttuynia cordata* injection using GC-MS fingerprint: A standardization approach. *J. Ethnopharmacol.* 105:436–440.

25. Satthakarn, S., Hladik, F., Promsong, A., Nittayananta, W. 2015. Vaginal innate immune mediators are modulated by a water extract of *Houttuynia cordata* Thunb. *BMC Complement. Altern. Med.* 15:183.

26. Liu, F. Z., Shi, H., Shi, Y. J., Liu, Y., Jin, Y. H., Gao, Y. J., Guo, S. S., Cui, X. L. 2010. Pharmacodynamic experiment of the antivirus effect of *Houttuynia cordata* injection on influenza virus in mice. *Yao Xue Xue Bao.* 45:399–402.

27. Lu, H. M., Liang, Y. Z., Yi, L. Z., Wu, X. J. 2006. Anti-inflammatory effect of *Houttuynia cordata* injection. *J. Ethnopharmacol.* 104:245–249.

28. Lu, H. M., Wu, X. J., Liang, Y. Z., Zhang, J. 2006. Variation in chemical composition and antibacterial activities of essential oils from two species of *Houttuynia* Thunb. *Chem. Pharm. Bull.* 54:936–940.

29. Lau, K. M., Lee, K. M., Koon, C. M., Cheung, C. S., Lau, C. P., Ho, H. M., Lee, M. Y. et al. 2008. Immunomodulatory and anti-SARS activities of *Houttuynia cordata*. *J. Ethnopharmacol.* 118, 79–85.

30. Cui, X. H., Wang, L., Deng, S. L. Li, T. Q. Shang, H. C. 2011. Efficacy of *Houttuynia cordata* injection for respiratory system diseases: A meta-analysis. *Chin. J. Evid. Based Med.* 11:786–798.

31. Wang, L., Cui, X. H., Cheng, L., Yuan, Q., Li, T. Q., Li, Y. P., Deng, S. L., Shang, H. C., Bian, Z. X. 2010. Adverse events to *Houttuynia* injection: A systematic review. *J. Evid. Based Med.* 3:168–176.

32. Yi, Y., Liang, A. H., Liu, T., Zhao, Y., Cao, C. Y. 2008. Analysis of causes for adverse reaction of *Yuxingcao* injection. *Chin. J. Chin. Mater. Med.* 33:2439–2442.

33. Yuan, L. P., Ma, L. M. 2008. Aerosol inhalation of sodium houttuyfonate injection for treatment of pneumonia: A systematic review. *China Pharm.* 19:1652–1654.

34. Yuan, L. P., Zhou, X., Li, H. J., Wei, J. Y., Ma, L. M. 2011. Aerosol inhalation of sodium houttuyfonate injection: A systematic review. *Chin. J. New Drug* 20:284–292.

35. Lin, H. Y., Zeng, J., Fu, Y. P. 2001. Comparison of curative effects of herba *Houttuynia*e injection by spray inhalation and by intravenous drip on respiratory tract infection. *Chin. Tradit. Patent. Med.* 23:727–728.

36. Lan, H. Y., Huang, R. P., Huang, S. Z., Chen, Z. J., Lu, Z. S., Tan, X. L. 1998. Efficacy comparison between ultrasonic nebulized and intravenous infused *Yuxingcao* injection treatment of children with respiratory tract infection. *J. Youjiang Med. Coll. Natl.* 20:591.

37. Wang, X. L., Liu, C. Y. 1989. Efficacy comparison between ultrasonic nebulized and intramuscular dosed *Yuxingcao*. *Hubei J. Tradit. Chin. Med.* 11:22–23.

38. Zheng, X. Y. 2002. *Guiding Principle of Clinical Research on New Drugs of Traditional Chinese Medicine*. Chinese Medicine Science and Technology Press, Beijing, China.

39. Zhang, H. Y., Hu, P., Luo, G. A., Liang, Q. L., Wang, Y. L., Yan, S. K., Wang, Y. M. 2006. Screening and identification of multi-component in *Qingkailing* injection using combination of liquid chromatography/time-of-flight mass spectrometry and liquid chromatography/ion trap mass spectrometry. *Anal. Chim. Acta.* 577:190–200.

40. Yue, S. J., Li, Q. J., Luo, Z. Q., Tang, F., Feng, D., Deng, S., Yu, P. 2005. The neuro-protective effects and its mechanisms of *Qingkailing* injection on bacterial meningitis induced by E. coli in rabbits. *Chin. J. Integr. Tradit. West. Med.* 25:633–636.

41. Tian, Q. M., Bi, H. S., Cui, Y., Guo, D. D., Xie, X. F., Su, W. H., Wang, X. R. 2012. *Qingkailing* injection alleviates experimental autoimmune uveitis in rats via inhibiting Th1 and Th17 effector cells. *Biol. Pharm. Bull.* 35:1991–1996.

42. Li, D., Huang, J. H., Zhang, S. H., Yang, F. J. 2009. Study on anti-bacterial activity of *Qingkailing* freeze-dried powder for injection in vivo. *Res. Prac. Chin. Med.* 21:53–55.

43. Xiao, H., Gu, X., Li, L., Yang, F. J. 2009. Study on anti-viral activity of *Qingkailing* freeze-dried powder for injection in vivo. *Pharm. Clin. Chin. Mater. Med.* 25:53–54.
44. Gao, X. Y., Guo, M. X., Peng, L., Zhao, B. S., Su, J. K., Liu, H. Y., Zhang, L., Bai, X., Qiao, Y. J. 2013. UPLC Q-TOF/MS-based metabolic profiling of urine reveals the novel antipyretic mechanisms of *Qingkailing* injection in a rat model of yeast-induced pyrexia. *Evid. Based Complement. Alternat. Med.* 2013:864747.
45. Wu, J. R., Zhang, X. M., Zhang, B. 2014. *Qingkailing* injection for the treatment of acute stroke: A systematic review and meta-analysis. *J. Tradit. Chin. Med.* 34:131–139.
46. Zhang, L. G., Zhao, W. P., Yang, K. 2011. A systematic review about treating pneumonia with *Qinkailing* injection. *Gansu J. TCM.* 24:18–24.
47. Liu, Y., Lu, J. Q., Liu, Z. Q. 2010. A meta-analysis on treating respiratory system infections with *Qinkailing* injection. *Chin. Hosp. Pharm. J.* 30:519–521.
48. Zhou, Y. L., Chen, H. M., Lu, H. 2007. Systematic evaluation of adverse drug reactions of *Qingkailing* injection from documents. *Chin. Pharm.* 16:50–52.
49. Hao, Y., Kong, X. Y., Wu, T. X. 2010. Assessment of the safety of *Qingkailing* injection: A systematic review. *Chin. J. Evid. Based Med.* 10:162–175.
50. Zhang, Q. L., Wang, Z., Jin, Z. W., Yang, W. B. 2015. Study on 5800 cases of post-marketing safety intensive hospital monitoring of *Qingkailing* injection. *Chin. J. Pharmacovigil.* 12:417–423.
51. Lei, Y., Lei, J., Zhao, J. D., Chen, R. 2005. Investigation on clinical effect of *Qingkailing* injection for parainfluenza virus by aerosol inhalation or inject. *J. Dali Univ.* 4:51–53.
52. Yu, H. G., Cai, C. J. 2006. Efficacy comparison of the treatment of *Qingkailing* injection for pediatric respiratory system infection via different administration routes. *Prac. Clin. J. Integr. Tradit. Chin. West. Med.* 6:56.
53. Sun, L., Wei, H., Zhang, F., Gao, S. H., Zeng, Q. H., Lu, W. Q., Chen, W. S., Chai, Y. F. 2013. Qualitative analysis and quality control of traditional Chinese medicine preparation *Tanreqing* injection by LC-TOF/MS and HPLC-DAD-ELSD. *Anal. Methods* 5:6431–6440.
54. Zhu, L. Q., Bai, M., Li, J. Y., Xu, Y. G., Gao, Z. Y. 2008. Meta-analysis of the efficacy *Tanreqing* injection on infections of respiratory system. *Chin. Hosp. Pharm. J.* 28:464–467.
55. Zhong, Y. Q., Mao, B., Wang, G., Fan, T., Liu, X. M., Diao, X., Fu, J. J. 2010. *Tanreqing* injection combined with conventional Western medicine for acute exacerbations of chronic obstructive pulmonary disease: A systematic review. *J. Altern. Complement. Med.* 16(12):1309–1319.
56. Jiang, H. L., Mao, B., Zhong, Y. Q., Yang, H. M., Fu, J. J. 2009. *Tanreqing* injection for community-acquired pneumonia: A systematic review of randomized evidence. *J. Chin. Integr. Med.* 7:9–19.
57. Li, Y. H., Zhu, H. J. 2011. Systematic assessment on randomized controlled trials for treatment of acute exacerbation of chronic obstructive pulmonary disease by *Tanreqing* injection. *Prac. Pharm. Clin. Remed.* 14:281–285.
58. Tang, Q. L., Sun, Y. X., Kang, A. R., Li, K. Q., Lu, C. X. 2015. Analysis of clinical application of *Tanreqing* injection in children based on real world research. *Chin. J. Hosp. Pharm.* 16:1488–1490.
59. Yang, X. F., Dong, Z., Lu, X. Q., Zhu, S. B. 2015. Analysis of 376 adverse drug reactions of *Tanreqing* injection in Chongqing. *Chin. J. New Drugs Clin. Rem.* 34:239–242.
60. Zhang, Y., Yang, Y. H., Liu, F., Zhai, S. D. 2010. Aerosol inhalation of *Tanreqing* injection in the treatment of respiratory system diseases: A systematic review. *Eval. Anal. Drug Use Hosp. Chin.* 10:483–487.

61. Li, Y. F., Ren, H. X., Zhang, W., Zhuang, S. N., Wang, D., Wang, X. X., Wang, J., Wang, H. C., Wang, J. Y., Zhao, L. P. 2015. Effect of nebulized *Tanreqing* injection on the inflammation of patients with acute exacerbation chronic obstructive pulmonary diseases. *Ningxia Med. J.* 37:555–557.

62. Nong, D. M., Jiang, F. Z., Wu, X. L., Huang, S. Q., Hu, X. D., Liu, R. S. 2009. The clinical effects of bronchiolitis treated by *Tanreqing* injection in different ways. *Chin. Modern Doc.* 47:34–35.

63. Zou, S. Y., Gu, X. Y. 2013. Efficacy of *Tanreqing* injection in different administration routes in the treatment of bronchitis. *Chin. J. Pharm. Econom.* 8:243–244.

64. Jarukamjorn, K., Nemoto, N. 2008. Pharmacological aspects of *Andrographis paniculata* on health and its major diterpenoids constituent andrographolide. *J. Health Sci.* 54:370–381.

65. Kumar, R. A., Sridevi, K., Kumar, N. V., Nanduri, S., Rajagopal, S. 2004. Anticancer and immunostimulatory compounds from *Andrographis paniculata*. *J. Ethnopharmacol.* 92:291–295.

66. Jayakumar, T., Hsieh, C. Y., Lee, J. J., Sheu, J. R. 2013. Experimental and clinical pharmacology of *Andrographis paniculata* and its major bioactive phytoconstituent andrographolide. *Evid. Based Complement. Alternat. Med.* 2013:846740.

67. Sun, S. G., Shi, Y. F., Li, Y., Wang, R., Wang, S. H., Sun, X. D. 2015. *Xiyanping* injection in treatment of viral pneumonia in children: A meta-analysis of random control trials. *Chin. Herb. Med.* 7:173–178.

68. Liu, L., Jiang, D., Chen, F., Xu, W. F., Du, X. H., Sun, Q. R., Jia, P. 2013. The efficacy and safety of *Xiyanping* injection in treating bronchiolitis: A systematic review. *West Chin. J. Pharm. Sci.* 28:650–652.

69. China Food and Drug Administration. 2011. *Adverse Drug Reaction Information Bulletin*. http://www.sda.gov.cn/WS01/CL0078/72891.html. Accessed August 25, 2016.

70. Wang, Y. P., Jiao, K., He, Z. F. 2011. Systematic evaluation of adverse drug reactions of *Xiyanping* injection from documents. *Chin. J. Exp. Tradit. Med. Form.* 17:236–239.

71. Yang, H. G. 2014. Clinical observation of the treatment of pediatric respiratory tract infection in 500 children. *Chin. Health Ind.* 35:129–130.

72. Geng, L., Fang, B. X., Chen, S. M., Zhu, J., Li, P. 2014. Meta-analysis of different administrative route of *Xiyanping* injection for treating respiratory tract infection in children. *Modern J. Integr. Tradit. Chin. West. Med.* 23:3214–3216.

73. Liu, G. F., Zou, Y. F., Liu, G. H., Bai, J. R., Zhang, Y. F., Zhang, X. Y. 2013. The efficacy of radioactive pneumonia treated by *Lianbizhi* injection in intravenous and inhalation for adjuvant therapy. *Hebei Med. J.* 35:854–855.

74. Liu, A. H., Lin, Y. H., Yang, M., Guo, H., Guan, S. H., Sun, J. H., Guo, D. A. 2007. Development of the fingerprints for the quality of the roots of Salvia miltiorrhiza and its related preparations by HPLC-DAD and LC-MS^n. *J. Chromatogr. B.* 846:32–41.

75. China Food and Drug Administration. 2012. *Adverse Drug Reaction Information Bulletin*. http://www.sda.gov.cn/WS01/CL0078/70155.html. Accessed August 25, 2016.

76. The United Nations Environment Programme. 2012. Report of the technology and economic assessment panel. http://ozone.unep.org/Assessment_Panels/TEAP/Reports/TEAP_Reports/teap-progress-report-may2012.pdf. Accessed August 25, 2016.

77. Wang, Y. H., Xu, K. J., Jiang, W. S., Lu, F. Z., Hu, M. Y., Zhe, Z. K., Gao, F., Zhang, J. W., He, X. L., Hong, F. Y. 1996. Clinical and experimental study on treatment of acute respiratory tract infection with *Shuanghuanglian* Aerosol. *Chin. J. Integr. Tradit. West. Med.* 2:162–165.

78. Yang, J. J., Liu, C. Y., Quan, L. H., Liao, Y. H. 2012. Preparation and in vitro aerosol performance of spray-dried Shuang-Huang-Lian corrugated particles in carrier-based dry powder inhalers. *AAPS PharmSciTech.* 13:816–825.

79. Han, R., Ye, J. X., Quan, L. H., Liu, C. Y., Liao, Y. H. 2011. Evaluating pulmonary toxicity of *Shuanghuanglian in vitro* and *in vivo*. *J. Ethnopharmacol.* 135:522–529.
80. Ma, Z. Q., Lu, J. J., Xu, W. S., Chen, X. P., Hu, H., Wang, Y. T. 2013. Analysis of traditional Chinese medicine injections used in the treatment of respiratory system-related diseases based on the Chinese market. *Global J. Res. Med. Plant. Indigen. Med.* 2:499–508.
81. Ye, J. X., Wang, W., Quan, L. H., Liu, C. Y., Liao, Y. H. 2010. An LC-MS/MS method for the simultaneous determination of chlorogenic acid, forsythiaside A and baicalin in rat plasma and its application to pharmacokinetic study of Shuang-huang-lian in rats. *J. Pharm. Biomed. Anal.* 52:625–630.

10 Bronchoprovocation Tests for the Evaluation of Drug Efficacy in Asthma

*John Paul Oliveria, Brittany M. Salter,
and Gail M. Gauvreau*

CONTENTS

INTRODUCTION

Asthma is a chronic disease of the airways, which is characterized by increased sensitivity of the airways, variable airflow obstruction, and inflammation. Increased sensitivity of the airways is an exaggerated bronchoconstrictor response to physical, chemical, or pharmacologic stimuli and can be assessed by measures of airway hyperresponsiveness and hyperreactivity or both. Increased airway hyper-responsiveness is observed by a steeper slope of the dose–response curve, whereas airway hyperreactivity is observed by a greater maximal response to a stimulus (Figure 10.1).

Inhalation challenges are commonly used as a tool for diagnosis and characterization of airway disease. Measurements of airway hyperresponsiveness (AHR) are also extremely valuable for understanding the pathobiology of asthma and are increasingly employed to monitor response to therapy as well as to test efficacy of asthma therapies (Juniper et al. 1978; Fowler et al. 2000; Inman et al. 1998; Gauvreau 1999a; Woolcock et al. 1988). This chapter will summarize the most common inhalation challenges utilized for assessing airway sensitivity.

INDIRECT VERSUS DIRECT AIRWAY CHALLENGES

Bronchoconstriction in the asthmatic airways can be induced by various stimuli through direct or indirect mechanisms. Direct stimuli include endogenous mediators (histamine, leukotrienes, and prostaglandins) or synthetic agonists (methacholine) that bind specific receptors on airway smooth muscle to cause contraction (Figure 10.2). Indirect tests, on the other hand, cause airway narrowing through

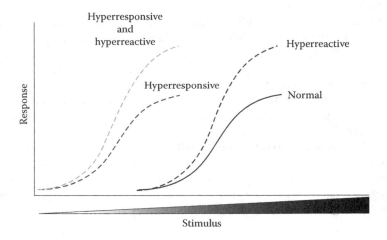

FIGURE 10.1 Dose–response curve to bronchoconstrictor agent showing the response in a normal individual and the shift observed in individuals with airway hyperresponsiveness, airway hyperreactivity, and both.

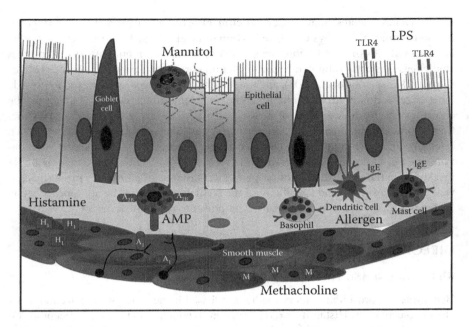

FIGURE 10.2 Cross section of an asthmatic airway showing inhaled agonists (mannitol, lipopolysaccharide, allergen, histamine, adenosine monophosphate, and methacholine), and their cell targets and respective receptors (A = adenosine, H = histamine, IgE = immunoglobulin E, M = muscarinic, TLR4 = toll-like receptor 4).

intermediate pathways, leading to activation of inflammatory cells and their release of endogenous mediators in the airways to cause contraction of airway smooth muscle. Physical stimuli, such as exercise and eucapnic voluntary hyperpnea, can also activate airway inflammatory cells by increasing the osmolarity of the airway surface, and subsequent mediator release leads to constriction of airway smooth muscle. Indirect challenges with osmotic aerosols such as mannitol and hypertonic saline were introduced in pulmonary function laboratories as a simpler alternative to exercise testing and thus can be used for clinical diagnosis of asthma. Adenosine monophosphate (AMP) and aeroallergens are other examples of indirect chemical stimuli but are not as widely used for diagnostic purposes.

Direct and indirect challenges provide tests of airway narrowing that can be used for clinical applications to assist with the diagnosis of asthma. Although airway hyperresponsiveness is most often assessed using direct challenges with methacholine as the provocative stimulus, the advantages of using indirect airway provocation tests for the measurement of airway hyperresponsiveness are becoming increasingly recognized. Indirect airway challenges elicit airflow limitation by acting on multiple inflammatory and epithelial cells, or nerves, thereby stimulating the release of mediators that induce smooth muscle contraction. Since many of the natural asthma triggers act through indirect pathways, it is widely believed that indirect airway responsiveness relates more closely to clinical asthma, where asthma is triggered by environmental or physical stimuli (Inman et al. 1998; Gauvreau et al. 1999a; Fowler et al. 2000). In addition, the sensitivity of the asthmatic airways to indirect challenges is greatly inhibited by anti-inflammatory treatment with inhaled cortico-steroids (ICSs) (Joos et al. 2003), and thus indirect challenges are believed to provide a better reflection of airway inflammation versus the direct airway challenges. The choice of test for assessments of airway sensitivity varies across pulmonary func-tion laboratories, and each test has particular advantages and disadvantages. When selecting the most appropriate test to evaluate efficacy of a therapeutic interven-tion, one must take into consideration the mechanism of action of the therapy under investigation (i.e., bronchodilator properties versus anti-inflammatory properties), as well as the sensitivity and specificity of the challenge to select the appropriate study design and sample size to enable sufficient power to detect differences.

DIRECT AIRWAY CHALLENGES

METHACHOLINE AND HISTAMINE CHALLENGES

Histamine is a pro-inflammatory mediator released by activated mast cells and baso-phils in the airways. Histamine exerts its actions by binding to histamine receptors. Of the four G protein–coupled histamine receptors that have been discovered in humans, designated H1 through H4, the binding of histamine to H1 receptors on airway smooth muscle and endothelium causes bronchoconstriction and vasodilation (Figure 10.2).

Methacholine is a synthetic derivative of acetylcholine delivered as a wet aero-sol. Methacholine acts as a nonselective muscarinic receptor agonist in the para-sympathetic nervous system and is highly active at all of the muscarinic receptors. Methacholine induces bronchoconstriction primarily through a direct binding to muscarinic receptors on smooth muscle within the airways (Figure 10.2). Acetyl-p-methylcholine chloride (Provocholine) is available as a dry crystalline powder and approved by the U.S. Food and Drug Administration for testing in humans (Juniper et al. 1978; Fowler et al. 2000).

During inhalation challenges, increasing concentrations of methacholine (or histamine) from 0.031 to 16 mg/mL are administered in an aerosolized form by tidal breathing or by dosimeter in doubling concentrations (i.e., 2, 4, 8 mg/mL). The forced expiratory volume in 1 s (FEV_1) is measured at 30, 90, and 180 s after each concentration and the test is terminated when there is a 20% reduction in FEV_1. The methacholine (or histamine) provocative concentration causing a 20% fall in the FEV_1 (PC_{20}) is calculated by linear interpolation. Responses to histamine and methacholine are highly reproducible (coefficients of determination [r^2] = 0.994 and 0.990, respectively) (Juniper et al. 1978). A positive test is commonly considered as a PC_{20} of less than 8 mg/mL. A test >16 mg/mL is considered to be negative, while tests of 4–16 mg/mL should be interpreted with caution.

Target Population

Methacholine challenge testing is used clinically in adults, often when spirometry or reversibility to bronchodilator has not been able to establish a diagnosis of asthma.

Since the negative predictive power of methacholine testing is large, the test can be more helpful to exclude a diagnosis of asthma.

Contraindications

Contraindications may compromise the quality of the overall inhalation challenge and output measurements, as well as the safety of the patient. Substantial falls in FEV_1 may occur during a methacholine inhalation challenge, and those individuals with low-baseline lung function are at risk (Martin et al. 1997). In general, the predicted accepted baseline FEV_1 of <65% should be used as a cutoff for conducting a methacholine inhalation challenge. In addition, low-baseline spirometry measurements are indicative of airway obstruction, thus making it difficult to interpret positive methacholine inhalation challenge results. This is due to a strong correlation between airway hyperresponsiveness and the degree of baseline airway obstruction that is a characteristic of chronic obstructive pulmonary disease (COPD). However, if baseline spirometry indicates airway obstruction that can be significantly reversed following use of a bronchodilator (>12% and >0.2 L increases in FEV_1 or FVC), then the diagnoses of asthma can be confirmed, thereby eliminating the need to do a methacholine inhalation challenge. Additional contraindications include cardiovascular problems. Cardiovascular events can be exacerbated in patients with uncontrolled hypertension or recent heart attack or stroke, following the added cardiovascular stress brought on by bronchospasms during an inhalation challenge. In particular, bronchospasms can induce ventilation–perfusion mismatching, which may in turn lead to arterial hypoxemia and compensatory changes in blood pressure, cardiac output, and heart rate (Stewart et al. 1989; Rodriguez-Roisin et al. 1991; Roca and Rodriguez-Roisin 1992; Goldman et al. 1995).

Safety Considerations

Methacholine provocative tests have several advantages over other tests of airway hyperreactivity. First, a relatively low dose of methacholine is needed to exert an airway response, with no limit to the dose that can be administered. In addition, methacholine inhalation is safe, with few side effects at low concentrations, and can easily be conducted in outpatient clinics. Methacholine and histamine inhalation challenges induce bronchoconstriction at relatively equivalent concentrations (Bhagat and Grunstein 1984; Toelle et al. 1994). However, methacholine is more commonly used as an inhalation challenge agent as opposed to histamine (Scott and Braun 1991), due to histamine being associated with more systemic side effects and less reproducibility (Juniper et al. 1978; Chatham et al. 1982; Higgins et al. 1988). For example, Juniper et al. reported that following inhalation challenge with histamine or methacholine, there appeared various side effects including throat irritation, flushing, and headache. On the other hand, these symptoms were notably more frequent with histamine than methacholine and were dose related (Juniper et al. 1978).

Outcomes and Interpretation of Results

Generally, a methacholine PC_{20} of <8 mg/mL provides a rationale to use asthma therapy but is not in itself diagnostic of asthma. Methacholine-responsive patients have a significantly lower % predicted FEV_1 and higher dose of ICSs, and thus the response to methacholine has indeed been related to asthma severity (Fowler et al. 2000).

While the methacholine test has some limitations for asthma diagnosis, it is extremely useful for evaluating the effects of asthma triggers and/or asthma therapy on airway hyperresponsiveness (Inman et al. 1998). The methacholine test is used to track responses to environmental triggers, such as occupational sensitizers, inhaled allergen, and respiratory viral infections, which significantly reduce the methacholine PC_{20} (Gauvreau et al. 1999a).

Studies have shown that airway hyperresponsiveness to both histamine and methacholine is associated with the presence and magnitude of atopy (Crockcroft et al. 1984; Fowler and Lipworth 2003). The early asthmatic response (EAR) to allergen described as the allergen PC_{20} (provocation concentration causing a 20% FEV_1 fall) is dependent on the levels of the patients' allergic sensitization and airway smooth muscle hyperresponsiveness (Killian et al. 1976; Cockcroft et al. 1979; Hill et al. 1982). The allergen PC_{20} can be predicted within 2–3 doubling concentrations, from the skin prick test end point and the histamine PC_{20} (Cockcroft et al. 2005). The relationship between the skin test end point and the methacholine PC_{20} can provide value in safely determining a starting inhalation concentration for allergen, thereby avoiding long allergen challenge protocols.

The effect of corticosteroid treatment in symptomatic asthmatic subjects improves the PC_{20} of methacholine by shifting the PC_{20} up to four doubling doses (i.e., from 1 to 16 mg/mL) (Woolcock et al. 1988) (Figure 10.3), suggesting that at least some of the response to methacholine is related to inflammation. The magnitude of shift in the methacholine/histamine PC_{20} to corticosteroids is variable (Koskela et al. 2003) and dependent upon factors such as steroid dose, duration of treatment, and severity of asthma.

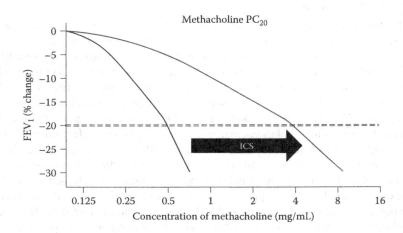

FIGURE 10.3 Percent change in forced expiratory volume in 1 s (FEV_1) at doubling concentrations of methacholine (mg/mL) in patients with asthma without treatment (left) and following treatment with inhaled corticosteroids (ICSs) (right). The provocative concentration of methacholine causing a 20% fall in FEV_1 (PC_{20}) shifts approximately 4 doubling concentrations higher with ICS treatment.

Methacholine challenges are most useful for assessing functional antagonism of beta-2 agonists on airway smooth muscle (Parameswaran et al. 1999). Shifts in the provocative concentration of methacholine can be used to establish optimum drug doses and to evaluate the onset and offset of drug activity in the airways. In a more recent study by O'Byrne et al., administration of a novel long-acting beta agonist (BI 1744 CL) at varying doses (2, 5, 10, 20 mcg) significantly increased the methacholine PC_{20} in a dose-dependent manner. In addition, the PC_{20} was elevated by a 30 min postdosing and remained elevated over a 32 h period (O'Byrne et al. 2009b). In contrast, leukotriene antagonist and mast cell stabilizers have no effect on AHR to direct stimuli (O'Byrne et al. 2009a).

It is important to note that the effectiveness of using the methacholine challenge to monitor drug activity within the airways is limited by prior administration of muscarinic antagonists. For example, the compound ipratropium bromide is a potent antagonist of muscarinic agonists, including methacholine (Crimi et al. 1992; Crapo et al. 2000). Inhaled ipratropium bromide has been shown to significantly inhibit methacholine-induced airway hyperrepsonsiveness; however, its duration of action is still unclear. There have been conflicting results as to the duration of bronchoprotection that ipratropium bromide may provide against methacholine. It is recommended by the American Thoracic Society to withhold the use of inhaled ipratropium bromide 24 h prior to a methacholine challenge (Crapo et al. 2000). Conversely, Illamperuma et al. demonstrated that ipratropium bromide promotes bronchoprotection for up to 6 h but none by 12 h (Illamperuma et al. 2009). This lends support to conducting methacholine inhalation challenges 12 h after the last dose of ipratropium bromide as opposed to 24 h. Interestingly, other compounds such as leukotriene modifiers are to be withheld for a recommended 24 h prior to methacholine challenge testing. However, Davis et al. demonstrated that montelukast sodium administered orally at either 1 or 25 h before methacholine challenge testing did not affect the outcomes of the test. These findings demonstrate that while some compounds can negatively affect methacholine outcomes, others have little to none effect (Davis and Cockcroft 2005).

The histamine challenge has also been used to assess the efficacy of various biological agents for the treatment of asthma. For example, Purokivi et al. used histamine challenge–induced cough to assess the efficacy of ICS treatment in asthmatics (Purokivi et al. 2010). Treatment with corticosteroids showed improvements in histamine PC_{20} and histamine challenge–induced couch, thereby demonstrating that these outcome measurements can be used as sensitive markers to assess treatment with corticosteroids. On the other hand, Leckie et al. monitored the effects of an IL-5 blocking monoclonal antibody to treat asthma and reported that although the mean blood eosinophil count was lowered following treatment, there was no effect on airway hyperresponsiveness to histamine (Leckie et al. 2000). Bryan and colleagues carried out a double-blind, randomized parallel group study, in which patients with mild allergic asthma were given subcutaneous recombinant IL-12 or placebo. They then assessed airway hyperresponsiveness using the histamine challenge. They found a decrease in peripheral blood eosinophil counts 24 h postinjection compared to the placebo but no change in the airway hyperresponsiveness to histamine (Bryan et al. 2000).

Last, Salome et al. determined the effect of aerosol and oral fenoterol as both a histamine and methacholine challenge in asthmatic subjects. They found that the dose–response curves to both histamine and methacholine shifted to the right with aerosol fenoterol; however, no significant change was seen with oral administration. Thus, this study used airway hyperresponsiveness challenges to determine that aerosol administration of fenoterol was more effective than oral. These studies highlight that both histamine and methacholine challenges can be used to assess drug treatment and pathogenesis of asthma.

INDIRECT AIRWAY CHALLENGES

MANNITOL INHALATION CHALLENGE

Mannitol is a sugar alcohol that is inhaled orally from a dry powder inhaler device. Inhaled mannitol induces acute bronchoconstriction and can be used as a measure of AHR.

The precise mechanisms through which inhaled mannitol causes bronchoconstriction are not well characterized. Mannitol is known to induce bronchoconstriction by a hypertonic mechanism, that is, drawing water out of cells and into the airways, which is similar to the actions of hypertonic saline that is also used as an indirect airway challenge (Jones et al. 2001). While this mechanism of action may assist in the clearance of mucus from airways, mannitol also activates local inflammatory cells, causing the release of inflammatory mediators from mast cells and basophils (Brannan et al. 2003) (Figure 10.2).

Mannitol doses are administered as doubling doses, starting with 5 mg, then 10 mg, followed by 20, 40, 80, and 160 mg, and then two more inhalations of 160 mg. The FEV_1 is measured 1 min after each dose and the challenge is stopped when the FEV_1 falls by 15% or if the cumulative dose of 635 mg is reached. A positive test occurs when a 15% fall in FEV_1 is reached at a dose of ≤635 mg mannitol (Spector et al. 2009) and the response to inhaled mannitol is reported as the PD_{15}, the provocative dose causing a 15% reduction in FEV_1.

Target Population

Mannitol challenges are used to assess airway hyperresponsiveness in adults and children 6 years of age and older. The mannitol challenge is as sensitive as methacholine for diagnosing asthma and has positive/negative predictive values of 79%/48% in a population without clearly diagnosed asthma (Spector et al. 2009; Stickland et al. 2011). The test can also be used to evaluate subjects with COPD (de Nijs et al. 2011).

Safety Considerations

The mannitol challenge can be safely carried out in adults and children using only a simple dry powder inhaler device. Mannitol is recognized to cause cough, which can be severe in some patients (Brannan et al. 2005).

Outcomes and Interpretation of Results

The mannitol challenge model has been a helpful clinical tool for assessing changes in AHR following intervention. Reproducibility of the test is suitable (Anderson et al. 1997), and the standardized test kit purchased from the supplier provides identical

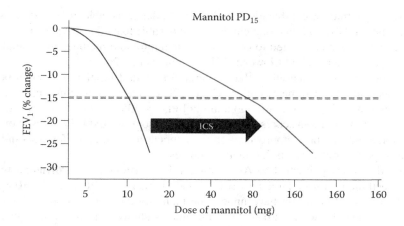

FIGURE 10.4   Percent change in forced expiratory volume in 1 s (FEV_1) during inhalation challenge with doses of mannitol (mg) in patients with asthma without treatment (left) and following treatment with inhaled corticosteroids (ICSs) (right). The provocative dose of mannitol causing a 15% fall in FEV_1 (PD_{15}) shifts approximately 4 doubling doses higher with ICS treatment.

methodology for use in multicenter clinical trials. To date, there have been several airway therapeutics tested using mannitol challenges. After regular treatment with corticosteroids, the response to mannitol is significantly reduced (Figure 10.4) and in some patients inhibited completely (Koskela et al. 2003). The response to mannitol is also significantly reduced by sodium cromoglycate and nedocromil sodium (Anderson et al. 2010), which suggests that mannitol responsiveness reflects activation of airway.

In a study by Lipworth, mannitol inhalation challenge and the measurement of airway hyperresponsiveness were utilized as tools to titrate ICSs (ciclesonide) to improve asthma control and reduce airway inflammation (Lipworth 2012). The results of the study demonstrated that mannitol inhalation challenge and the associated increases in AHR facilitated the exposure of primary care patients to higher doses of ICS (Lipworth 2012). Furthermore, the levels of eosinophil cationic protein (ECP) and the fraction of exhaled nitric oxide (FE_{NO}) were lowered in the patients exposed to mannitol compared to the control group. This study suggested that mannitol challenge was tolerated well in mild to moderate asthmatics in the primary care setting; however, larger trials utilizing mannitol need to be conducted to evaluate severe asthmatics to further validate and explore the utility of mannitol.

Another study by Torok et al. utilized the mannitol inhalation challenge to determine the effects of budesonide and montelukast treatment on the pediatric population undergoing an exercise challenge (Torok et al. 2014). The main outcome of this study was to evaluate AHR after mannitol and exercise challenge. Torok et al. found that combination therapy with budesonide (bronchodilator) and montelukast (mast cell stabilizer) decreased AHR to both exercise and mannitol challenge compared to no treatment or budesonide alone (Torok et al. 2014). This highlights the utility of mannitol in evaluating the efficacy of drug therapeutics in the treatment of asthma.

Although mannitol inhalation (indirect) challenge is able to evaluate AHR, methacholine (direct) inhalation challenge is also able to evaluate AHR, and several studies have been completed to compare the mannitol and methacholine inhalation challenges (Anderson and Lipworth 2012; Lemiere et al. 2012).

Lemiere et al. compared methacholine and mannitol inhalation tests in people with occupational asthma (Lemiere et al. 2012). When comparing subjects with methacholine $PC_{20} \leq 4$ mg/mL and mannitol $PD_{15} \leq 635$ mg, there were no striking differences in symptom scores, FE_{NO}, sputum eosinophils, and FEV_1. Based on this, direct and indirect bronchoprovocation tests appear to yield no differences in bronchial responses or airway inflammatory indices.

Another study published by Anderson and Lipworth compared different severities of asthmatics (mild, moderate, severe) and the ICS dose, FE_{NO} levels, FEV_1, and ECP levels for those who have undergone mannitol and methacholine challenges (Anderson and Lipworth 2012). Mild asthmatics showed similar values in FEV_1 and ECP levels in both the mannitol and methacholine challenge groups; however, FE_{NO} was lower in the mannitol group, while ICS dose was lower in the methacholine group. Moderate asthmatics showed similar values in ICS dose, FE_{NO} levels, FEV_1, and ECP levels in both the mannitol and methacholine challenge groups. Severe asthmatics showed similar values in FEV_1 and ECP levels; however, FE_{NO} was lower in the methacholine group, while ICS dose was lower in the mannitol group. Generally, the values of ICS dose, FE_{NO} levels, FEV_1, and ECP level were consistent across disease severity groups (Anderson and Lipworth 2012). In the mannitol group, FE_{NO} levels increased as disease severity increased, and methacholine PC_{20} decreased as disease severity increased. However, in the methacholine group, FE_{NO} levels decreases as disease severity increased (opposite result compared to the mannitol group), and mannitol PD_{15} increased as diseases severity increased (same result compared to the methacholine group) (Anderson and Lipworth 2012). The different trends seen in FE_{NO} may be due to the difference in challenge targets (directs versus indirect); however, more studies comparing methacholine and mannitol are warranted in order to make any definitive conclusions.

ADENOSINE MONOPHOSPHATE INHALATION CHALLENGE

AMP (or 5'-adenylic acid) is a ubiquitous nucleic acid used for many processes in the human body. AMP is a component of ribonucleic acid, which is used for the translation of DNA into proteins. AMP is also a precursor of adenosine triphosphate, which powers living cells. Inhalation of AMP induces bronchoconstriction in asthmatics.

Inhaled AMP is rapidly converted to adenosine and has been thought to elicit bronchospasm by binding to and activating adenosine receptors on primed mast cells. This binding causes cells to degranulate, releasing mediators such as prostanoids and eicosanoids that cause smooth muscle constriction and mucosal edema (Joos et al. 2003). AMP is also thought to act on A2b receptors in vascular beds and neurosecretory cells to induce mucosal edema directly (Polosa and Holgate 1997).

By targeting inflammatory cells, it has been proposed that AMP may be a more sensitive marker of inflamed airways in asthma as compared to direct agents such as methacholine and histamine. AMP responsiveness is closely associated with measurements of airway inflammation such as sputum eosinophils and eosinophil products including ECP (Polosa et al. 2000). Adenosine has also been proposed to involve C fibers and parasympathetic reflexes (Figure 10.2).

AMP challenges deliver nebulized solution by tidal breathing or by using a modified dosimeter method. Doubling concentrations of AMP are inhaled until the required fall in FEV_1 is reached or until the highest concentration of 800 mg/mL is administered (Polosa and Holgate 1997). The response to AMP is determined by measuring the provocative concentration of inhaled AMP causing the FEV_1 to decrease by 20%. The exact cutoff point between normal and abnormal PC_{20} AMP remains controversial; however, the most commonly designated cutoff is 160 mg/mL.

Target Population

AMP challenges have been utilized in both adults and children. The test is highly specific and therefore can be used to discriminate between asthma and COPD.

Safety Considerations

AMP is ubiquitous in the human body, and inhalation challenges are not associated with side effects. However, doses administered to subjects are 50–100-fold higher compared to methacholine, thus reaching a dose plateau where subjects cannot be pushed further. Whether or not AMP inhalation induces airway eosinophilia is debatable (van den Berge et al. 2004).

Outcomes and Interpretation of Results

AMP challenges have been used for clinical research to assess the effects of asthma medications on airway responsiveness (Figure 10.5). Nonsteroidal

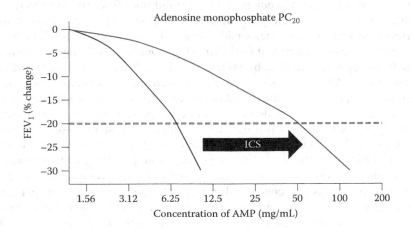

FIGURE 10.5 Percent change in forced expiratory volume in 1 s (FEV_1) at doubling concentrations of adenosine monophosphate (AMP) (mg/mL) in patients with asthma without treatment (left) and following treatment with inhaled corticosteroids (ICSs) (right). The provocative concentration of AMP causing a 20% fall in FEV_1 (PC_{20}) shifts approximately 4 doubling concentrations higher with ICS treatment.

therapeutic agents, including the anti–immunoglobulin E (IgE) antibody, omalizumab, have been shown to shift the PC_{20} to AMP (Currie et al. 2003; Prieto et al. 2006). Studies of this nature demonstrate the usefulness of AMP to assess asthma therapies but also provide evidence of IgE and thus mast cell/basophil involvement in the pathophysiology of airway constriction induced by AMP. Lee et al. evaluated the effectiveness of single and short-term dosing regime of a histamine H_1 receptor antagonist on AMP PC_{20}. Treatment with levocetirizine significantly increased AMP PC_{20} values compared to the placebo, without effecting prechallenge FEV_1 (Lee et al. 2004). The leukotriene receptor antagonist, montelukast, has also been shown to be a valuable add-on therapy for asthmatics not well controlled by ICSs due to genetic susceptibility to β2-receptor genotype (Sims et al. 2003). The effectiveness of montelukast in this subject group was assessed using AMP PC_{20}, given that it is thought to be a more sensitive method to detect ICS inflammatory effects as opposed to methacholine(O'Connor et al. 1992; van den Berge et al. 2001).

Interestingly, other intervention studies with ICSs verify that changes in airway hyperresponsiveness to indirect stimuli such as AMP provide more information on airway inflammatory control than symptoms and lung function or airway reactivity to direct stimuli like methacholine or histamine. For example, O'Connor et al. demonstrated that inhaled glucocorticosteroids decreased airway hyperresponsiveness to AMP to a significantly greater extent than it reduces airway hyperresponsiveness to methacholine in subjects with mild asthma. They proposed that this might represent a reduction in mast cell numbers and activity (O'Connor et al. 1992). Ketchell et al. expanded on these findings to demonstrate that following inhalation of fluticasone propionate (100–1000 µg) in mild stable asthma, there was a reduction in airway hyperresponsiveness to AMP, whereas a single inhalation of fluticasone propionate 1000 µg did not affect airway hyperresponsiveness to histamine (Ketchell et al. 2002). Wilson et al. reported that 4 weeks of treatment with 160 mcg ciclesonide once daily in subjects with mild persistent asthma significantly increased the AMP PC_{20} from 13 to 140 mg/mL, compared to only 17 mg/mL with placebo (Wilson et al. 2006). This eightfold increase in mean PC_{20} to AMP was associated with a decrease in sputum eosinophils and significant improvements in exhaled nitric oxide levels. Similarly, Taylor and colleagues reported that ICSs decreased airway hyperresponsiveness to AMP in a dose-dependent manner, which was in line with a decrease in sputum eosinophils (Taylor et al. 1999). On the other hand, Green et al. showed that after 4 weeks of treatment with twice the equivalent dose of budesonide (800 µg/day), there was only a 0.4 doubling dose reduction of airway hyperresponsiveness to methacholine from baseline, which was associated with a 1.6-fold reduction in sputum eosinophils (Green et al. 2006). Young children have also been included in studies comparing responses to both methacholine and AMP. These studies have reflected that AMP responsiveness is more likely to be associated with atopy, IgE, and inflammatory markers including blood eosinophils compared with methacholine (Bakirtas and Turktas 2006; Choi et al. 2007). These findings suggest that airway responsiveness to AMP appears to provide better reflection of changes in inflammatory markers than responsiveness to methacholine.

ALLERGEN INHALATION CHALLENGE

Allergens are natural stimuli that when inhaled by sensitized individuals can induce three hallmarks of allergic asthma: bronchoconstriction, airway inflammation, and AHR. The mechanism by which allergens induce asthmatic responses is an active area of study with established animal and human allergen challenge models. Inhaled allergens can be administered to subjects with allergic asthma to provoke controlled asthma exacerbations for the evaluation of the immunobiology and pathophysiology of allergic asthma, and also to test the efficacy of novel therapeutics for the treatment of asthma (Diamant et al. 2013).

The pathogenesis of allergic asthma is driven by allergen exposure and subsequent activation of the innate and adaptive immune responses. The inhaled allergen is a pro-inflammatory stimulus that activates immune cells in the airway, resulting in asthmatic symptoms of wheezing, shortness of breath, chest tightness, and cough. More specifically, the innate immune system detects inhaled allergens through pattern recognition receptors, such as toll-like receptors (TLR4, TLR9), which leads to the release of pro-inflammatory cytokines (IL-1, IL-6, IL-25, IL-33) and thymic stromal lymphopoietin (TSLP) (Willart et al. 2012; Chu et al. 2013). IgE bound on the surface of mast cells and basophils are able to bind and cross-link allergen, which results in the induction of their activation and the release of inflammatory mediators (histamines, leukotrienes, prostaglandins) (Gould and Sutton 2008; Stone et al. 2010; Dullaers et al. 2012).

The adaptive immune response mediated by antigen-presenting cells (APCs), specifically dendritic cells, T cells, and B cells, which drives an adaptive immune response against allergens. Dendritic cells (professional APCs) process and present antigens to Th2 cells (CD4+ T cells), thus initiating the Th2 response, a characteristic of allergic disease (Mempel et al. 2004; Trivedi and Lloyd 2007; Dua et al. 2010). Furthermore, a myriad of cells (T cells, basophils, ILC2s) are able to produce IL-4 and IL-13 (Mandler et al. 1993; Ogata et al. 1998; Smith et al. 2015), which acts as a maturation factor for B cells that allow them to isotype-switch into IgE-producing plasma cells (Kasaian et al. 1995; Zuidscherwoude and van Spriel 2012). Specifically, Th2 cells present allergen peptides to B cells via T cell receptor and B cell receptor interactions (Robinson 2010), which initiates IgE isotype-switching of B cells, allowing B cells to mature into IgE-secreting plasma cells (Luger et al. 2009). Like T cells, B cells are also able to secrete cytokines, such as IL-4 and IL-13, which further propagates the Th2 response.

Allergic asthmatics typically respond to allergens in two phases, the EAR and the late asthmatic response (LAR), which are measured by a decline in the FEV_1. The EAR is characterized by an acute onset of bronchoconstriction, largely due to cross-linking of allergen-specific IgE bound to high-affinity IgE receptors (FcεRI) on mast cells and basophils (Figure 10.2), and subsequent activation and release of the bronchoconstrictor mediators including histamine, leukotrienes, and pro-inflammatory cytokines. The LAR is more a delayed bronchoconstriction occurring approximately 4–8 h postchallenge and is associated with cellular infiltration of the airways, which is predominantly eosinophilic in nature (Gauvreau et al. 2000; Gauvreau and Evans 2007).

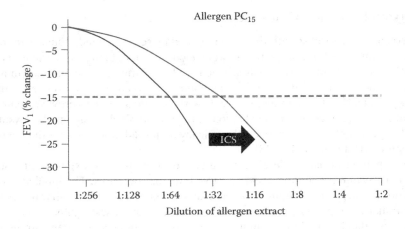

FIGURE 10.6 Percent change in forced expiratory volume in 1 s (FEV$_1$) at doubling titrations of sensitizing allergen extract in subjects with mild allergic asthma without treatment (left) and following treatment with inhaled corticosteroids (ICSs) (right). The provocative concentration of allergen causing a 15% fall in FEV$_1$ (PC$_{15}$) shifts approximately 1.5 doubling dilutions with higher ICS treatment.

During an allergen inhalation challenge, asthmatic subjects inhale an aeroallergen to which they are sensitized, as determined by skin prick testing. Common aeroallergens include house dust mite, cat dander, and pollens. Allergen extracts are diluted in saline, nebulized, and delivered by inhalation in increasing (often doubling) dilutions. The FEV$_1$ is measured 10 min after each inhalation, and the challenge is stopped when a 20% fall in FEV$_1$ is reached (Gauvreau and Evans 2007; Diamant et al. 2013). In the PC$_{15}$ model of allergen challenge, the acute response to allergen is expressed as a PC$_{15}$, that is, the concentration of allergen causing a 15% decline in FEV$_1$ (Figure 10.6). In the EAR/LAR model of allergen challenge, a predefined amount of allergen is inhaled and spirometry is measured regularly for 7–10 h to capture both the EAR and LAR. In such cases, responses to allergen can be expressed as the maximum percent fall in FEV$_1$ or as the area under the curve (AUC) of the EAR and LAR. A positive EAR is defined as a $\geq$20% fall in FEV$_1$ and a positive LAR is defined as a $\geq$15% fall in FEV (Figure 10.7).

Target Population

Individuals with stable, mild, allergic asthma and using only intermittent short-acting bronchodilators for the treatment of their asthma are suitable subjects for inhaled allergen challenges. Those requiring regular medications for the treatment of their asthma are not an appropriate population to test, because most classes of asthma drugs interfere with the allergen-induced responses.

Safety Considerations

Allergen challenges are conducted safely in laboratories with highly trained and experienced staff. Results from skin tests and airway responsiveness to

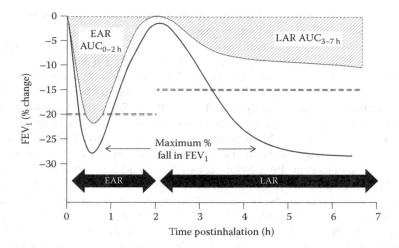

FIGURE 10.7   Percent change in forced expiratory volume in 1 s (FEV_1) after allergen inhalation challenge in subjects with mild allergic asthma with placebo treatment (lower curve) and following treatment with an effective antiasthma therapy (upper hatched curve). The magnitude of the early asthmatic response occurring acutely postchallenge and the late asthmatic response beginning at 3 h postchallenge are compared between active treatment and placebo control.

methacholine/histamine can be used to accurately predict the allergen PC_{20} (Cockcroft et al. 2005), and a stepwise approach to administering allergens will prevent overdose. Administering allergen can lead to loss of asthma control in those with more severe disease; thus, these challenges are not recommended for patients with moderate-to-severe asthma.

Outcomes and Interpretation of Results

The allergen challenge model has been valuable in human asthma research for assessing the mechanisms of variable airflow obstruction, airway hyperresponsiveness, and cellular inflammation. Measurements of airway tone are evaluated by examining the magnitude of the EAR and LAR expressed as percent fall in FEV_1 from prechallenge baseline. The EAR and LAR can also be expressed as AUC of the percent fall in FEV_1 × time curve. Inhaled allergen is shown to shift the dose–response to direct stimuli such as methacholine and histamine, and this is likely related to the allergen-induced accumulation of inflammatory cells, including eosinophils, basophils, and mast cells in the airways, which can also be counted in the bronchial biopsies, bronchoalveolar lavage, and samples of induced sputum (Gauvreau et al. 2000a; Gauvreau and Evans 2007; Diamant et al. 2013).

The high reproducibility and clinical relevance of allergen-induced airway responses has positioned the allergen challenge model as an invaluable tool for assessing the efficacy of current and investigational anti-inflammatory therapies for the treatment of asthma (Boulet et al. 2007). In a crossover study design, as few as 8 subjects can be used to detect a 50% inhibition of the EAR and LAR (Inman et al. 1995; Gauvreau et al. 1999b). The allergen challenge model was initially used to demonstrate the efficacy of commonly used asthma treatments, including ICSs, antileukotrienes, and short-acting beta agonists.

Many studies have been conducted to evaluate the effects of anti-inflammatory therapies on allergen-induced responses. Early studies demonstrated very clear inhibition of the LAR with single dose or regular treatment with inhaled budesonide (Gauvreau et al. 1996; Kidney et al. 1997), and ICSs have also been shown to significantly shift the allergen PC_{15} (Cockcroft et al. 1995). Subsequent studies sought to utilize the allergen challenge model to investigate the anti-inflammatory properties of ICSs, finding that in addition to inhibition of the EAR and LAR, ICSs reduced the number of eosinophils and their progenitors in the airways, circulation, and bone marrow (Gauvreau et al. 1996; Sehmi et al. 1997; Wood et al. 1999, 2002; Gauvreau et al. 2000b) (Figure 10.7). The allergen challenge model has been used to generate steroid dose–response (Inman et al. 2001), to compare other therapies to corticosteroids as "gold standard" (Leigh et al. 2002; Duong et al. 2007), and to evaluate new therapeutics acting through the glucocorticoid receptor (Gauvreau et al. 2015).

In the studies of bronchodilators, surprising results were discovered when evaluating the effects of short-acting beta agonists on allergen-induced responses. In a study conducted by Cockcroft, salbutamol treatment, a regularly inhaled β_2 agonist to reverse bronchoconstriction, was tested using the allergen inhalation challenge model. Since allergen is a more relevant environmental stimulus compared to chemical stimuli such as AMP, histamine, and methacholine, the inhaled allergen model was a highly relevant model to test the treatment effects of regular dosing of salbutamol compared to placebo in allergic asthmatics (Cockcroft 1993). Cockcroft reports that following regular salbutamol treatment, there was a significant decrease in the protective effect on both the methacholine and allergen PC_{20}, where the allergic asthmatics tolerated lower levels of methacholine and allergen after salbutamol treatment compared to placebo (Cockcroft 1993). These findings highlight the detrimental effects of continual, regular use of inhaled β_2 agonist. In support, Gauvreau et al. also showed that that allergen-induced LAR was far worsened in allergic asthmatics treated with albuterol after allergen inhalation challenge compared to placebo (Gauvreau et al. 1997). Further supporting the notion that regular use of inhaled β_2 agonist has detrimental effects on allergen sensitivity, Gauvreau et al. showed that in albuterol-treated asthmatics, but not placebo, there were increased airway hyperreactivity (decreased methacholine PC_{20}), increased sputum eosinophilia, and increased sputum ECP levels after allergen inhalation challenge. These studies demonstrated that regular use of salbutamol renders the airways more responsive to direct and indirect stimuli in terms of bronchoconstriction and inflammation.

In addition to testing the efficacy and inflammatory profiles of known asthma therapeutics using the allergen inhalation challenge model, novel therapeutics are also evaluated. Novel anti-inflammatory therapies such as anti-IL-13 have been tested in this model, where inhibition of the LAR by anti-IL-13 (Gauvreau et al. 2011) provides key information supporting further development of drugs targeting the IL-13 pathway. However, there are other biologic targets that have shown efficacy in the clinical treatment of allergic asthmatics, which have been tested using the allergen inhalation challenge model, including anti-IgE (omalizumab, also commercially known as Xolair) and anti-TSLP.

B cell production of IgE is an important therapeutic target, particularly in IgE-mediated disease, due to their involvement in initiating the allergic cascade (Platts-Mills 2001). Antibodies, like IgE, have been implicated in diseases since the 1890s and antibody-producing B cells were first reported in 1956 by Glick et al., when they found that cells from the bursa of Fabricius in young chickens produced antibodies early in their development to aid in disease resistance (Glick et al. 1956). As already established earlier, in the context of allergic asthma, IgE have large roles in disease pathogenesis (Smurthwaite et al. 2001). Historically, IgE was first reported on by Lichtenstein et al. (1966) and Ishizaka et al. (1966) in 1966. Over 50 years after the discovery of IgE, researchers have shown that IgE is increased in individuals with atopic diseases (Stone et al. 2010), especially in the airways and peripheral compartments after allergen inhalation challenge (Wilson et al. 2002; Gauvreau et al. 2014c). In a seminal study conducted by Boulet et al., anti-IgE treatment of allergic asthmatics was shown to have drastic improvements on allergen PC_1FEV_1 and free serum IgE. Furthermore, anti-IgE treatment demonstrated inhibitory effects on allergen-induced EAR, which made it a promising therapeutic to further study on allergic asthmatics, particularly using the allergen inhalation challenge model.

Several therapies have been developed to reduce the level of IgE, which have utilized the allergen inhalation challenge model as their proof of concept model. Currently, omalizumab is a monoclonal antibody against IgE that is able to bind free IgE in serum and on the surface of B cells (Holgate et al. 2005; Chan et al. 2013; Nyborg et al. 2015). In the allergen challenge model, it has shown efficacy in improving asthma symptoms and reducing exacerbations (O'Byrne et al. 1987; Fahy et al. 1997). In mechanistic studies using the allergen challenge model, the treatment with omalizumab inhibited both the EAR and LAR and decreased eosinophil levels in sputum (Fahy et al. 1997; Djukanović et al. 2004).

Due to the success of omalizumab, new systemic approaches for reducing circulating levels of IgE have been further pursued and evaluated. A novel anti-IgE therapeutic, ligelizumab (QGE031), has higher affinity for IgE compared to omalizumab, resulting in increased suppression of IgE-receptor complex formation (Arm et al. 2014) and providing enhanced protection compared to omalizumab (Oliveria et al. 2014). Furthermore, Gauvreau et al. showed that ligelizumab was superior to omalizumab at improving $PC_{15}FEV_1$ at both 72 and 240 mg doses of ligelizumab treatment (Gauvreau et al. 2014). In addition to the improvement in bronchial provocation testing, ligelizumab also demonstrated suppression of free serum IgE, surface IgE receptors on basophils (FcεRI), and skin prick test responses.

Unlike omalizumab and ligelizumab, there have been advances in specifically targeting IgE expressed on the surface of memory B cells. Gauvreau et al. used monoclonal antibody, which targeted M1-prime, a specific epitope on IgE bound on the surface of B cells, to specifically target the depletion of IgE+ B cells. The treatment with anti-M1-prime antibody (quilizumab) reduced total IgE and airway eosinophils, accompanied by blunted EAR, but not LAR to inhaled allergen (Gauvreau et al. 2014c).

In addition to omalizumab, ligelizumab, and quilizumab, there are also other approaches that have been tested using the allergen inhalation challenge model, which indirectly aim to reduce the synthesis of IgE by regulating B cell functions in subjects with allergic asthma. Briefly, the blockade of OX40L was found by Gauvreau et al. to decrease total and allergen-specific IgE in the circulation compared to placebo (Gauvreau et al. 2014), and these decreases were sustained over 250 days after treatment. Additionally, anti-OX40L treatment also reduced eosinophil levels in the sputum. However, there were no treatment effects on the EAR or LAR comparing anti-OX40L and placebo.

Elucidating the inflammatory pathways leading to the EAR and LAR using the allergen challenge model is crucial in discovering the critical pathways for the treatment of allergic asthma. For example, targeting TSLP, an upstream alarmin cytokine capable of initiating the inflammatory cascade, using a monoclonal antibody would be a promising upstream target with the potential of dampening downstream inflammatory processes (Dahlén 2014). A study by Gauvreau et al. evaluated allergen-induced asthmatic responses after treatment with anti-TSLP (AMG 157) (Gauvreau et al. 2014d). Remarkably, the treatment with anti-TSLP attenuated both the EAR and LAR compared to placebo (Gauvreau et al. 2014d). Furthermore, blood and sputum eosinophils and the fraction of exhaled nitric oxide (FE_{NO}) were also decreased after anti-TSLP treatment compared to placebo (Gauvreau et al. 2014d). Taken together, anti-TSLP attenuated allergen-induced bronchoconstriction and hallmark indices characterizing airway inflammation before and after allergen inhalation challenge.

As discussed earlier, the allergen challenge model is particularly useful for testing new therapeutics targeting type 2 inflammation. Overall, the allergen challenge model has an excellent negative predictive value for investigational therapies, which is an important consideration during drug development, thus highlighting the utility of the allergen inhalation challenge in early-phase clinical trials and the testing efficacy of a treatment in a disease.

CONCLUSION

Bronchoprovocation tests continue to play a valuable role clinically. While the preferred tests for clinical diagnosis and monitoring of asthma are chosen based largely on experience and recommended guidelines, limited access to some agents in different parts of the world may limit the options.

Bronchoprovocation tests, both direct and indirect, also play a valuable role in research laboratories for investigating the pathobiology of asthma. These tests are also recognized for their unequivocal potential in assessing efficacy of asthma treatments. In addition to the tests described herein, other inhalation challenges are being validated as models for drug development. One such test uses lipopolysaccharide (Figure 10.2) (Janssen et al. 2013), a derivative of bacterial endotoxin, which activates TLR4 on epithelial cells and induces a distinct neutrophilic inflammatory response in the airways.

When employing bronchoprovocation tests in clinical trials to determine the efficacy and/or proof of activity of asthma therapies, care must be taken to select a challenge most suitable to test the drug under investigation. Direct airway challenges have been central for the determination of optimal doses and duration of action when evaluating bronchodilator therapies, while indirect challenges, such as allergen, are valuable for assessing the effects anti-inflammatory therapies on the late-phase airway responses and accumulation of inflammatory cells. One must also be certain to allow sufficient recovery between tests, particularly tests that induce refractoriness (such as exercise challenge, not described here) or those that induce airway inflammation, such as allergen challenges.

Research investigations into the pathogenesis of asthma will continue to identify new therapeutic targets. An improved understanding of the mechanisms by which indirect airway challenges induce bronchoconstriction will enable the most appropriate model to be selected for testing of drugs in the early clinical development.

SUMMARY

- Asthma is a chronic disease of the airways, which is characterized by inflammation, variable airflow obstruction, and airway hyperresponsiveness, which is an exaggerated bronchoconstrictor response to physical, chemical, or pharmacologic stimuli.
- Airway hyperresponsiveness can be quantified by measuring the degree of bronchoconstriction to inhaled stimuli, using direct and indirect airway challenges.
- Direct airway challenges cause bronchoconstriction using agents such as methacholine and histamine, which act directly on receptors located on airway smooth muscle.
- Indirect airway challenges cause bronchoconstriction by acting on inflammatory cells or nerves to stimulate the release of mediators that induce smooth muscle contraction.
- Bronchoprovocation tests using direct and indirect airway challenges are valuable for testing the effects of asthma therapies on airway hyperresponsiveness.

REFERENCES

Anderson, SD, J Brannan, J Spring, N Spalding, LT Rodwell, K Chan, I Gonda, A Walsh, and AR Clark. 1997. A new method for bronchial-provocation testing in asthmatic subjects using a dry powder of mannitol. *American Journal of Respiratory and Critical Care Medicine* 156 (3 Pt 1) (September): 758–765.

Anderson, SD, JD Brannan, CP Perry, C Caillaud, and JP Seale. 2010. Sodium cromoglycate alone and in combination with montelukast on the airway response to mannitol in asthmatic subjects. *The Journal of Asthma: Official Journal of the Association for the Care of Asthma* 47 (4) (May): 429–433.

Anderson, WJ and BJ Lipworth. 2012. Relationship of mannitol challenge to methacholine challenge and inflammatory markers in persistent asthmatics receiving inhaled corticosteroids. *Lung* 190 (5): 513–521.

Arm, JP, I Bottoli, A Skerjanec, D Floch, A Groenewegen, S Maahs, CE Owen, I Jones, and PJ Lowe. 2014. Pharmacokinetics, pharmacodynamics and safety of QGE031 (ligelizumab), a novel high-affinity anti-IgE antibody, in atopic subjects. *Clinical and Experimental Allergy: Journal of the British Society for Allergy and Clinical Immunology* 44 (11) (November): 1371–1385.

Bakirtas, A and I Turktas. 2006. Determinants of airway responsiveness to adenosine 5'-monophosphate in school-age children with asthma. *Pediatric Pulmonology* 41 (6) (June): 515–521.

Bhagat, RG and MM Grunstein. 1984. Comparison of responsiveness to methacholine, histamine, and exercise in subgroups of asthmatic children. *The American Review of Respiratory Disease* 129 (2) (February): 221–224.

Boulet, L-P, G Gauvreau, M-E Boulay, P O'Byrne, DW Cockcroft, and Canadian Network of Centers of Excellence AllerGen Clinical Investigative Collaboration. 2007. The allergen bronchoprovocation model: An important tool for the investigation of new asthma anti-inflammatory therapies. *Allergy* 62 (10) (October): 1101–1110.

Brannan, JD, SD Anderson, CP Perry, R Freed-Martens, AR Lassig, B Charlton, and Aridol Study Group. 2005. The safety and efficacy of inhaled dry powder mannitol as a bronchial provocation test for airway hyperresponsiveness: A phase 3 comparison study with hypertonic (4.5%) saline. *Respiratory Research* 6: 144.

Brannan, JD, M Gulliksson, SD Anderson, N Chew, and M Kumlin. 2003. Evidence of mast cell activation and leukotriene release after mannitol inhalation. *The European Respiratory Journal* 22 (3) (September): 491–496.

Bryan, SA, BJ O'Connor, S Matti, MJ Leckie, V Kanabar, J Khan, SJ Warrington et al. 2000. Effects of recombinant human interleukin-12 on eosinophils, airway hyperresponsiveness, and the late asthmatic response. *The Lancet* 356 (9248): 2149–2153.

Chan, M, NM Gigliotti, AL Dotson, and LJ Rosenwasser. 2013. Omalizumab may decrease IgE synthesis by targeting membrane IgE+ human B cells. *Clinical and Translational Allergy* 3 (1) (January): 29.

Chatham, M, ER Bleecker, PL Smith, RR Rosenthal, P Mason, and PS Norman. 1982. A comparison of histamine, methacholine, and exercise airway reactivity in normal and asthmatic subjects. *The American Review of Respiratory Disease* 126 (2) (August): 235–240.

Choi, SH, DK Kim, J Yu, Y Yoo, and YY Koh. 2007. Bronchial responsiveness to methacholine and adenosine 5'-monophosphate in young children with asthma: Their relationship with blood eosinophils and serum eosinophil cationic protein. *Allergy* 62 (10) (October): 1119–1124.

Chu, DK, A Llop-Guevara, TD Walker, K Flader, S Goncharova, JE Boudreau, CL Moore et al. 2013. IL-33, but not thymic stromal lymphopoietin or IL-25, is central to mite and peanut allergic sensitization. *The Journal of Allergy and Clinical Immunology* 131 (1) (January): 187–200.e1–e8.

Cockcroft, DW. 1993. Regular inhaled salbutamol and airway responsiveness to allergen. *The Lancet* 342 (8875): 833–837.

Cockcroft, DW, BE Davis, L-P Boulet, F Deschesnes, GM Gauvreau, PM O'Byrne, and RM Watson. 2005. The links between allergen skin test sensitivity, airway responsiveness and airway response to allergen. *Allergy* 60 (1) (January): 56–59.

Cockcroft, DW, RE Ruffin, PA Frith, A Cartier, EF Juniper, J Dolovich, and FE Hargreave. 1979. Determinants of allergen-induced asthma: Dose of allergen, circulating IgE antibody concentration, and bronchial responsiveness to inhaled histamine. *The American Review of Respiratory Disease* 120 (5) (November): 1053–1058.

Cockcroft, DW, VA Swystun, and R Bhagat. 1995. Interaction of inhaled beta 2 agonist and inhaled corticosteroid on airway responsiveness to allergen and methacholine. *American Journal of Respiratory and Critical Care Medicine* 152 (5 Pt 1) (November): 1485–1489.

Crapo, RO, R Casaburi, AL Coates, PL Enright, JL Hankinson, CG Irvin, NR MacIntyre et al. 2000. Guidelines for methacholine and exercise challenge testing-1999. This official statement of the American thoracic society was adopted by the ATS board of directors, July 1999. *American Journal of Respiratory and Critical Care Medicine* 161 (1) (January): 309–329.

Crimi, N, F Palermo, R Oliveri, R Polosa, I Settinieri, and A Mistretta. 1992. Protective effects of inhaled ipratropium bromide on bronchoconstriction induced by adenosine and methacholine in asthma. *The European Respiratory Journal* 5 (5) (May): 560–565.

Crockcroft, DW, KY Murdock, and BA Berscheid. 1984. Relationship between atopy and bronchial responsiveness to histamine in a random population. *Annals of Allergy* 53 (1) (July): 26–29.

Currie, GP, DKC Lee, K Haggart, CE Bates, and BJ Lipworth. 2003. Effects of montelukast on surrogate inflammatory markers in corticosteroid-treated patients with asthma. *American Journal of Respiratory and Critical Care Medicine* 167 (9) (May 1): 1232–1238.

Dahlén, S-E. 2014. TSLP in asthma—A new kid on the block? *The New England Journal of Medicine* 370 (22) (May 29): 2144–2145.

Davis, BE and DW Cockcroft. 2005. Effect of a single dose of montelukast sodium on methacholine chloride PC20. *Canadian Respiratory Journal: Journal of the Canadian Thoracic Society* 12 (1): 26–28.

de Nijs, SB, N Fens, R Lutter, E Dijkers, FH Krouwels, BS Smids-Dierdorp, RP van Steenwijk, and PJ Sterk. 2011. Airway inflammation and mannitol challenge test in COPD. *Respiratory Research* 12 (January): 11.

Diamant, Z, GM Gauvreau, DW Cockcroft, LP Boulet, PJ Sterk, FHC De Jongh, B Dahlén, and PM O'Byrne. 2013. Inhaled allergen bronchoprovocation tests. *Journal of Allergy and Clinical Immunology* 132 (5): 1045–1055.

Djukanović, R, SJ Wilson, M Kraft, NN Jarjour, M Steel, KF Chung, W Bao et al. 2004. Effects of treatment with anti-immunoglobulin E antibody omalizumab on airway inflammation in allergic asthma. *American Journal of Respiratory and Critical Care Medicine* 170 (6) (September 15): 583–593.

Dua, B, RM Watson, GM Gauvreau, and PM O'Byrne. 2010. Myeloid and plasmacytoid dendritic cells in induced sputum after allergen inhalation in subjects with asthma. *The Journal of Allergy and Clinical Immunology* 126 (1) (July): 133–139.

Dullaers, M, R De Bruyne, F Ramadani, HJ Gould, P Gevaert, and BN Lambrecht. 2012. The who, where, and when of IgE in allergic airway disease. *The Journal of Allergy and Clinical Immunology* 129 (3) (March): 635–645.

Duong, M, G Gauvreau, R Watson, G Obminski, T Strinich, M Evans, K Howie, K Killian, and PM O'Byrne. 2007. The effects of inhaled budesonide and formoterol in combination and alone when given directly after allergen challenge. *The Journal of Allergy and Clinical Immunology* 119 (2) (February): 322–327.

Fahy, JV, HE Fleming, HH Wong, JT Llu, JQ Su, J Reimann, RB Fick, and HA Boushey. 1997. The effect of an anti-IgE monoclonal antibody on the early- and late-phase responses to allergen inhalation in asthmatic subjects. *American Journal of Respiratory and Critical Care Medicine* 155: 1828–1834.

Fowler, SJ, OJ Dempsey, EJ Sims, and BJ Lipworth. 2000. Screening for bronchial hyperresponsiveness using methacholine and adenosine monophosphate. relationship to asthma severity and beta(2)-receptor genotype. *American Journal of Respiratory and Critical Care Medicine* 162 (4 Pt 1) (October): 1318–1322.

Fowler, SJ and BJ Lipworth. 2003. Relationship of skin-prick reactivity to aeroallergens and hyperresponsiveness to challenges with methacholine and adenosine monophosphate. *Allergy* 58 (1) (January): 46–52.

Gauvreau, GM, L-P Boulet, DW Cockcroft, JM Fitzgerald, C Carlsten, BE Davis, F Deschesnes et al. 2011. Effects of interleukin-13 blockade on allergen-induced airway responses in mild atopic asthma. *American Journal of Respiratory and Critical Care Medicine* 183 (8) (April 15): 1007–1014.

Gauvreau, GM, L-P Boulet, DW Cockcroft, JM Fitzgerald, I Mayers, C Carlsten, M Laviolette et al. 2014a. OX40L blockade and allergen-induced airway responses in subjects with mild asthma. *Clinical and Experimental Allergy: Journal of the British Society for Allergy and Clinical Immunology* 44 (1): 29–37.

Gauvreau, GM, L-P Boulet, R Leigh, DW Cockcroft, BE Davis, I Mayers, JM FitzGerald et al. 2014b. Efficacy and safety of multiple doses of QGE031 (ligelizumab) versus omalizumab and placebo in inhibiting the allergen-induced early asthmatic response. *European Respiratory Journal* 44: A700306.

Gauvreau, GM, L-P Boulet, R Leigh, DW Cockcroft, KJ Killian, BE Davis, F Deschesnes et al. 2015. A nonsteroidal glucocorticoid receptor agonist inhibits allergen-induced late asthmatic responses. *American Journal of Respiratory and Critical Care Medicine* 191 (2) (January 15): 161–167.

Gauvreau, GM, J Doctor, RM Watson, M Jordana, and PM O'Byrne. 1996. Effects of inhaled budesonide on allergen-induced airway responses and airway inflammation. *American Journal of Respiratory and Critical Care Medicine* 154 (5) (November): 1267–1271.

Gauvreau, GM and M Evans. 2007. Allergen inhalation challenge: A human model of asthma exacerbation. *Contributions to Microbiology* 14: 21–32.

Gauvreau, GM, JM Harris, L-P Boulet, H Scheerens, JM Fitzgerald, WS Putnam, DW Cockcroft et al. 2014c. Targeting membrane-expressed IgE B cell receptor with an antibody to the M1 prime epitope reduces IgE production. *Science Translational Medicine* 6 (243) (July 2): 243ra85.

Gauvreau, GM, M Jordana, RM Watson, DW Cockcroft, and PM O'Byrne. 1997. Effect of regular inhaled albuterol on allergen-induced late responses and sputum eosinophils in asthmatic subjects. *American Journal of Respiratory and Critical Care Medicine* 156 (6): 1738–1745.

Gauvreau, GM, JM Lee, RM Watson, AM Irani, LB Schwartz, and PM O'Byrne. 2000a. Increased numbers of both airway basophils and mast cells in sputum after allergen inhalation challenge of atopic asthmatics. *American Journal of Respiratory and Critical Care Medicine* 161 (5) (May): 1473–1478.

Gauvreau, GM, PM O'Byrne, L-P Boulet, Y Wang, D Cockcroft, J Bigler, JM FitzGerald et al. 2014d. Effects of an anti-TSLP antibody on allergen-induced asthmatic responses. *The New England Journal of Medicine* 370 (22) (May 29): 2102–2110.

Gauvreau, GM, RM Watson, and PM O'Byrne. 1999a. Kinetics of allergen-induced airway eosinophilic cytokine production and airway inflammation. *American Journal of Respiratory and Critical Care Medicine* 160 (2) (August): 640–647.

Gauvreau, GM, RM Watson, TJ Rerecich, E Baswick, MD Inman, and PM O'Byrne. 1999b. Repeatability of allergen-induced airway inflammation. *The Journal of Allergy and Clinical Immunology* 104 (1) (July): 66–71.

Gauvreau, GM, LJ Wood, R Sehmi, RM Watson, SC Dorman, RP Schleimer, JA Denburg, and PM O'Byrne. 2000b. The effects of inhaled budesonide on circulating eosinophil progenitors and their expression of cytokines after allergen challenge in subjects with atopic asthma. *American Journal of Respiratory and Critical Care Medicine* 162 (6) (December): 2139–2144.

Glick, B, TS Chang, and RG Jaap. 1956. The bursa of fabricius and antibody production. *Poultry Science* 35 (1): 224–225.

Goldman, MD, M Mathieu, JM Montely, R Goldberg, JM Fry, JL Bernard, and R Sartene. 1995. Inspiratory fall in systolic pressure in normal and asthmatic subjects. *American Journal of Respiratory and Critical Care Medicine* 151 (3 Pt 1) (March): 743–750.

Gould, HJ and BJ Sutton. 2008. IgE in allergy and asthma today. *Nature Reviews Immunology* 8 (3) (March): 205–217.

Green, RH, CE Brightling, S McKenna, B Hargadon, N Neale, D Parker, C Ruse, IP Hall, and ID Pavord. 2006. Comparison of asthma treatment given in addition to inhaled corticosteroids on airway inflammation and responsiveness. *The European Respiratory Journal* 27 (6) (June): 1144–1151.

Higgins, BG, JR Britton, S Chinn, TD Jones, AS Vathenen, PG Burney, and AE Tattersfield. 1988. Comparison of histamine and methacholine for use in bronchial challenge tests in community studies. *Thorax* 43 (8) (August): 605–610.

Hill, DJ, MJ Shelton, and CS Hosking. 1982. Predicting the results of allergen bronchial challenge by simple clinical methods. *Clinical Allergy* 12 (3) (May): 295–301.

Holgate, ST, R Djukanović, T Casale, and J Bousquet. 2005. Anti-immunoglobulin E treatment with omalizumab in allergic diseases: An update on anti-inflammatory activity and clinical efficacy. *Clinical and Experimental Allergy: Journal of the British Society for Allergy and Clinical Immunology* 35 (4) (April): 408–416.

Illamperuma, C, BE Davis, ME Fenton, and DW Cockcroft. 2009. Duration of bronchoprotection of inhaled ipratropium against inhaled methacholine. *Annals of Allergy, Asthma & Immunology: Official Publication of the American College of Allergy, Asthma, & Immunology* 102 (5) (May): 438–439.

Inman, MD, AL Hamilton, HA Kerstjens, RM Watson, and PM O'Byrne. 1998. The utility of methacholine airway responsiveness measurements in evaluating anti-asthma drugs. *The Journal of Allergy and Clinical Immunology* 101 (3) (March): 342–348.

Inman, MD, R Watson, DW Cockcroft, BJ Wong, FE Hargreave, and PM O'Byrne. 1995. Reproducibility of allergen-induced early and late asthmatic responses. *The Journal of Allergy and Clinical Immunology* 95 (6) (June): 1191–1195.

Inman, MD, RM Watson, T Rerecich, GM Gauvreau, BN Lutsky, P Stryszak, and PM O'Byrne. 2001. Dose-dependent effects of inhaled mometasone furoate on airway function and inflammation after allergen inhalation challenge. *American Journal of Respiratory and Critical Care Medicine* 164 (4) (August 15): 569–574.

Ishizaka, K, T Ishizaka, and MM Hornbrook. 1966. Physico-chemical properties of human reaginic antibody. IV. Presence of a unique immunoglobulin as a carrier of reaginic activity. *Journal of Immunology* 97 (1): 75–85.

Janssen, O, F Schaumann, O Holz, B Lavae-Mokhtari, L Welker, C Winkler, H Biller, N Krug, and JM Hohlfeld. 2013. Low-dose endotoxin inhalation in healthy volunteers—A challenge model for early clinical drug development. *BMC Pulmonary Medicine* 13: 19.

Jones, PD, R Hankin, J Simpson, PG Gibson, and RL Henry. 2001. The tolerability, safety, and success of sputum induction and combined hypertonic saline challenge in children. *American Journal of Respiratory and Critical Care Medicine* 164 (7) (October 1): 1146–1149.

Joos, GF, B O'Connor, SD Anderson, F Chung, DW Cockcroft, B Dahlén, G DiMaria et al. 2003. Indirect airway challenges. *The European Respiratory Journal* 21 (6) (June): 1050–1068.

Juniper, EF, PA Frith, C Dunnett, DW Cockcroft, and FE Hargreave. 1978. Reproducibility and comparison of responses to inhaled histamine and methacholine. *Thorax* 33 (6) (December): 705–710.

Kasaian, MT, CH Meyer, AK Nault, and JF Bond. 1995. An increased frequency of IgE-producing B cell precursors contributes to the elevated levels of plasma IgE in atopic subjects. *Clinical and Experimental Allergy* 25 (8): 749–755.

Ketchell, RI, MW Jensen, P Lumley, AM Wright, MI Allenby, and BJ O'Connor. 2002. Rapid effect of inhaled fluticasone propionate on airway responsiveness to adenosine 5′-monophosphate in mild asthma. *The Journal of Allergy and Clinical Immunology* 110 (4) (October): 603–606.

Kidney, JC, LP Boulet, FE Hargreave, F Deschesnes, VA Swystun, PM O'Byrne, N Choudry et al. 1997. Evaluation of single-dose inhaled corticosteroid activity with an allergen challenge model. *The Journal of Allergy and Clinical Immunology* 100 (1) (July): 65–70.

Killian, D, DW Cockcroft, FE Hargreave, and J Dolovich. 1976. Factors in allergen-induced asthma: Relevance of the intensity of the airways allergic reaction and non-specific bronchial reactivity. *Clinical Allergy* 6 (3) (May): 219–225.

Koskela, HO, L Hyvärinen, JD Brannan, H-K Chan, and SD Anderson. 2003. Sensitivity and validity of three bronchial provocation tests to demonstrate the effect of inhaled corticosteroids in asthma. *Chest* 124 (4) (October): 1341–1349.

Leckie, MJ, A ten Brinke, J Khan, Z Diamant, BJ O'Connor, CM Walls, AK Mathur et al. 2000. Effects of an interleukin-5 blocking monoclonal antibody on eosinophils, airway hyper-responsiveness, and the late asthmatic response. *The Lancet* 356 (9248) (December): 2144–2148.

Lee, DKC, RD Gray, AM Wilson, FM Robb, PC Soutar, and BJ Lipworth. 2004. Single and short-term dosing effects of levocetirizine on adenosine monophosphate bronchoprovocation in atopic asthma. *British Journal of Clinical Pharmacology* 58 (1) (July): 34–39.

Leigh, R, D Vethanayagam, M Yoshida, RM Watson, T Rerecich, MD Inman, and PM O'Byrne. 2002. Effects of montelukast and budesonide on airway responses and airway inflammation in asthma. *American Journal of Respiratory and Critical Care Medicine* 166: 1212–1217.

Lemiere, C, D Miedinger, V Jacob, S Chaboillez, C Tremblay, and JD Brannan. 2012. Comparison of methacholine and mannitol bronchial provocation tests in workers with occupational asthma. *The Journal of Allergy and Clinical Immunology* 129 (2): 555–556.

Lichtenstein, LM, PS Norman, WL Winkenwerder, and AG Osler. 1966. In vitro studies of human ragweed allergy: Changes in cellular and humoral activity associated with specific desensitization. *The Journal of Clinical Investigation* 45 (7): 1126–1136.

Lipworth, BJ 2012. A randomized primary care trial of steroid titration against mannitol in persistent asthma. *CHEST Journal* 141 (3): 607.

Luger, EO, V Fokuhl, M Wegmann, M Abram, K Tillack, G Achatz, RA Manz, M Worm, A Radbruch, and H Renz. 2009. Induction of long-lived allergen-specific plasma cells by mucosal allergen challenge. *The Journal of Allergy and Clinical Immunology* 124 (4) (October): 819–826.e4.

Mandler, R, FD Finkelman, AD Levine, and CM Snapper. 1993. IL-4 induction of IgE class switching by lipopolysaccharide-activated murine B cells occurs predominantly through sequential switching. *Journal of Immunology* 150 (2) (January 15): 407–418.

Martin, RJ, JS Wanger, CG Irvin, BB Bartelson, and RM Cherniack. 1997. Methacholine challenge testing: Safety of low starting FEV1. Asthma Clinical Research Network (ACRN). *Chest* 112 (1) (July): 53–56.

Mempel, TR, SE Henrickson, and UH Von Andrian. 2004. T-cell priming by dendritic cells in lymph nodes occurs in three distinct phases. *Nature* 427 (6970) (January 8): 154–159.

Nyborg, AC, A Zacco, R Ettinger, MJ Borrok, J Zhu, T Martin, R Woods et al. 2016. Development of an antibody that neutralizes soluble IgE and eliminates IgE expressing B cells. *Cellular and Molecular Immunology* 13(3):391–400.

O'Byrne, PM, J Dolovich, and FE Hargreave. 1987. Late asthmatic responses. *The American Review of Respiratory Disease* 136 (3) (September): 740–751.

O'Byrne, PM, GM Gauvreau, and JD Brannan. 2009a. Provoked models of asthma: What have we learnt? *Clinical and Experimental Allergy: Journal of the British Society for Allergy and Clinical Immunology* 39 (2) (February): 181–192.

O'Byrne, PM, J van der Linde, DW Cockcroft, GM Gauvreau, JD Brannan, M Fitzgerald, RM Watson et al. 2009b. Prolonged bronchoprotection against inhaled methacholine by inhaled BI 1744, a long-acting beta(2)-agonist, in patients with mild asthma. *The Journal of Allergy and Clinical Immunology* 124 (6) (December): 1217–1221.

O'Connor, BJ, SM Ridge, PJ Barnes, and RW Fuller. 1992. Greater effect of inhaled budesonide on adenosine 5′-monophosphate-induced than on sodium-metabisulfite-induced bronchoconstriction in asthma. *The American Review of Respiratory Disease* 146 (3) (September): 560–564.

Ogata, H, D Ford, N Kouttab, TC King, N Vita, A Minty, J Stoeckler et al. 1998. Regulation of interleukin-13 receptor constituents on mature human B lymphocytes. *The Journal of Biological Chemistry* 273 (16) (April 17): 9864–9871.

Oliveria, JP, H Campbell, S Beaudin, K Howie, J MacLean, S Kotwal, A Smith, JM Harris, H Scheerens, and GM Gauvreau. 2014. Characterization of IgE memory B cell subsets following whole lung allergen challenge in patients with mild asthma. *American Journal of Respiratory and Critical Care Medicine* 189: A2237.

Parameswaran, KN, MD Inman, BP Ekholm, MM Morris, E Summers, PM O'Byrne, and FE Hargreave. 1999. Protection against methacholine bronchoconstriction to assess relative potency of inhaled beta2-agonist. *American Journal of Respiratory and Critical Care Medicine* 160 (1) (July): 354–357.

Platts-Mills, TA. 2001. The role of immunoglobulin E in allergy and asthma. *American Journal of Respiratory and Critical Care Medicine* 164(8 Pt 2): S1-5.

Polosa, R, I Ciamarra, G Mangano, G Prosperini, MP Pistorio, C Vancheri, and N Crimi. 2000. Bronchial hyperresponsiveness and airway inflammation markers in nonasthmatics with allergic rhinitis. *The European Respiratory Journal* 15 (1) (January): 30–35.

Polosa, R and ST Holgate. 1997. Adenosine bronchoprovocation: A promising marker of allergic inflammation in asthma? *Thorax* 52 (10) (October): 919–923.

Prieto, L, V Gutiérrez, C Colás, A Tabar, C Pérez-Francés, L Bruno, and S Uixera. 2006. Effect of omalizumab on adenosine 5′-monophosphate responsiveness in subjects with allergic asthma. *International Archives of Allergy and Immunology* 139 (2): 122–131.

Purokivi, M, H Koskela, T Koistinen, K Peuhkurinen, and KM Kontra. 2010. Assessment of inhaled corticosteroid treatment response in asthma using hypertonic histamine challenge-induced cough. *The Clinical Respiratory Journal* 4 (2) (April): 67–73.

Robinson, DS. 2010. The role of the T cell in asthma. *The Journal of Allergy and Clinical Immunology* 126 (6) (December): 1081–1091; quiz 1092–1093.

Roca, J and R Rodriguez-Roisin. 1992. Asthma, allergen challenge and gas exchange. *The European Respiratory Journal* 5 (10) (November): 1171–1172.

Rodriguez-Roisin, R, A Ferrer, D Navajas, AG Agusti, PD Wagner, and J Roca. 1991. Ventilation-perfusion mismatch after methacholine challenge in patients with mild bronchial asthma. *The American Review of Respiratory Disease* 144 (1) (July): 88–94.

Schafroth T, TM Salome, D Miedinger, A Jochmann, LJ Zellweger, S Sauter, A Goll et al. 2014. An open-label study examining the effect of pharmacological treatment on mannitol- and exercise-induced airway hyperresponsiveness in asthmatic children and adolescents with exercise-induced bronchoconstriction. *BMC Pediatrics* 14 (1): 196.

Scott, GC and SR Braun. 1991. A survey of the current use and methods of analysis of bronchoprovocational challenges. *Chest* 100 (2) (August): 322–328.

Sehmi, R, LJ Wood, R Watson, R Foley, Q Hamid, PM O'Byrne, and JA Denburg. 1997. Allergen-induced increases in IL-5 receptor alpha-subunit expression on bone marrow-derived CD34+ cells from asthmatic subjects. A novel marker of progenitor cell commitment towards eosinophilic differentiation. *The Journal of Clinical Investigation* 100 (10) (November 15): 2466–2475.

Sims, EJ, CM Jackson, and BJ Lipworth. 2003. Add-on therapy with montelukast or formoterol in patients with the glycine-16 β2-receptor genotype. *British Journal of Clinical Pharmacology* 56 (1) (July 9): 104–111.

Smith, SG, R Chen, M Kjarsgaard, C Huang, J-P Oliveria, PM O'Byrne, GM Gauvreau et al. 2016. Increased numbers of activated group 2 innate lymphoid cells in the airways of patients with severe asthma and persistent airway eosinophilia. *The Journal of Allergy and Clinical Immunology* 137(1): 75–86.

Smurthwaite, L, SN Walker, DR Wilson, DS Birch, TG Merrett, SR Durham, and HJ Gould. 2001. Persistent IgE synthesis in the nasal mucosa of hay fever patients. *European Journal of Immunology* 31 (12): 3422–3431.

Spector, S, SD Anderson, B Charlton, JM Weiler, and S Nichols. 2009. Mannitol inhalational challenge. *Proceedings of the American Thoracic Society* 6: 331.

Stewart, IC, A Parker, JR Catterall, NJ Douglas, and DC Flenley. 1989. Effect of bronchial challenge on breathing patterns and arterial oxygenation in stable asthma. *Chest* 95 (1) (January): 65–70.

Stickland, MK, BH Rowe, CH Spooner, B Vandermeer, and DM Dryden. 2011. Accuracy of eucapnic hyperpnea or mannitol to diagnose exercise-induced bronchoconstriction: A systematic review. *Annals of Allergy, Asthma & Immunology: Official Publication of the American College of Allergy, Asthma, & Immunology* 107 (3): 229–234.e8.

Stone, KD, C Prussin, and DD Metcalfe. 2010. IgE, mast cells, basophils, and eosinophils. *The Journal of Allergy and Clinical Immunology* 125 (2 Suppl. 2) (February): S73–S80.

Taylor, DA, MW Jensen, V Kanabar, R Engelstätter, VW Steinijans, PJ Barnes, and BJ O'Connor. 1999. A dose-dependent effect of the novel inhaled corticosteroid ciclesonide on airway responsiveness to adenosine-5'-monophosphate in asthmatic patients. *American Journal of Respiratory and Critical Care Medicine* 160 (1) (July): 237–243.

Toelle, BG, JK Peat, CM Salome, J Crane, D McMillan, J Dermand, W D'Souza, and AJ Woolcock. 1994. Comparison of two epidemiological protocols for measuring airway responsiveness and allergic sensitivity in adults. *The European Respiratory Journal* 7 (10) (October): 1798–1804.

Trivedi, SG and CM Lloyd. 2007. Eosinophils in the pathogenesis of allergic airways disease. *Cellular and Molecular Life Sciences* 64(10) (May): 1269–89.

van den Berge, M, HAM Kerstjens, DM de Reus, GH Koëter, HF Kauffman, and DS Postma. 2004. Provocation with adenosine 5'-monophosphate, but not methacholine, induces sputum eosinophilia. *Clinical and Experimental Allergy: Journal of the British Society for Allergy and Clinical Immunology* 34 (1) (January): 71–76.

van den Berge, M, HA Kerstjens, RJ Meijer, DM de Reus, GH Koëter, HF Kauffman, and DS Postma. 2001. Corticosteroid-induced improvement in the PC20 of adenosine monophosphate is more closely associated with reduction in airway inflammation than improvement in the PC20 of methacholine. *American Journal of Respiratory and Critical Care Medicine* 164 (7) (October 1): 1127–1132.

Willart, MM, K Deswarte, P Pouliot, H Braun, R Beyaert, BN Lambrecht, and H Hammad. 2012. Interleukin-1α controls allergic sensitization to inhaled house dust mite via the epithelial release of GM-CSF and IL-33. *The Journal of Experimental Medicine* 209 (8) (July 30): 1505–1517.

Wilson, AM, M Duong, B Pratt, M Dolovich, and PM O'Byrne. 2006. Anti-inflammatory effects of once daily low dose inhaled ciclesonide in mild to moderate asthmatic patients. *Allergy* 61 (5) (May): 537–542.

Wilson, DR, TG Merrett, EM Varga, L Smurthwaite, HJ Gould, M Kemp, J Hooper, SJ Till, and SR Durham. 2002. Increases in allergen-specific IgE in BAL after segmental allergen challenge in atopic asthmatics. *American Journal of Respiratory and Critical Care Medicine* 165 (1) (January 1): 22–26.

Wood, LJ, R Sehmi, S Dorman, Q Hamid, MK Tulic, RM Watson, R Foley et al. 2002. Allergen-induced increases in bone marrow T lymphocytes and interleukin-5 expression in subjects with asthma. *American Journal of Respiratory and Critical Care Medicine* 166 (6) (September 15): 883–889.

Wood, LJ, R Sehmi, GM Gauvreau, RM Watson, R Foley, JA Denburg, and PM O'Byrne. 1999. An inhaled corticosteroid, budesonide, reduces baseline but not allergen-induced increases in bone marrow inflammatory cell progenitors in asthmatic subjects. *American Journal of Respiratory and Critical Care Medicine* 159 (5 Pt 1) (May): 1457–1463.

Woolcock, AJ, K Yan, and CM Salome. 1988. Effect of therapy on bronchial hyperresponsiveness in the long-term management of asthma. *Clinical Allergy* 18 (2) (March): 165–176.

Zuidscherwoude, M and AB van Spriel. 2012. The origin of IgE memory and plasma cells. *Cellular & Molecular Immunology* 9 (5) (September): 373–374.

Index